O's Guide to Life

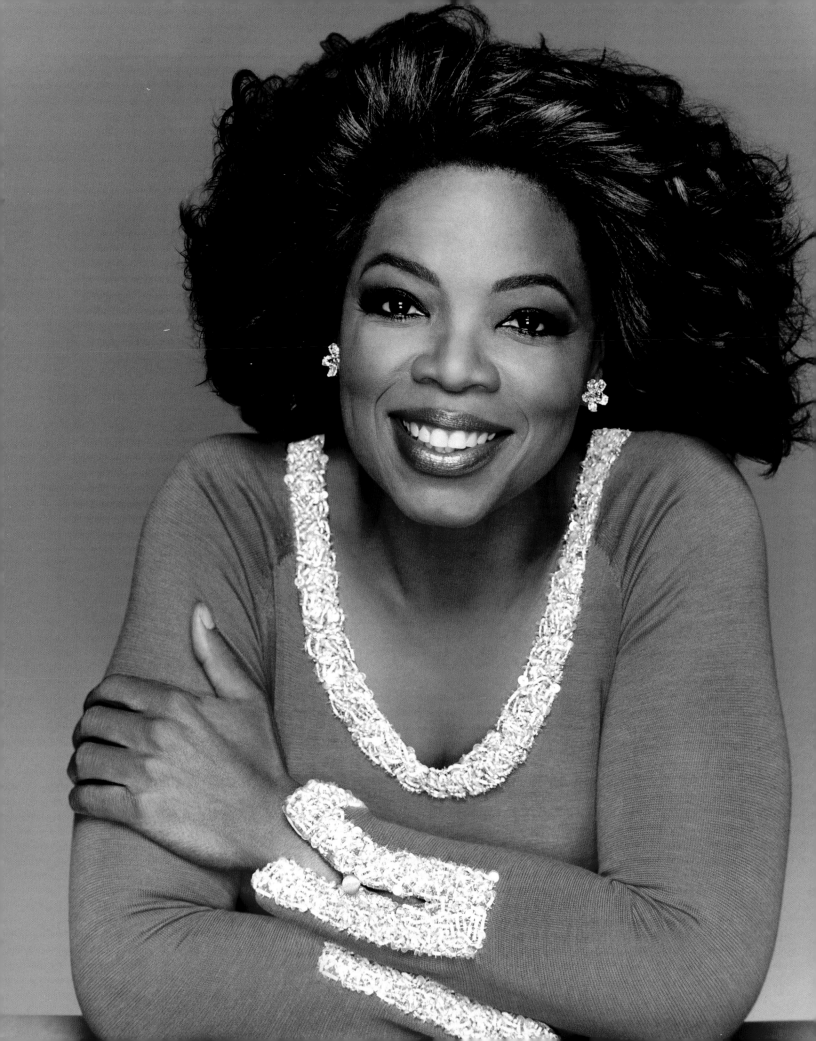

O's Guide to Life

The Best of *O, The Oprah Magazine*
(Wisdom, Wit, Advice, Interviews and Inspiration)

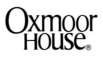
Oxmoor House®

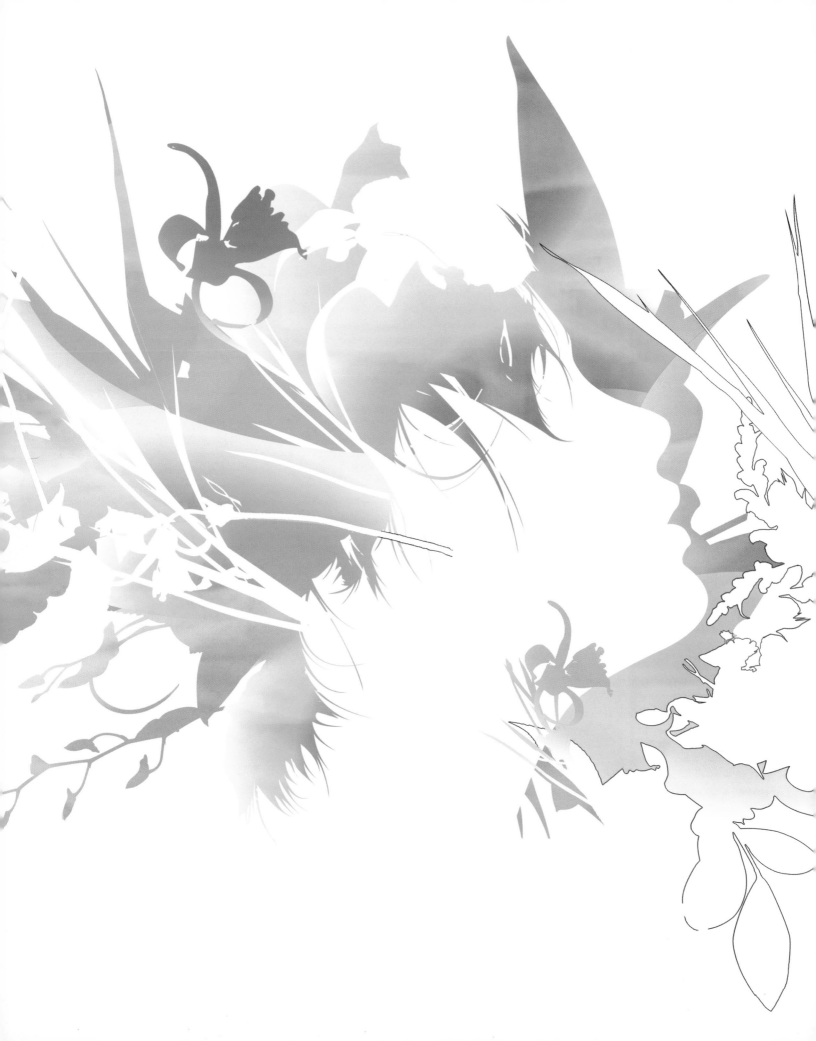

Contents

"Here's to pleasures
great and small,
connections delicate
and strong, love given
and received.
Here's to living your
very best life!"

Here We Go

Welcome to *O's Guide to Life,* with more than 100 of my favorite articles culled from the pages of *O, The Oprah Magazine.* Our plan was to give you a greatest-hits collection in one knockout of a book you can reach for whenever you find yourself craving another perspective, a few laughs, a little expert advice, a great big dream, or maybe just a terrific conversation with an old friend.

We've set out to talk—*really talk*—about everything under the sun. We want to challenge a couple of assumptions ("What Men Wish You Knew About Them," page 173); bust a few myths ("You Need 8 Glasses of Water a Day…and Other Rules to Blow Off," page 40); speak truth to wrinkles ("Beauty Over 40: Seven Things Nobody Ever Tells You About Aging," page 148); pull you through the bad times ("Take Two Risks and Call Me in the Morning," page 100); and celebrate when those bad times turn out to yield some fantastic surprises ("Astonished by Love," page 179).

We've spent the last seven years attempting to cover all 360 degrees of a woman's life. That means we've done a whole lot of thinking about how to get comfortable with everything from what you've got in your bank account to what you see in your mirror. The section called "Your Personal Best" takes you on a grand tour of life as we've all come to know it—whether at home ("Overhelpers Anonymous," page 67), at the office ("How to be Wildly Successful," page 130), or out there on your own ("What Never to Say to a Single Woman Over 35," page 124). We went in search of excellent health, a doable diet, spirituality, beauty, balance, a burst of happiness, and a great read—for me, those last two are one and the same!

Our "Relationships" section is filled with the good, the bad, and the "he-did-*what?*" of couplehood. See if you don't relate ("Looking Out For #2," page 185), learn ("How to Get Through to a Man," page 211), and make a copy for your significant other ("The Love Breakthrough," page 163). Of course, you can't talk about relationships without talking about friends, family, and sex—rest assured, we've got plenty to say on all three subjects.

Finally, I'd like you to meet a few people who are trying to push the planet into better shape. I don't think anybody can read what Archbishop Desmond Tutu, Christiane Amanpour, Paul Rusesabagina, and the other miracle workers in our "Living in the World" section have to say without feeling absolutely enchanted and utterly inspired.

That's what it's all about. We aim to dazzle, to delight, to defy expectations, and to dare everybody who picks up this book to shoot for the stars. Here's to pleasures great and small, connections delicate and strong, love given and received. Here's to living your very best life!

Oprah

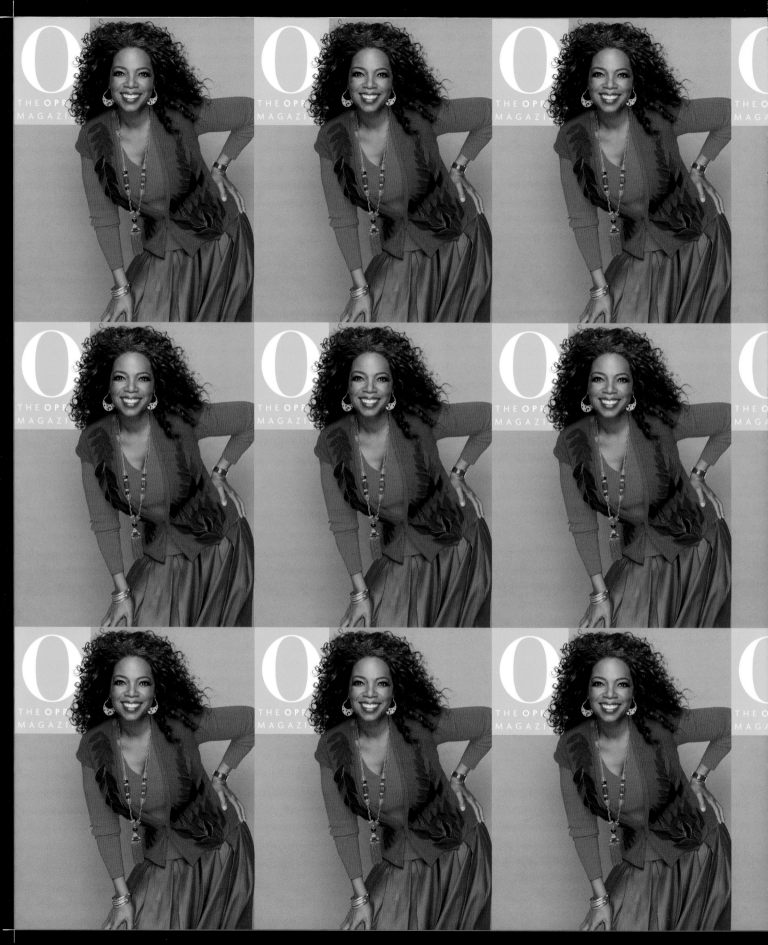

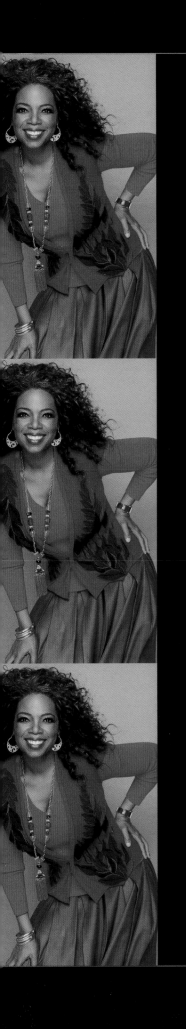

Your Personal Best

Your best possible life starts with feeling and looking great . . .
and uncovering what you want and how to get there. By defining
your purpose, you're that much more likely to succeed.

Diet & Exercise

10 Easy Food Switches
for an Extra 10 Good Years

BY DAVID L. KATZ, MD

Milk chocolate → Dark chocolate	1. **DARK CHOCOLATE** (look for at least 60 percent cocoa) is a concentrated source of antioxidants, which protect cells from age-related damage; milk chocolate contains significantly smaller amounts. And chocolate's fat doesn't raise cholesterol. Preliminary results from my lab show benefits to blood vessels two hours after eating dark chocolate or drinking it in cocoa. Nibble an ounce, sip a small cup—the calories still add up.
White wine → Red wine	2. **COMPARED WITH WHITE**, red wine, like dark chocolate, provides more antioxidants, in this case from the skin of grapes. And alcohol in general can keep platelets from sticking together, possibly preventing blood clots. Moderation is the key here, too; one glass of wine a day, according to studies, appears optimal for most women.
White bread → Whole grain bread	3. **WHENEVER YOU REPLACE** white flour with whole grains—in bread, cereal, pasta—it's a strike against aging. Soluble fiber, found in oats and barley, has been linked to lower levels of insulin and bad cholesterol (think: diabetes and heart disease), and insoluble fiber in whole wheat reduces risk of gastrointestinal maladies like diverticulosis. Check out bread made with the new albino whole wheat—it tastes like the real white thing.
Soda → Tea	4. **A CUP OF TEA** infuses you with antioxidants instead of the wallop of sugar you get in a can of soda. Green, black, and especially white—drink it hot or iced: All offer the powerful nutrients and a boost of caffeine.
¼ of the sugar in a baking recipe → The same amount of nonfat powdered milk	5. **REDUCING SUGAR** in cakes, cookies, and bread will start retraining your taste buds to prefer less sweetness in your entire diet—a good antiaging goal, because in addition to weight gain and diabetes, chronically high intake of sugar can lead to glycosylation. This is a process in which sugar molecules adhere to protein molecules, potentially damaging cells, increasing inflammation, and contributing to the blockage of arteries.
Diet soda → Water	6. **THERE IS NO BETTER** beverage than water to help you stay hydrated, which is important in keeping body systems running well. Diet soda quenches thirst, but some experts still worry that its artificial sweeteners—officially considered safe—may be linked to cancer. My main concern with them is that they propagate a sweet tooth, which leads to more sugar intake and the overall deterioration of the diet.
¼ of your meat → Lentils	7. **SATURATED FAT** (which meat tends to have a lot of) can gum up arteries and speed you toward heart disease. Too little fiber (meat has zero) can accelerate the aging of the gastrointestinal system. Beans and lentils are the opposite of meat: lots of fiber and no saturated fat—and they provide protein. How can you lose?
Regular yogurt → Low-fat or fat-free yogurt	8. **DAIRY FOODS** are a great source of calcium and vitamin D, which help keep bones from thinning. But the saturated fat in whole milk, cheese, and yogurt contributes to artery clogging. Switching to low- or no-fat dairy gives you all the benefits without the risks.
¼ of your meat → Fish	9. **FISH IS AN IDEAL** lean protein source, low in saturated fat. Certain varieties such as salmon are also high in omega-3 fatty acids—vital for heart and possibly brain health. Unfortunately, some species also contain contaminants: If possible, eat wild versus farm-raised salmon and limit albacore (white) tuna to one meal a week. If you're pregnant or nursing, check out the guidelines at epa.gov/ost/fishadvice/advice.html.
Bag of potato chips → Slices of apple	10. **AN APPLE HAS NO FAT**, few calories, lots of soluble fiber, and antioxidants. What does a potato chip offer? Pretty nil on the valuable nutrients score, and it's a great source of oil, calories, and salt. A good rule of thumb is to go with foods that come packaged by Mother Nature, i.e., apple (skin) versus chips (plastic bag), banana (peel) versus candy bar (wrapper). Both you and the environment will be around longer to enjoy each other. ◖

I'm Doing Everything Right— Why Can't I Lose Weight?

Out of the 100-plus women who e-mailed us this very complaint, we chose three and had a team of no-nonsense experts—a nutritionist, a trainer, a life coach—take them on. What were our subjects really eating? More important, what was eating them? Three months (and a total of 47 lost pounds) later, the answers are in. BY EMILY YOFFE

Take your plate of food, go to the wastebasket, and throw it away."

This is Martha Beck's politely delivered command to the three women sitting down for lunch in a New York City hotel conference room in June 2004. The women are here because they've written to *O* in frustration, claiming they can't lose weight despite doing everything right. Wagering that some part of their "right" is probably wrong (and if the suspense is killing you, it turns out we're onto something), the magazine has put together an ace makeover squad: *O* columnist and life coach Martha Beck, nutritionist Rovenia Brock, PhD, and exercise consultant Jorge Cruise. Today the team is getting together with the women for the first time to find out what's really going on and come up with a targeted (and truth-telling) three-month plan to take off the extra pounds.

Meet the women:

Michelle Williams, 37. Height: 5'3". Weight: 150 pounds. Goal: 130 pounds. Financial analyst; Colorado Springs, Colorado. Married with two children. Problem (as defined in her original e-mail): "I have tried continuously to lose weight and can't. I exercise two to three times a week, my diet is relatively healthy, and I eat many low-fat foods. I am very active because I have two very active boys."

Dorine Mooney, 43. Height: 4'10". Weight: 147 pounds. Goal: 127 pounds. Baby-clothing designer; Newport Beach, California. Married with two children. Problem: "I had a baby last April and gained 60 pounds during the pregnancy. No matter what I do, I cannot, and I mean cannot, lose that last 20 pounds. It's very crushing. I've tried dieting, I walk five miles every day; nothing is working!"

Susan Schwartz, 52. Height: 5'4". Weight: 156 pounds. Goal: 126 pounds. Branding consultant; San Mateo, California. Single, no children. "I've been 20 pounds overweight most of my adult life. I have given up bread, pasta, all white flour, and most dairy. I exercise 30 to 45 minutes a day, but my body doesn't respond."

Back at the hotel, the Park Central, the three women give Martha Beck skeptical looks. Is she kidding about tossing their lunch? "Studies are very clear that the ability to throw away food is a great indicator of an ability to lose weight,"

says Martha. To Michelle's plaintive, "That's wasteful," Martha replies with a knowing smile, "It's going to waste if it goes to your thighs, belly, and upper arms."

Michelle gets it. "I want to lose the 20 pounds," she says, and dumps the contents of her plate into the garbage. The others follow. Martha asks them to go back to the catering trays and get much more food than they could possibly want. Tiny Dorine returns with three sandwiches. Martha then instructs the women to leave on their plates just the amount of lunch they feel they need to satisfy their hunger. The rest they are, again, going to throw away.

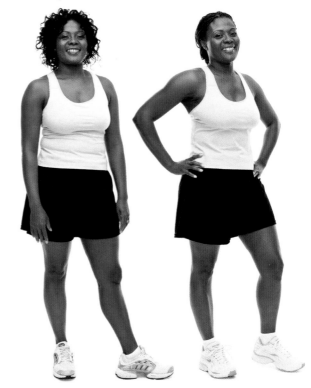

BEFORE
Michelle Williams, 37, at 150 pounds, when she often ate Snickers instead of a real lunch (why not— the bars were the same calories).

AFTER
Having learned that candy and fruit juice make her hungry for more sweets, she brings carrots and nuts to work and is 15 pounds lighter.

Susan, sounding almost childlike, asks, "What if I'm okay now and two minutes later I'm hungry?"

"Susan, why are you concerned?" Martha replies. "When was the last time you began to waste away because there wasn't enough to eat?"

Martha is doing radical therapy on these women because she has only a short time to peel away their layers of self-defense around the issue of food. She knows all about the self-loathing and delusion of destructive eating. Now fit and healthy, she tells the women that earlier in her life she swung through dangerous eating disorders. "As a teenager, I ate 600 calories a day and ran 100 miles a week. Then I couldn't leave the house without eating 2,000 calories." While none of the three women has as serious a problem as Martha did, they could all use some reeducation about listening to the long-muffled signals of what it feels like to be hungry and what it feels like to be full.

The day started with a breakfast meeting conducted by nutritionist Rovenia Brock, a former host on Black Entertainment Television and the author of the no-nonsense eating guide *Dr. Ro's Ten Secrets to Livin' Healthy* (Bantam). When Brock, who goes by the name Dr. Ro, first entered the conference room and discovered the hotel's spread of cake and Cokes, she asked the staff to take it away and come back with yogurt, cereal, skim milk, and berries. She isn't a carb counter; instead she advocates balanced meals of mostly unrefined foods.

Before the meeting, Dr. Ro had each woman send her a week's food diary. As she reviews their entries with them over breakfast, their "I'm doing everything right" defense quickly collapses. She ticks off the evidence. To Dorine she says, "A glaring thing for me is the glass or glasses of wine at every dinner. The second glass will never give you the feeling the first one does. I want you to limit your wine to four ounces, once or twice a week." That reduction alone will eliminate more than 1,000 empty calories from Dorine's weekly consumption.

"I used to sell wine for a living!" says Dorine, hoping for a reprieve.

"You don't have to be so loyal," Dr. Ro answers amiably. She notes that yogurt is a good snack, but Dorine eats custard-style yogurt and piles it in a sugar cone.

"It was a treat," says Dorine, as if that gives it some magical calorie-reducing powers.

Dr. Ro suggests how to make it a healthier treat: switch to no- or low-fat yogurt, put it in a bowl, and top it with a table-spoon of low-fat granola.

She turns to Michelle, who says her downfall is not planning. "If I'm in a meeting and rushing to do something, I'll skip a meal and have a Snickers," she explains. The calories are the same as a real lunch, Michelle rationalizes, and, as she puts it, "I need this candy bar." But Dr. Ro points out the self-sabotage. Good food would provide nutrition and a feeling of fullness that lasts all afternoon. Michelle, however, is going for a quick "cheap thrill"—a rush of sugar-fueled energy that will leave her hungry again in about an hour.

Dr. Ro tells Michelle to take Baggies of food to work that she can turn to when the cravings hit: slices of chicken, strips of bell peppers, strawberries. "And try a protein bar as opposed to 32 ounces of fruit punch," she advises.

"Did I have that?" Michelle asks, appalled.

"It's right here."

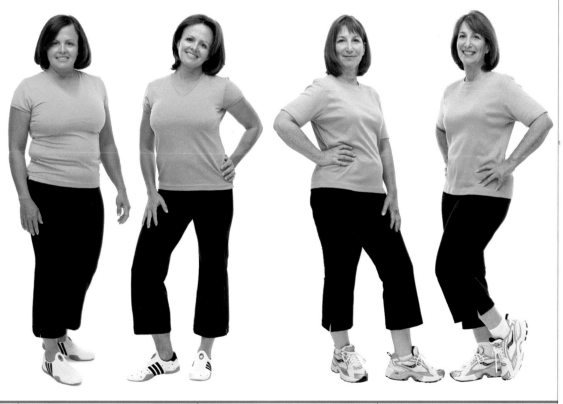

BEFORE	AFTER	BEFORE	AFTER
Dorine Mooney, 43 and 147 pounds, walked five miles a day and dieted (well, except for the wine at dinner and frequent midnight fridge raids).	Dorine minus 22 pounds: Once she realized why she was comforting herself with food, the excess weight almost evaporated.	Susan Schwartz, 52, gave up bread, pasta, and dairy and worked out 30 to 45 minutes a day—so why couldn't she lose some of her 156 pounds?	More honest about what she's really eating (especially when life gets testy) and how much exercise she's doing, Susan has lost ten pounds.

Thirty-two ounces of fruit punch is a sugary 480 calories. A protein bar is about 200 calories, and a high-quality one can contain ten to 30 grams of protein with only a few grams of fat—a vast improvement over a candy bar.

Susan is next. She doesn't go for a lot of sweets, but Dr. Ro observes that she often eats alone and reads through the meal. That makes it possible to consume large amounts without being aware of it. With Susan's attention on the words she's reading, not the food, says Dr. Ro, she's "eating mindlessly. You're full way before that last bite, but you don't notice." She suggests that Susan put away the magazines and set the table for herself.

"I barely get it onto a plate," Susan says of the prepared food she brings home in cartons.

"Portion control is key for you," Dr. Ro says firmly.

Her diet advice for all is refreshingly gimmick-free: Step up the fruits and vegetables; eat some lean protein (egg whites, low-fat dairy, skinless poultry, beans) at each meal; and replace doughnuts, bagels, and candy with complex carbohydrates like whole grains and cereals. She believes in snacks, just healthy ones like a handful of nuts or a small bag of carrots. And she wants the women to cut back on their calories but not go so low that their bodies think there's a famine. Starving will only encourage the retention of fat around the waist and hips, she explains. It's all right once or twice a week to satisfy a sweet tooth, but her idea of a treat is a small slice of angel food cake topped with berries or a scoop of frozen yogurt.

Dr. Ro recognizes that for these diet-savvy women, losing weight isn't simply a matter of getting a written food plan. "You know the right choices," she tells them, "but if something upsets you, you go off course." That's why she feels Martha Beck's role in exposing their emotional eating triggers is so important. Without self-knowledge, all the nutritional information in the world won't do any good, because every time the women need to relieve stress or salve an emotional wound—in other words, deal with life—they'll probably resort to food. And life, she says, happens every day.

Dorine wants to make one thing clear to Jorge Cruise when the women meet with him after breakfast. "I'm not running unless someone is after me with a gun," she says. That's fine with Jorge. "I don't run either," he replies.

Jorge is AOL's online weight loss coach and the author of the popular 8 Minutes in the Morning book series (published by HarperResource and Rodale). His basic program consists of just two exercises of high-intensity strength training a day, six days a week.

The threesome is dubious that eight minutes a day can accomplish anything much, but he assures each of them that if they do his routine properly, they will reshape their bodies and charge up their metabolism. He says a lot of people waste time at the gym resting too long between sets and not using heavy enough weights. "Strength training is like a house's foundation," he says. "It's the structural support."

"What about aerobics?" one of the women asks. He tells her that aerobics are great, but you need a lot more than eight minutes to get the benefit. "And if you have an unrealistic plan, you won't follow it," he says.

The key to his program's success, he explains, is that it's excuse-proof: No one can convincingly claim she can't carve eight minutes out of her day to get in shape. The exercises can be done at home; the only equipment you need is a pair of dumbbells. He recommends a set of graduated weights for the women to start with, ranging from three to 15 pounds. "The most important thing in resistance training is intensity," he says (his own dumbbells are 30 pounds). He tells the women that as they gain strength, they will increase the weight they use.

He leads the group to the New York Health & Racquet Club to demonstrate the daily exercises. Monday: chest and back. Tuesday: shoulders and abdominals. Wednesday: biceps and triceps. Thursday: hamstrings and quadriceps. Friday: calves and rear end. Saturday: inner and outer thighs. Sunday is the day they can rest—and the only day they should weigh themselves.

"I refuse to give up my scale," says Susan, who gets on it at least once a day.

"You like stress?" Jorge asks. "You're adding stress to your life."

"I refuse to give up my scale," she says more insistently. Jorge continues to try to convince her but finally shrugs. She'll have to work this one out for herself.

When the women return to the hotel for lunch—Dr. Ro has ordered salads, sandwiches on whole wheat, and bowls of fruit—it's time for their session with Martha Beck, author of *The Joy Diet* (Crown) and *Expecting Adam* (Berkley). "I believe losing weight is about telling the truth," says Martha. She means a kind of truth beyond admitting, say, that before bed you tend to devour a pint of chocolate chip–cookie dough ice cream.

Her theory is that we all have an "essential self" who wants to live our "right life." But so often our real life is not our right life. If work or intimate relationships are keeping us from what we really want and need, she says, "the essential self kicks up a fuss through eating, addiction, and getting sick."

Martha has already had private phone consultations with the women, and after the food-toss exercise, as they finally start to eat, she focuses her attention on them one by one and tries to figure out what is kicking up the fuss inside of each.

For Dorine, it's fear. With a husband, who is in recovery for substance abuse, and two young children to care for, she sometimes feels crushed by her financial and emotional burdens. "We're programmed to fear that there won't be enough," says Martha, "enough food, money, love." She explains that this kind of anxiety goes back to the time when we were hunter-gatherers and in constant peril of starvation. "You feel, *I'm in danger.* So you calm yourself by eating."

> Though all the women wanted the experts to tell them what to do, they didn't always want to obey the instructions.

"That's amazing," says Dorine. "I never saw it that way."

Martha moves on to Michelle. "You're thinking, *I'm sick and tired of having other people tell me what to do and not having it work.*" Michelle nods. Martha encourages her to talk about what it's taken for a black woman to succeed in corporate America. "I think you've experienced severe racism. Your anger is enormous and appropriate. I want you to celebrate every bit of it."

Michelle's cool exterior cracks, and she begins to cry. "It's hard, working in the corporate world. My family in the South had inherited land that was taken from my grandparents by a white person.... I'm aware every time I'm discounted and overlooked because of my race. I will not accept it."

Martha asks, "What are white people thinking?"

Michelle takes a moment. *"You're not good enough. Who do you think you are?"*

Martha says, "I want you to own that you are pissed."

Michelle wipes her tears and nods.

When Martha gets to Susan, she reminds her of something she seems to have forgotten, that she is in charge of her own life. "You are free. For you this is a real issue," Martha says. Susan is divorced, lives and works alone, and is the main caretaker for her mother. Martha sees her as someone who has thwarted her own desires in order to do what's proper and fulfill her obligations. "Susan, you are a bohemian dancer, a free spirit who is cut off from your heart," she tells her. "The part that is not cut off says, *Please feed me something.*" Now it's Susan's turn to cry.

"When you started tearing up, you turned away from your food," Martha observes. She explains that when the women are actually addressing the reasons they are feeling fear or anger or frustration, they won't feel hungry. "If you're processing that mountain of emotional energy, you can't eat. Your relationship with food is an amazing passage to your deepest issues."

Martha's two goals are to help these women find their essential selves and reach the point where they don't need the advice of the experts. "The instructions are inside you," she says. "They don't need to come from an authority figure. Your body knows what it needs to eat."

After one long New York day, Dorine, Michelle, and Susan head home. They are told to check in with each other and with the experts weekly over the next three months and to start trying to really "do everything right."

There may be some women in America who don't know that eating junk food by the bucket and getting no exercise is the reason they can't fit into their old pants, but Dorine, Michelle, and Susan are not among them. As they embarked on their various programs, they all found it helpful to have their dietary pitfalls outed and structure brought to their previously erratic workouts. But once they returned to the stresses and conflicts of normal life, each acknowledged that the core of her weight struggle was emotional.

For Dorine, talking with Martha was like a jolt from a defibrillator applied to her psyche. In their first phone conversation, Dorine hadn't mentioned her husband's substance abuse problem, for which he is now in recovery, but Martha intuited it after ten minutes. When Martha told her, "You can't hold him up," it clicked. Dorine returned to California and realized she was trying to solve his problem and live his life for him. She had gained weight from waking up in the middle of the night and—discovering him gone from their bed—going to raid the kitchen. In a fruitless search for comfort, she had turned her body into one she didn't even recognize. Dressing in black for her was not a fashion statement but an expression of her self-image. "I was dead," she says now, looking back on herself.

Dorine's awakening was so profound that her weight started dropping immediately, as if she were zipping off clothing that no longer fit. She saw that filling her emotional needs with food she didn't want was just one more way of making her life wrong. She couldn't fix her husband; she could only fix herself.

The wine stopped, the late-night scavenging stopped, the fast food and treats stopped. She realized how unaware she'd been. "I was eating stuff I don't even like. I don't like pepperoni pizza, but Dr. Ro pointed out it was on my list. I don't even know if I was tasting it." Once she got back from New York, she never had to beat down a craving. "No. I just had no interest."

Her husband's recovery is ongoing. "But I'm dealing with it in a different way," Dorine says now. "When I took back responsibility for me, everything kind of fell into place."

Michelle, too, had an epiphany with Martha. Her weight problem was not, she felt, specifically a response to racism. But she realized that whenever she had confronted racism in life, her reaction was always to work harder and ultimately succeed. She'd applied the same determination in giving her best to her husband and kids. Martha helped her see that she just needed to be the same forceful, tenacious Michelle in losing weight as she was at work and with her family. As that lesson sank in, it occurred to Michelle that she could not wait for the magical moment when her life was without pressure to change her habits. As she wrote in an e-mail on July 19, 2004, "So many things have been going on (traveling, my

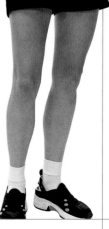

"The bottom line issue of weight control is picking up authority for your own life. The instructions are inside you. Your body knows what to eat."
—*Martha Beck, Life coach*

> "Strength training is like a house's foundation. It's the structural support. And you can do it in eight minutes a day. If you have an unrealistic plan, you won't follow it." —*Jorge Cruise, Exercise consultant*

---

mother has been in the hospital, a friend of ours passed away, a coworker has been ill, etc.), and with all of this, I have still managed to eat healthier and do my daily exercises."

For Susan, change was not as easy. She grappled with the experts and with herself. In an e-mail from San Mateo, she wrote bluntly, "It's not what I'm eating, it's what's eating me. But I don't feel I have the strength to clear out all the crud that stands in the way of opening the dam to let the fat flow/whoosh out of my little holding places."

More than the other two, she insisted that despite doing everything right—really right this time—she wasn't seeing the results she expected. "Since New York, I have cut down on the juice I was drinking, upped my water, added vitamins, increased my exercise, and still nothing," she complained. There were hints, however, that her self-assessment had some blind spots. She admitted that when she was upset over anything, her impulse was: "Let me go look in the fridge." She also confessed that she calmed unruly emotions by eating something sweet.

Her daily weigh-ins, as Jorge had promised, increased her stress. She wrote, "Yesterday: 153. Today: 154. This is frustrating in the extreme! How can it take me a month to drop two pounds, and then that only lasts for a day?"

In several conversations with Martha in which Susan despaired about the weight ever coming off, Martha asked her to describe a typical day's eating. One day the food totaled only about 800 calories. Martha didn't believe her. Another, more typical day, Susan's consumption came out to about 2,000 calories. As Martha explained to her, eating that much and getting minimal exercise would result in a woman of Susan's height gaining weight. Still Susan resisted the idea she could make any more changes. "It seems like the more I pay attention to everything I'm eating," she wrote in an e-mail, "the more I want to eat." She acknowledged her reluctance to keep a food diary: "The amount

of time I waste resisting is much more than the time it would actually take me to write it down." And despite her frequent claims that her diet couldn't be more spartan, she had to admit that when she did keep the diary, it revealed "I haven't been very good—at all good—the last three days."

America's love of makeovers is tied up in the fantasy that "before" flips to "after" as easily and instantly as switching the TV channel (you just need the right diet, expertise, surgeon's knife...). The real process of losing weight, however—even when successful—means slogging through doubts, frustration, and failure, and is deeply (and unglamorously) difficult not only for the person attempting it but also for those trying to help. That was certainly the case for this group.

Though all the women wanted the experts to tell them what to do, they didn't always want to obey the instructions. Like teenagers going through the dance of needing their parents, resenting them, and finally learning to be independent of them, each woman found herself demanding advice and then taking only some of it—and occasionally totally rejecting it—in the process of ultimately striking out on her own.

Martha says this dynamic found a healthy expression in Michelle. "A lot of her resistance was coming from anger. She got mad at the coaches—'Aren't they going to do it for me?' The answer was no, she had to do it herself. She started finding her own power in every situation, and her anger went away."

For Susan, Jorge recommended at least 30 minutes of cardio three times a week. She concurred but then realized, "When I try to push myself to do something, I go into very strong and immediate resistance. And then all efforts are off." It's no wonder Susan's weight was stuck. As Martha put it, she might as well have been standing there shouting, "I'm not doing anything you suggested—and the weight loss plan is not working!"

Dorine started out completing Jorge's eight minutes but quickly discovered her body was craving more. Having been a trainer herself in the past, she began working out vigorously at least an hour a day, alternating Pilates, weight lifting, and bicycling. She decided to drop out of the weekly phone check-ins with Jorge and didn't want to be pressured to do his program. She wrote, "If this means I'm out of the article, then I'm out. To me, it's about taking charge and being responsible for my own success."

Three months after their first meeting, the women flew back to New York and reconvened in the Park Central lobby. Dorine showed up wearing a tight gray sweater and a matching miniskirt. "I'm a cheerleader gone bad," she said with a laugh. In the first six weeks of the program, she lost 22 pounds—surpassing her goal—and kept it off for the remaining six weeks. She dropped from a size 10 to a size 4. "And I went from all black to colors," she said. "This was the summer of pink."

Dorine also discovered what could be a new law of physics: As her weight decreased, her free time increased. She not only found an extra hour a day for working out, she also began preparing the kinds of meals Dr. Ro had suggested, drastically reducing her dependence on less-healthy frozen food entrées and dinners out: "In the morning, I have yogurt and granola. For a snack, I'll have a protein bar. Lunch is salad with grilled chicken. Afternoon snack is a banana or an apple. For dinner, I'll have baked chicken with a vegetable and a potato."

She says of her three-month journey, "We came to New York with the hope that we'd be given a magical answer. There isn't one. Nobody sat us down and said, 'Eat this at this time.' It was more like: 'Get a grip.'"

Dorine is confident that the personal struggles ahead will not send her back to her old ways. (After returning home from New York, she continued to shed weight. At last report, she'd lost 26 pounds.) "Before," she says, "I was in such a fog I didn't realize things were as serious as they were. At least I'm present right now, not absent."

Michelle, wearing a red sweater and white pants (yes, white, the color that hides nothing!), had lost 15 pounds and achieved her goal of going from size 12 to size 8—sometimes even a 6. For years, her husband, an exercise fanatic, would invite her to go to the gym with him early in the morning. "I'd say, 'I'll meet you,'" she recalls, "and then I never would." Now she gets there. Thanks to Dorine's recommendation, Michelle has also taken up Pilates. In the evenings, instead of relaxing on the couch, the whole family goes for a walk with the dog, and Michelle will say, "Let's take a longer route." (She, too, kept dropping weight after the reunion, going down to 128 for a total of 22 pounds lost.)

> ## "When you eat mindlessly, you're full way before that last bite, but you don't notice."
> — *Dr. Ro, Nutritionist*

On Dr. Ro's advice, Michelle started bringing healthier snacks to work so she could bypass the vending machine. "This morning it was carrots," she says. She also packs nuts and eats just a handful or small boxes of raisins. "Once or twice a week, I treat myself," she says of her love for sweets. "But I don't go overboard the way I used to."

She also followed Martha's advice on not automatically finishing everything on her plate. And there was something else. Thinking about her first e-mail to *O*, she admits, "I was a liar. I wasn't doing everything right." She knew what to do, she says; she just wasn't doing it.

Susan came in an olive sweater and pants—last winter's pants, which were so loose they almost fell to the floor when she tugged at the waistband. She had lost ten pounds. That means she broke through a personal weight barrier, the Berlin Wall on her scale—the 150-pound mark—getting down to 146. She stuck religiously to Jorge's eight minutes. "It's like brushing my teeth now," she says.

As befits Susan's nature, she simultaneously feels heartened by her accomplishment while expressing frustration that she didn't do better. "This," she says, putting her hands on Dorine's shoulders, "is where I'm going to get."

Why did her weight finally start to come off? For one thing, she got honest with herself. "I really felt I had done everything I could and that losing weight was impossible," she says. "Now I feel I'm not doing everything I can." Susan knows she needs more exercise. And because she's no longer running to the kitchen every time something hurts, she can admit that she used to. She mentions that she recently heard about her ex-boyfriend moving in with another woman. News like that normally would have resulted in "a month of nibbling." This time it didn't.

She has freed herself from having a specific goal on the scale. "The weight is creeping down the way it crept up. A few months from now I will have lost a few more pounds."

As it had been for the others, the admonition to throw away food was a turning point for Susan. She realized how much her overeating was connected to her irrational fear that there won't be enough. She describes having lunch not long ago with a friend who encouraged her to have the last bite of dessert. Susan declined, saying there would always be another opportunity to enjoy dessert.

"Not this dessert," the friend tempted.

"There'll be another one," Susan repeated firmly.

Another insight from Martha that Susan found helpful was seeing eating patterns as a path to self-understanding. "It's not so much about getting the food right as getting the rest of your life right," Susan says. Acting on Martha's reminder that she is free to live her life as she wishes, Susan enrolled in massage school, something she'd wanted to do for 14 years but didn't because she felt the people in her life wouldn't have accepted it. She's doing it now, she says, "because that's what my soul wants."

At their first meeting in New York, Martha told Dorine, Michelle, and Susan, "Dieting is just the beginning. Pushing away that food is like pushing away your drug—you will be left with your feelings." And once those feelings were exposed, the process of getting honest began. The women lost weight because they became truthful about the fact that they weren't doing "everything right" and straight about the reasons why. Martha left them with the knowledge that their success had little to do with reducing the circumference of their thighs and everything to do with discovering what had been going on inside their minds and hearts to keep them from reaching their goals. "I want you to have bodies you love," she said. "But more important, I want you to have lives you love." They are on their way. ◘

Oprah's Boot Camp

Thanks to a fierce diet-and-exercise program, OPRAH got herself a new body. But she still wants to lose another ten pounds. So to share what she's learned and to build some crucial buddy-system support, she's chosen a team to join her in a 12-week blitz. You're invited to follow along.

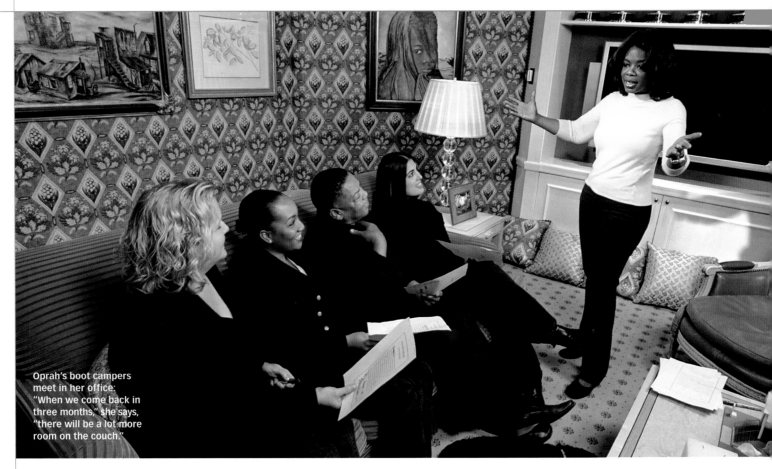

Oprah's boot campers meet in her office: "When we come back in three months," she says, "there will be a lot more room on the couch."

I was standing on the front porch of my new home in California, the one I've worked on for three years as a gift to myself. I was looking at the mountains folding over on themselves and my yard filled with oak, pine, and redwood trees, thinking how this property is really graced by God, a promised land, and I suddenly said to myself: *I do not want to be an unhealthy fat person standing in the doorway of this beautiful house.*

That's when everything really clicked.

I'm not struggling anymore. I've lifted the veil. Because when you're wrestling with your weight and not being the person you know you can be, you are living behind a veil. And every person who is buried in fat knows that. When I turned 50, I made a vow to myself that I would live only in the space of moving forward. I wasn't feeling my biological clock ticking; what I felt was my life

clock chiming, "Is that all there is?" The answer is, no! There's always more—you just have to open yourself to the possibility of being transformed by it all.

So after many years of my weight going up and down—of saying on Monday "I'm going to do it" and by Wednesday failing—I realized that the commitment to do well and to be well is a lifetime of choices that you make daily. The space to live in is not "I'll try." Not "I want to." Not "I really want to." It's "I have decided."

I've known all of this intellectually for a while, but the click came as an emotional and spiritual awakening.

Now I live straight through the center of myself, which means telling the truth about everything. No more games. Every day I make the choice to live as well as I possibly can. And that starts with exercise. I do not have the genetics or the body type to

YOUR PERSONAL BEST

function without it. So I stopped vacillating between "Maybe I'll work out" and "Maybe I'll take the day off." I do it the way I bathe. And guess what: I do not hate it anymore. Don't get me wrong—you won't see me jumping up and down going, "Oh, jeez, exercise is great," but I no longer dread it. And that is nothing less than a revolution.

I do at least 30 minutes of aerobics a day, regardless, and when I'm feeling especially sassy—Tina's pumping on the stereo, or Stevie Wonder—I can do up to 45 minutes. I call it a Party for One. Instead of *Oh God, this is so hard* (because that just negates the whole process of trying to move forward), I tell myself, *I have the incline up as high as it will go—I can't believe it!* Three days a week I add resistance training. I also started doing Pilates two to three times a week—this is mostly a spiritual act for me. I use the Pilates principles of moving out from the center, awareness, harmony, balance, and control to help me embody where I'm going with my life. The benefit is that you end up walking taller, feeling stronger, and looking leaner; but if you're doing it just for those reasons, you'll get frustrated because the process is very slow.

With food, what works for me is treating refined and processed carbohydrates as though they were poison. I've given myself four to six times a year when I'm allowed to indulge. And you can bet, next Christmas morning I'll be having my Williams-Sonoma croissant—you know the frozen ones they ship to your door, and when you heat them up the whole house smells like bread? The difference is, in the past, I took an entire tray of those croissants on the plane to South Africa, and we ate them all the way to Sweden. I'm no physician, but I know that the more sugar you consume, the more your body wants. You think your craving is a lack of willpower, but what you've really got is a chemical imbalance.

The biggest imbalance for many of us, though, is in the amount of thought we devote to food and weight. If I could add up the time I've spent worrying about what I just ate and what I shouldn't have just eaten, feeling guilty about it, and getting down on myself about why I'm not where I want to be, it would probably be several years of my life. And you can't get those years back.

I am not wasting any more time. And by no longer dwelling on all of these negative thoughts, I have opened up a whole new energy field for myself. It's amazing. I feel as if I'm living on a higher frequency, a stronger, brighter charge. The voltage got turned up. People stop me all the time and ask, "What have you done to look so different?" This is the answer.

I've also stopped seeing every big occasion as a license to eat. I used to go to parties thinking, *Oh boy, I hope they have good hors d'oeuvres.* Now I wonder who might be interesting to meet there. And I've changed my behavior to avoid what are food triggers for me. Before, I'd get home, put down my purse, and go straight to the refrigerator. Now, I come in the door, put down my purse, and head for the bedroom to change into my pajamas—those five minutes get me past the fridge impulse. Same thing at work: I'd

come up the stairs, go into my little room, and think, *I've got to eat some potato chips because I just finished the show and I deserve it.* Now I walk all the way around the other side of the building to get to my office, so I break the pattern.

The real key for me is to decide before a meal or an event what I'm going to eat—and if I do have some dessert, I just move on. One piece of anything isn't going to kill you; it's the seconds and thirds and fourths that become a problem. At my own 50th birthday celebration, I made a choice not to have a piece of the incredible cake everybody saw on the show. I appreciated the love that went into that cake. And it sure was pretty. But I did not have any. I didn't even think about it. And to go, "You're not going to eat the cake" and stick to it...what can I say? It felt absolutely fabulous.

I still want to lose ten pounds, though, maybe 12. I'm a size 10, 5'6½", and 163 pounds (the tabloids have said 140, but I haven't been that low since seventh grade, okay?). My goal is to get into the "safe zone"—where I'm not just a meal or vacation away from slipping to the other side and having to fight my way back. For me that's in the 150s. I don't have an exact number, but I'll know it when I get there.

To do this, I decided to start my own personal three-month boot camp. Riffing off my trainer, Bob Greene, and his book, *Total Body Makeover,* I've put together an eating and exercise plan based on what I've found to work. And for extra motivation, I've asked four people at Harpo—all of whom I've seen struggling—to do it

> "The reason you're fat is that you give more to other people than you give to yourself."

with me. I've been so psychologically shackled by my weight for most of my adult life, I view my ability to help others break free as a part of what I'm supposed to do. When you learn, you teach. Here's what I have to tell you: There's no easy way out. If there were, I would have bought it. And believe me, it would be one of my favorite things!

The first thing I told my team was, "I want you to think about why you're overweight. But let me save you a lot of time: The reason you're fat is that you give more to other people than you give to yourself, because you don't feel you're worth it." The bottom line is, you cannot lose weight until you make yourself enough of a priority to do the things you need to do to make it happen. People always say, "I'm too busy to exercise," "I have to be there for the kids," "I've got too much work." You know what? These are little lies you're telling yourself, and they go against the laws of self-preservation, because the more whole and healthy you are, the more fully you can give to other people. And that's the truth. I'm not asking anyone to abandon her children. I'm just saying: Put yourself at the top of the list so you can treat your body with as much care and respect as you'd give to someone else's—and when anyone needs something from you, you will be operating from a full cup.

I'm so pleased to be living from a full cup instead of a half-empty one—and kicking it up as I go. As I celebrate another birthday, I want to assure you, getting older is not the end. It's the beginning of my life deepening to a level I had never even imagined was there. ▶

Profiles of the Challenged

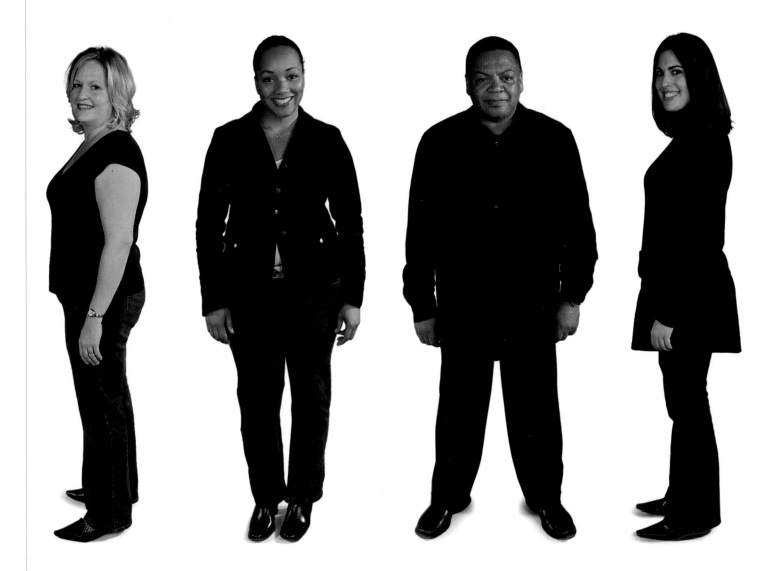

NAME: Kathleen Penny
AGE: 42
OCCUPATION: Production manager for creative services
STARTING WEIGHT: 209 pounds
WANTS TO LOSE: 30 pounds
WHY SHE'S DOING IT: "I have high cholesterol and need to lower it. I also want to set a good example for my daughter."

NAME: Stacey Moses
AGE: 32
OCCUPATION: Supervisor of music licensing for legal and business affairs
STARTING WEIGHT: 171 pounds
WANTS TO LOSE: 25 pounds
WHY SHE'S DOING IT: "I want to be healthier and feel good in my own skin."

NAME: Reggie Wells
AGE: 57
OCCUPATION: Makeup artist
STARTING WEIGHT: 233 pounds
WANTS TO LOSE: 25 pounds
WHY HE'S DOING IT: "I am at the age where I'm concerned about my health. I want to conquer my weight before there are any problems."

NAME: Dana Leavitt
AGE: 23
OCCUPATION: Researcher
STARTING WEIGHT: 174 pounds
WANTS TO LOSE: 20 pounds
WHY SHE'S DOING IT: "I need the extra push because I can't motivate myself to do this. Now I have to!"

Twelve Weeks to a Better Body: The Plan

Eight eyes bulge in unison, their owners squished together on the couch. *Not even a sunflower seed?*

Oprah is laying out the rules for the next 12 weeks to four anxious-looking Harpo staffers. They are about to embark on a total body makeover (in the job description? No, but perhaps an occupational hazard of working for the country's most famous food addict), and the rule about "zero food for three hours before bed—not even a grape or a seed" is creating what you might call a nuh-huh moment.

"Am I on *Fear Factor*?" asks Oprah's makeup artist, Reggie Wells, looking around as if he showed up at the wrong studio.

Everyone laughs, relaxing a bit.

Oprah has settled on these staffers only after securing their deadbolt commitment—falter, she tells them, and they're out. She will be feeling their pain because she's doing the program with them.

THE FOOD

Overall, eat lean protein, two fruits a day, and all the green vegetables you want. Keep the fat low (for salad dressing, you can use a little olive oil with lemon and garlic). And no alcohol. The main rule is, eliminate the white stuff—bread, pasta, potatoes, rice—as well as candy, pastry, cookies, cake. ("A few people might get evil on me," Oprah says, knowingly—sugar deprivation can turn even a saint nasty.) For the first month, also stay away from whole grains (brown rice, oatmeal, whole wheat cereals, and breads). After that, you can slowly add them back.

The other big rule: You must stop eating three hours before bedtime. Do just this, Oprah says, and you'll lose weight. "If you were to write down everything you put in your mouth after 7:30 P.M., just knickknacking around the house—a handful of nuts here, a cracker there—you'd be shocked at how it all adds up."

During the 12 weeks, you get to choose three days when you can allow yourself either alcohol (a glass of wine, maybe two; a cocktail) or some refined carbs (one piece of cake, one slice of bread, one bowl of pasta. The key word is *one*).

THE EXERCISE

You have eight workouts a week with one day of rest. Six days a week, you do 20 minutes of resistance training using dumbbells. Choose a weight that's heavy enough to tire the muscle by the 12th rep—most women begin with five to ten pounds (Oprah's using 15 pounds for the biceps and 12 for all the other moves; everyone else is starting with eight). If you already weight-train, go through your upper-body exercises (or see oprah.com/makeover). Each session includes a cardio workout. Start with 30 minutes, five days a week, and on the sixth day, double the time to an hour. But here's the trick: The more comfortable a workout is, the less effective, so the aerobics are designed to constantly up the metabolic ante. Oprah and her team are using treadmills and increasing the challenge every two minutes by raising the speed, incline, or both. The idea is to continually push yourself a little further than you thought you could go, until you get to the point where you can talk but don't want to. And every day, take it up a notch; staying at the same level is the biggest mistake people make. Don't be afraid to jack up that incline, says Oprah. "I remember being a fat person on the StairMaster with two dots on my monitor. And next to me this girl had her whole screen full of dots. I was a two-dotter. And there she was in her little string thing, wearing lipstick, with all those dots, and not even sweating."

In addition to keeping the intensity up, every week, extend the aerobics sessions by two minutes (week two would be 32 minutes and 64 on the long workout). So by the end of the three months, you'll be doing almost an hour a day, and double that on the sixth session. On top of all of this, you do a second half-hour workout two days a week. This session is a combination of cardio and strength training that Oprah learned from John Travolta's trainer, Steve Maye: Every five minutes, you alternate between the treadmill and a series of floor moves: situps, squats, and biceps curls and lateral raises with the hand weights. "You sweat a lot," she says. "I wouldn't do this if I wasn't in boot camp." Before taking even one step, you must sign a contract with yourself that reads: "I, [print your name], hereby commit to 12 weeks of regular vigorous exercise—that's eight workouts a week—and to self-control when it comes to eating. I will be focused on challenging my abilities in the pursuit of elevating my physical performance. In addition, with the exception of three days, I will not indulge in any alcoholic beverages during the 12-week period, regardless of the nature of the temptation. I will also terminate my consumption of all food three hours prior to my bedtime. I will endeavor to be conscious of when and why I eat and will, to the best of my ability, eat simply to satisfy my nutritional needs as opposed to my emotional needs. I will also do my best to make healthful food choices. I realize that this contract is solely with myself and that it carries no rewards, penalties, or punishments other than those associated with the reflection of the strength of my character." Sign and date it. Stick it on your fridge.

For Oprah's group, the contract is also a commitment to the team. And there's one more detail. They have to weigh in periodically. On TV. "I want you to own the number," says Oprah. Now this is from a woman who has tried every trick in the book to get one over on the scale. "I'd put *alllll* my weight on the right foot and lift the left foot a little. That gives you about three pounds. I'd take off my pantyhose, because you can get an ounce per leg." But the truth, she says, is essential if you want to succeed.

"KP," she says, turning to Kathleen Penny, a production manager, "how many times have you tried to lose weight?"

"I'm always thinking about it," Kathleen replies.

"Well that's going to end," Oprah says. "You've got more important things to think about." She stresses that the only way this program will work for good is to approach it not as another diet but as a choice to redefine your life—because as you lose the weight and lift the veil, you will see yourself differently, and others will, too. And you have to be willing to accept what comes with that.

Oprah winds up the prep session. They start tomorrow: 6 A.M. at the gym.

"When we come back in three months," she says with a grin, "there will be a lot more room on the couch." ⓞ

Oprah's Boot Camp, Part 2:
She Answers Your Questions

Ever since Oprah grabbed four Harpo staffers for her 12-week weight loss boot camp—eight workouts a week, strict eating rules, no wine, no excuses—two things have happened. The four have turned into lean, mean fat-fighting machines (turn to page 25 to track their progress). And the thousands of readers who followed along online (at oprah.com) have bombarded us with e-mails about the program. Here, Oprah replies to a batch of the most pressing and frequently asked questions.

SELF-SABOTAGE

For some reason, the minute I start feeling and looking good and getting compliments, I sabotage myself. How do I find out what's keeping me from liking myself?

—Michi, 46, Lakewood, California

Michi from Lakewood, that is a really good question you're asking. Obviously, you have some shadow beliefs that you are not worthy of happiness and true success. That's the only reason you would keep sabotaging yourself.

When I started working out with my group, I said to them, "We're going to peel back the layers. You need to ask yourselves a lot of questions about why you've put on the weight and why you've dieted time and time again. But I can already tell you what the answer is: You didn't feel worthy of being loved."

The "Am I good enough?" question plagues millions of people and, if you ask me, is the root of many evils. To get a handle on it, I'd try to figure out at what age this started to form as a reality for you.

One thing that helped me was realizing that I am not just Vernon and Vernita's daughter but God's child, so I am worthy of the abundance that the universe has to offer. Nobody who has struggled with her weight achieves a significant loss without some kind of spiritual and emotional component. And that spiritual component always, always comes down to: Am I worthy of being loved? Am I worthy of the best?

BATTLING DEPRESSION

I am very overweight, and so is my oldest daughter. We both suffer from depression and eat to cover up our pain. How do you handle weight when dealing with depression?

—Linda Beasley, 43, Hogansville, Georgia

I'm not a therapist, so I can't tell you how to treat your depression. And eating for emotional reasons is such a big issue, it deserves a whole book (my trainer Bob Greene's book *Get With the Program!* is great on the subject). But I do know that if you just start moving, you *will* feel better. My motto to my boot campers has been "Do the thing you think you cannot do." In other words, force yourself to get up and walk a mile or go to the gym, even though it's the last thing you want to do. After ten or 20 minutes—for me it's about seven—the endorphins kick in and your spirits lift. In fact, we did a piece called "Shortcut to Bliss" (on page 32) about how exercise can be as helpful as antidepressants. And during our boot camp, a study came out saying three half-hour workouts a week relieved depression by almost 50 percent. But this is the deal: You can't sit around and wait for the mood to strike—"Oh, wouldn't a workout be nice?"—because it's not going to happen. You know what? I *never* feel like it. You do it although you don't feel like it—that's what discipline is. You just have to walk through the wall. And start slow. Many a day, I ease my way in—getting on the treadmill at three mph, going up a tenth of a point every minute, and before you know it, I'm kicking it at seven.

THE WHITE STUFF

When you say you stay away from refined carbs and sugars, can you tell me specifically what you mean? Anything white?

—Linda Boyd, 39, Lockport, Illinois

I do often say "the white stuff," but what I mean is any carbohydrates that have been processed. Potato chips. Crackers. White bread. White pasta. White rice. Cookies. Cake....

TEAM SPIRIT

I started a wellness program for the staff at Hellgate High School in Missoula. About 50 of us are "steppin' to Chicago to see Oprah," which is 1,589.4 miles away, by keeping track on a pedometer. I have a map up and a chart of how everyone is doing. Our goal is to reach you by the end of the school year.

—Lynn, 43, Montana

Bravo. That's how you do it. Listen, I've worked out by myself, with a trainer, with a group—it's definitely more fun with a group. So I'm applauding you. Can you hear me applauding you all the way from Chicago?

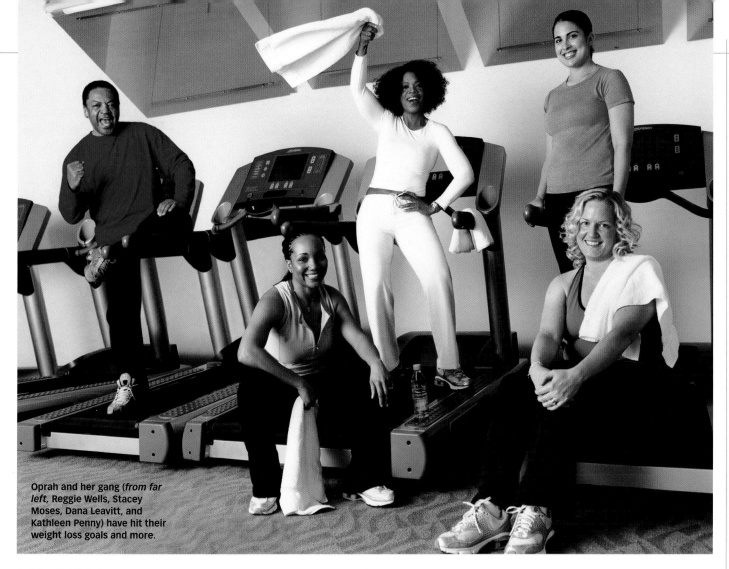

Oprah and her gang (*from far left,* Reggie Wells, Stacey Moses, Dana Leavitt, and Kathleen Penny) have hit their weight loss goals and more.

DOING IT FOR YOURSELF

When I met my husband, Cory, I was 125 pounds. Two years later, I weigh in at about 205. We used to be intimate, but now we hardly do anything. I promised him that I would be back down to what I looked like when we met by our anniversary, but I can't stick to my diet. I don't want to lose Cory to a good-looking girl. I will do anything if I can get your help. Please.

—*Christina DeMille, 19, Washington, Utah*

Fuhggedit. *F.u.h.g.g.e.d.i.t.* It will never, ever work. Christina, you can't lose weight for Cory. You didn't put the weight on because of Cory, and you won't be able to take the weight off because of Cory. If you want to look like you did two years ago, the decision—and it must be an emotional, spiritual decision—can come only from you and be only for you. From you. For you. Nothing to do with Cory.

WHAT TO EAT

I want to join the boot camp. But I have a few questions: (1) Can you have any dairy? (2) Eggs? (3) Yams or sweet potatoes? (4) Any vegetables besides green ones?

—*Syneetra Hill, 25, Newark, New Jersey*

In our boot camp, we didn't do any dairy. But you could. I'd just keep it to eight ounces of low-fat or fat-free milk or yogurt per day. And yes, you can have eggs. Now the yams and sweet potatoes, that's a no, not while you're in the boot camp phase. When you get into maintenance, you can add them back in. As for other vegetables, you can have all of them except corn, potatoes, and beets. So yes on tomatoes, yes on squash. You can even have carrots. Nobody ever got fat eating carrots.

HOW ABOUT SPLENDA?

Can I use Splenda in my oatmeal once I get past the first month?

—*Stephanie Berry, 33, Jennings, Missouri*

Yes, and this is one of my favorite ways of doing it: Take your oatmeal (I use steel-cut because it's crunchier), add 1 Splenda, 1 Tbsp. of hazelnut coffee creamer; mix in a handful of blueberries, then sprinkle 6 chopped almonds on top. Da-lish! Tastes better than a sundae. I like it so much, sometimes I'll have it for lunch.

THE PLATEAU

Oprah! I need your help. At my peak, I was 257 pounds. I am now 195 and have hit a wall. I just can't seem to get past it. How have you gotten over plateaus?

—*Carissa Taft, 24, Auburn, Washington*

The way to get past a plateau is to move faster and harder. People think they can do the same old workout every day, but your body

23

gets used to it and stops losing weight. That's what happened with one of my boot campers, Stacey. Before we started, I'd see her in the gym year in, year out, doing the treadmill, StairMaster, weights…treadmill, StairMaster, weights—it never changed. One day when I thought, *Dear God, there she is again!*, I said, "Do you want me to help you?" It wasn't until boot camp, where we pushed ourselves further every day, that she lost 25 pounds. So if you are stuck, gradually add more speed and intensity to your workout and you should start losing weight again. And by the way, to anybody reading the paper on the StairMaster, I say, "May I offer you a cocktail, too? Would you like a lemon with that?"

PORTION CONTROL

Can you help me with the amounts of food I should eat on the plan?

—*Patty Karfs, 46, Belleville, Illinois*

This is the way I look at it: When you consider that your stomach is about the size of your fist, no portion should be larger than what can fit into the palm of your hand. So if you're having steak, the piece must be only as big as your palm—not the palm, wrist, and extended thumb and fingers. The same with each of the other foods you're eating with that steak. You should be able to cup the peas in one hand without them spilling all over the place, you know what I mean? That's how I measure portions.

SUGAR ADDICT

I am a carb addict. What do you eat to feed the sweet cravings so you don't blow all the hard work you've accomplished?

—*Wendy Oakley, 32, Ozark, Missouri*

What saves me when I'm craving—because I have a huge chocolate thing—are sugar–free Fudgsicles. The sugar-free Popsicles hit the sweet spot, too. With diet drinks, I limit myself to two a day. I say two because if you have more, you're going to feel bloated. Also, I know people who guzzle diet soda all day long, and that cannot possibly be good for you.

FINDING SUPPORT

I am a teen who has been dealing with constant weight battles. Every day I go home crying to my mother about how much I get teased. Since my hometown is small, I can't seem to find help; I'm not sure where to turn.

—*Sierra Cummings, 18, Lottsburg, Virginia*

Why don't you join our boot camp online at oprah.com/makeover? We're just starting a special walking program for people who can't get to the gym. If you do the program, you'll lose weight. Guaranteed. You could also organize your own boot camp group where you live. I've struggled with my weight for years, but I finally realize it's not that hard. The key is making up your mind that you want to do this for yourself. You also need to get the right information about food and exercise—and then follow it. When people say, "I've tried every diet and not one of them has worked," I ask, "And how many did you stick with?" All diets work if you follow them.

NO TIME

I've been trying most of my life to lose weight, but when I do, I can't keep it off. Now I can't stand to look at myself in the mirror. I work full-time and go to school, so it's hard to get to the gym. Could you tell me what has helped you, besides hiring a personal trainer, which I can't afford?

—*Maribel Jiminez, 27, Texas*

You say you can't bear to look at yourself in the mirror. I can relate. I felt that way every day I was more than 200 pounds. But I also know that you do not need a personal trainer or a gym to get fit. You need a decision. A decision on your part to take action, which means educating yourself about what to eat and making a commitment to start moving—a half mile, then a mile, two miles, one step at a time. My point is this: If you can't find time to work out, then you don't want to lose the weight. It's simply a matter of physics. So ask yourself what you're willing to do. And if you aren't prepared to exercise and cut down on your volume of food as a way of life, stop wasting time feeling bad about your weight and move on to something else.

ABUSE AND WEIGHT

I was abused as a child and am just beginning to face it at 40 years of age. Now for the first time I find myself comfort-eating (desserts seem to be the only thing that make me happy). How do you deal with the pain? I'm sad and worn-out from trying to confront my past. What worked for you, and do you think it could work for me? I want to lose 40 pounds.

—*Cheryl Carr Johnson, 40, Wichita, Kansas*

First, let me commend you for your courage. I was abused, I was ignored, I felt abandoned, my single greatest emotion growing up was feeling alone. And for me, a big moment was recognizing that I'd come through it all, that I'm still here. A book that helped me a lot and that I highly recommend is *The Power of Now,* by Eckhart Tolle. It's basically about how the only time that matters is the present and the way you choose to use it. What I'd say to you, Cheryl, is this: Remember, you were able to overcome unimaginable horrors you had no control over. Now you do have control (even over those desserts). To really let go of the pain, you've got to give up the hope that the past could have been different. So move forward with the strength you've been given to live an undefeated life.

STARTING FROM SCRATCH

My mother and I need a weight loss plan (she's at least 300 pounds, and I'm 260). We want to support each other, but we have no idea where to start. Please point us in the right direction.

—*Kerri Olds, 24, Waco, Texas*

You can start a mother-daughter boot camp by walking together (see oprah.com/makeover). At first you may only make it two blocks or one lap around the track. When I was 237 pounds, I could do only half a mile, but in eight months I was able to run a 26-mile marathon. I would also recommend eliminating "the white stuff" from your diet—for me that's the easiest way to lose weight. You'll probably feel lethargic as you detox from the sugar, which can be like a drug. But after the third day, you should come out of it.

Reggie, my makeup artist and a doughnut freak, got off sugar in our boot camp, and it took him only three days. Oh, I tell you, though, that second day, he looked like he'd been in a boxing match with Mike Tyson, and I mean Tyson in his prime.

FEEDING THE FAMILY

I am 5'4" and weigh more than 250 pounds. It is *so* hard to make healthy items for me and meet my family's meat-and-potatoes needs when I barely have the energy to work out and still cook. Any suggestions?
—*Kelly Kritz, 41, Wauwatosa, Wisconsin*

Food doesn't have to be artery clogging in order for it to taste good. "The Incredibles" from the April 2005 issue really are incredible. I live on everything from that article, and it's all nutritious, delicious, quick, and simple to make. A bowl of garlic-wilted spinach? My God, it's unbelievable! The wild salmon and soybeans—fantastic. The broccoli and roasted-walnut soup, that's a favorite as well. Find those recipes at www2.oprah.com/omagazine/200504/omag_200504_food.jhtml. Or you can find a lot of healthy and easy recipes in Art Smith's *Kitchen Life: Real Food for Real Families—Even Yours!* I've eaten everything in that book. And if your family still has to have their meat and potatoes, serve yourself a smaller portion of the beef or pork and go easy on the spuds. Losing weight permanently is about integrating the way you eat into your lifestyle.

OPRAH'S OWN QUESTION

Okay, it's my turn to ask myself a question: What did I gain—and lose—from this boot camp? In a way, this was the most perfect experiment because four out of four lost weight. My boot campers confirmed for me how hard work and persistence pay off. And I got to see my favorite motto—"Always go higher than you think you can go"—in action. We'd be in the gym, and I'd say, "Okay, is everybody out of breath? You think you can't take another step? All right, let's take two more." Two steps later: "So, you did two. Now let's take four."

I always work and play better if I can be the teacher. It's been that way since the time I was standing on my grandmother's front yard teaching the children Bible stories, telling them who Nicodemus was. And I learn along with my students. Our youngest teammate, Dana, for example, was working harder than any of us and losing the least. One day she was complaining that she'd lost only 11 pounds. So I went and filled a bag with pork fat and hogs' intestines. "Here's 'only' 11 pounds," I said. "That's what you were lugging around before—you want it back?" The idea was not to get caught up with the number on the scale but to focus on how your body feels. She totally got it. And that's something I've been thinking about as well.

At the beginning of boot camp, I weighed in with everybody else. I was 163, and I wanted to get down to the 150s because somewhere in there is my fighting weight. But I can't tell you how much I've lost because I haven't stepped on a scale since.

During these 12 weeks, I've come to a decision: I'm not going to live in my 50s as a weight or a size. My whole life—anytime I've looked at a video or picture of myself—I could tell you to a pound, "There I was size 18...that one, a 22...oh, here I am a size 6 (for two hours)...yup, cover of *Vogue* at 160." I just don't want to do that to myself anymore.

I'm still working on getting to the point where I'm tight and performing optimally on all cylinders—moving from my center in Pilates, carrying my body so that I completely honor myself. I'm not there yet. But I will be.

For now I know that this obsession we have with thinness is diminishing to us all. So my new obsession is going to be with fullness. I can't tell you if I'll ever get on a scale again. In the next phase of life, I am determined to fully own myself as a woman, in a way that is not associated with my size or weight but with how I feel in my skin. That's what I'm looking for. Let me just say, the possibility is thrilling. **O**

The Boot Campers: How'd They Do?

REGGIE WELLS, Makeup artist, 57; weight lost: 30 pounds
BIGGEST BREAKTHROUGH: "I think I got the eating and the exercise part down pat. Now I realize it's continuing this lifestyle that's important. I'm hoping I get to the point where I can relax and take a piece of bread now and then because that doggone no-carbs thing can drive you insane."
BONUS: "When I started, my blood pressure was 180 over 100. I was very afraid when I saw those numbers. Now it's 122 over 78—almost normal."

STACEY MOSES, Supervisor of music licensing for legal and business affairs, 32; weight lost: 25 pounds
BIGGEST BREAKTHROUGH: "Oprah says to do the things you think you cannot do. So every time I wanted to give up, I'd just tell myself, *I have to walk a little farther, a little faster,* and I'd do it. And that was huge."
BONUS: "I feel so much better, and the workouts are a lot easier."

DANA LEAVITT, Researcher, 23; weight lost: 14 pounds
BIGGEST BREAKTHROUGH: "I discovered that if I just get up and take a little walk whenever I'm feeling trapped or overwhelmed, I don't turn to food. Making tea or doing a minute of breathing also helps."
BONUS: "I've gone down two sizes and learned to like my body more. I've also learned how to push myself, and the boot camp gave me the confidence to know I can do it."

KATHLEEN PENNY, Production manager for creative services, 42; weight lost: 19 pounds
BIGGEST BREAKTHROUGH: "The 7:30 P.M. food cutoff time was my toughest challenge. I used to come home and eat dinner around 9 as the reward at the end of the day. I was taking in so many calories in the evening. So now I get home and eat, and the reward is to lie down on the couch or watch TV."
BONUS: "After 12 weeks, I forget the pain and how hard it is."

I Can't Believe I Ate the Whole Thing

We crunch. We stuff. We say, "Seconds, please." And most of the time, we haven't the faintest idea how much we're eating—or why. But social scientist Brian Wansink's discoveries might very well change your life. PATRICIA VOLK listens hungrily.

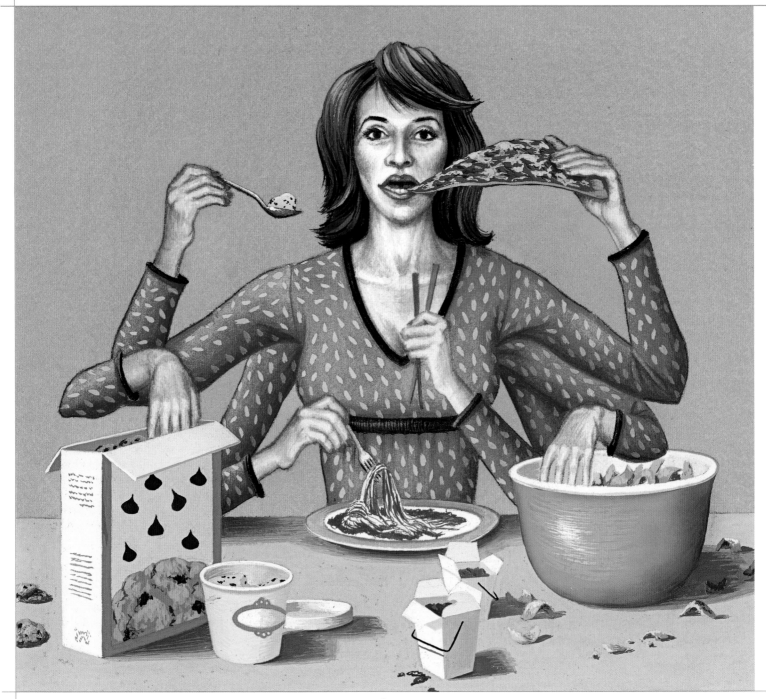

I'm watching behind a two-way mirror. A woman serves herself lunch. She scoops two ladles full of pasta into a 17-ounce bowl. She's in a state-of-the-art yet homey kitchen. A man takes her tray and adds a soda to it. The tray "slips" from his hands. Pasta cascades into the sink.

"Sorry, Vicky," he says. This time he hands her a 34-ounce bowl. This time she ferries four ladles into it.

The bigger the plate, the more you will eat.

I ATE *THAT?*

Professor Brian Wansink, PhD, is the author of *Mindless Eating: Why We Eat More Than We Think.* Director of the Food and Brand Lab at Cornell University, Brian has conducted more than 250 experiments proving that people have no idea how much they're putting in their mouths or for what reason. Everyone, he tells me, makes about 250 food decisions a day: Should I have coffee? Should I put milk in it? Whole or skim? Sugar? Splenda? Do I pour my orange juice into a short, wide glass (you'll drink more) or a tall, narrow glass (you'll drink less)?

After finishing her pasta, Vicky is debriefed. She thought she was participating in a taste test. She's shocked to learn that her second bowl contained twice as much as her first. She had no idea she'd plopped in four ladles. Brian reports: "In the thousands of debriefings we've done for hundreds of studies, more than 90 percent of the people didn't realize that the words on a label, the size of a package or plate, or the lighting in a room had any effect on how much they consumed."

According to the Centers for Disease Control, 32.2 percent of American adults are obese. Brian Wansink wants to help. "If we knew why we ate the way we do, we could eat a little less, eat a little healthier, and enjoy it a lot more," he says. He is targeting that bag of chips your hand keeps dipping into while you watch TV. That 13-inch plate you load whether you're hungry or not (you'll eat 92 percent of what's on it anyway). That second helping of pie because the pie plate is on the table.

His kitchen with two-way mirrors can be converted into a dining room or living room in three hours. Scales lurk beneath plates. A table is rigged so two diners get normal soup bowls. The other two have bowls with holes in the bottom linked to hoses that pump in more tomato soup as they eat. Guess who spoons up more soup? Guess who has no idea they did?

EXPERIMENTS IN EATING

Since opening in 1997, the Food Lab has proved that the more variety we have, the more we eat. If you offer people a bowl of mixed jelly beans, they'll take a bigger portion than if there's only one flavor.

> "Everyone makes about 250 food decisions a day: Should I have coffee? Should I put milk in it? Whole or skim? Sugar? Splenda?"

We don't know when we're *not* hungry. In one study, moviegoers who'd had a meal within the previous hour were given a free bucket of popcorn, either giant-size or medium. Although everyone had just eaten, and half the participants were given two-week-old popcorn, they all dug in. Those with larger buckets consumed significantly more, even if they had a stale batch. Their cue was the size of the container. "Cues can short-circuit a person's hunger and taste signals, leading them to eat even if they're not hungry and even if the food doesn't taste good," Brian says.

Shoppers think famous brands are better than store brands. But they can't pick which brand is the one they prefer when they can't see the label. Offered a free glass of inexpensive wine (Charles Shaw, a.k.a. Two-Buck Chuck), diners who were told it was from a California vineyard drank more and lingered ten minutes longer at the table. People told the wine was from North Dakota drank less, ate less, and finished eating in record time.

You will consume more gâteau du chocolate au ganache than the identical dessert called chocolate cake. My dad was in the restaurant business in New York. Ever the poet, he was famous for his chicken soup, listed as "Essence of Young Fowl" on the menu.

A HUNGRY BOY

Brian grew up in Sioux City, Iowa. Rangy, 6'1", with a shock of blond hair and cornflower blue eyes, he is what Iowa looks like. When I arrive in Ithaca to spend the day with him, we stop at a fast-food place so he can have breakfast number two. Up at 5 A.M. to work, he had a bowl of cereal and shared a can of tuna with Kirby, his cat, for breakfast number one. Now Brian orders a 32-ounce diet soda (he prefers his caffeine without coffee), a yogurt parfait, and eggs he drowns in ketchup.

Food wasn't always this plentiful. Whenever Brian's father was laid off, there wasn't enough. "If we have only two pieces of bread," his mother reassured him, "you will have one and your brother will have one."

"Is your brother thin, too?" I ask.

"My brother," Brian's eyes fill, "is very big."

Brian says everyone has a comfort food. I ask what his is. He names the classic stretchable meal: "Casseroles."

"Do you ever mindlessly eat?"

"If I'm at a reception, I don't pay attention. I'll eat fruit and veggies till they're gone. They're what I call free foods. I'll eat those instead of pizza."

THE MINDLESS MARGIN

Brian believes you can lose weight as thoughtlessly as you gain it. If you eat 30 percent less, he says, you'll notice. If you eat 20 percent less, you probably won't. Making a 100 to 200 calorie change a day, you won't feel deprived. There are 3,500 calories in a pound. Add or subtract 250 calories a day, and that's a half pound more or less each week, or 26 pounds a year. One less Snickers a day equals a weight loss of almost 30 pounds a year, one less soda is 14 pounds. Walk one extra mile a day, you can burn 100 extra calories, good for a ten-pound loss per year. Give up your daily Snickers, too, and you've lost about 40 pounds by this time next year. I love when Brian says, "Cutting out our favorite foods is a bad idea. Cutting down on how much of them we eat is mindlessly doable."

LITTLE THINGS MEAN A LOT

During our day together, Brian gives two lectures, one to academics, one to students. He also describes addressing PTAs to teach parents of overweight kids how to painlessly reeducate a sweet tooth: "If they like chocolate ice cream, try switching to strawberry ice cream. Then serve sliced strawberries on vanilla ice cream. And then a bowl of sliced strawberries with no ice cream."

Brian tells me his wife, Jennifer, is visiting her father in Taiwan with Audrey, their 1-year-old.

"What does Audrey eat?" I ask.

"Everything."

Mindful Eating

7 ESSENTIAL TIDBITS FROM BRIAN WANSINK

1. **PEOPLE WHO STOCK UP AT DISCOUNT STORES** eat up to 48 percent more. If you buy in bulk, put pretzels and other snacks in portion-size Baggies. Never, never, ever eat out of the box.

2. **THE LONGER YOU SIT AT THE TABLE,** the more you'll eat. Dine with one friend, you'll eat about 35 percent more. With a group of seven, you'll eat 96 percent more. If you're trying to lose weight, eat alone or with the smallest group possible and pace yourself with the lightest eater.

3. **IF YOU PRE-PLATE YOUR FOOD IN THE KITCHEN,** you'll eat 14 percent less than if you serve yourself a smaller portion at the table and then take seconds.

4. **BRIAN'S RULE OF TWO:** When eating at a buffet, put only two items at a time on your plate. Even if you make repeated trips, you'll eat a lot less.

5. **ALWAYS EAT IN THE SAME ROOM OF YOUR HOUSE** (but not in front of a TV or computer). You won't snack as much.

6. **DON'T LEAVE SERVING DISHES ON THE TABLE** unless they're filled with vegetables.

7. **A BUTTERFINGER OR A HUG?** What do you really want? Physical hunger builds gradually. Emotional hunger develops suddenly.

"Anchovies?"

"White anchovies."

Late in the afternoon, Brian fine-tunes a new experiment with his staff. Before I catch my plane home, we stop for dinner at his house. The food looks gorgeous—deviled eggs, ratatouille over pasta, a tomato and cuke salad with goat cheese and balsamic vinaigrette, and another salad with mozzarella, prepared by Ganael Bascoul and Carolina Werle, PhD candidates visiting from France. Brian is a generous host. He fills our wineglasses with precious Château Mouton Rothschild 1945. We clink. All of us agree the wine is superb. Dessert is warm-from-the-oven homemade apple tart with vanilla ice cream. I mindlessly scarf it. Then Brian reaches for the empty wine bottle. He peels off the label. It is a Romanian cheapo called Werewolf.

Brian belongs to a band. "Will you play your saxophone?" I ask. He shakes his head. "When Audrey was three days old, I played 'You Belong to Me' for her and she cried so hard I haven't played much since."

"Could you do the chocolate ice cream–strawberries experiment with her?"

"What do you mean?"

"Start her on John Coltrane played low, then Coltrane played louder, then you playing John Coltrane."

THE POWER OF THREE

At the beginning of every month, Brian makes three changes in his life. As a social scientist, he believes that "if you repeat a behavior for 28 days, it becomes a new habit. You can change your default behavior to something else."

"What three things are you doing now?" I ask.

"I'm drinking two glasses of water for every glass of soda I drink. I'm eating French fries only on weekends. And no candy unless it's something I've never had before."

"What's a new candy?"

"Reese's caramel peanut butter cups. White chocolate M&M's."

I decide I'll try the power of three, too. For the next 28 days, no old-fashioned M&M's, no bagels, and...*what?* "Does it have to be food related?" I ask.

"No. I gave up nail-biting on my wedding day."

He holds out a perfect hand.

In recent months, Brian has used the power of three to include a protein at breakfast, have any snack he wants but *only* after eating a piece of fruit, and give his wife a unique compliment (one he's never given before) every day.

So for my third thing, I'm going to make the bed when I get out of it, not right before I get into it at night.

It has been 21 days since I met Brian Wansink. No M&M's have crossed these lips. You could bounce a quarter on my bed by 8 A.M. And the bagels? Those dripping-butter, crusty, crunchy, toasted New York cinnamon raisin bagels I covet with my coffee? Those bagels I think I can stockpile in the freezer and somehow not touch? I know I have a bagel problem. I know it's serious. So for my next power of three, I'm starting with "When you get to the block with the bagel store, cross the street." ◘

9 Things Weight Loss Winners Know (That You Don't)

It's not chocolates or potato chips that sabotage diets (try fear, old attitudes, tempting environments). PHILLIP C. McGRAW, PhD, shows what works.

In 30 years of working with weight loss patients, I've seen a lot of people achieve physical transformations they never thought they were capable of. They'd all tried different approaches, had individual challenges, and were ultimately guided by their own philosophies and personalities. But no matter what strategy ended up working for them, the majority of people whom I've seen reach and maintain their goals learned to accept certain core ideas that kept them solidly on the path

> Food is the most powerfully addictive substance in the world because you can't abstain from it.

to success. Below I've outlined these fundamentals, which are also found in my book *The Ultimate Weight Solution*. They've been mastered by weight loss winners the world 'round, some of whose stories you'll read here. Commit to them, and you will count yourself among the successes. You will achieve weight loss freedom once and for all.

1. FEELING GOOD IS YOUR GOD-GIVEN RIGHT. People who succeed feel they're entitled to be healthy—mentally, physically, emotionally, and spiritually. It's part of their personal truth. They've abandoned any tendencies to martyrdom and accepted that their families are better off with a healthy and happy mother, wife, or sister. They've acknowledged that they've got a right to feel good, live long, and be happy, even if it means being "selfish" with their time and claiming an hour a day to walk the mall or hop on the exercise bike. So start by saying to yourself—and believing it—*I'm doing this for me. I will accept nothing less because I deserve it.*

2. FEAR IS THE FIRST OBSTACLE. Do thoughts like these ever enter your head? *I'm not worthy of losing weight. Being slim and feeling good is for other people—not for me.* Do you believe your time is better spent in taking care of others, to the detriment of your own health? Have you ever thought your weight is in control of you, and you'll never conquer it?

All of these ideas are just excuses—they work as a decoy to prevent you from facing your fears. What fears? Well, perhaps you've tried so many times to lose weight that the thought of failing one more time is too scary. Or maybe it's the actual weight loss process that's frightening. You think you'll suffer deprivation, pain, hunger, or depression. Some fear life after they've slimmed down because being sexually relevant will be a new experience and there may be new social pressures. It's natural to find solace in inertia, because requiring nothing of yourself isn't as scary as instigating change. But smart people who've tried and tried and finally succeeded have learned that monsters live in the dark and that when they're brought into the light, they can be faced head-on. Identify your fears, find their sources, and acknowledge that you can handle them. Against any kind of scrutiny, they just won't stand up.

3. **THE NUMBERS ON THE SCALE ARE MEANINGLESS.** Everything you have to do to lose weight and maintain it depends on behavioral choices, so it makes sense to focus on behavior. The scale is fickle. Your menstrual cycle alone could cause the dial to go up a bit (that's before you even think about satisfying the cravings that come along with it). People who succeed say to themselves, *I'm not going to worry about what that number says from one day to the next. I'm going to start behaving like a healthy person, and then the number will come. I've got to change the way I live, what I focus on, and what I do.* You can't be overweight if you don't behave overweight. So stop talking about diets, and start thinking about being a healthy person and living in a way that will generate the results you want.

4. **FOOD IS AN ADDICTION.** Recognize that you have become addicted psychologically and physiologically. Food is the most powerfully addictive substance in the world because you can't abstain from it. You can quit alcohol or drugs, but you've got to eat. Understand also that you have been programmed by a marketing machine. You've seen too many fast food commercials with people laughing and talking and being part of a jovial group while they all hold a hamburger. That's manipulation of the highest order. You'll notice that you hardly ever see people in those commercials actually eating, because it's simply not fun or attractive to look at someone grinding up dead animals. Instead you see celebration and community. When you realize that your need to belong and be accepted is not going to control you, you won't want to give your power away again.

5. **BEFORE A PERSON CAN CHANGE, HER ENVIRONMENT HAS TO.** Unsuccessful dieters think that cleaning up their cupboards means simply getting the junk food out of the house and steering clear of the fast food lane. Successful losers take it one step further. They realize: *If I'm hungry, I'm going to eat, so I need to fill my environment with stuff that's good for me.* Don't put yourself in a position where you've got nothing at all in the house, you're starving, and you make an "emergency" hamburger run, or you feel so deprived at work that you have to sprint to the vending

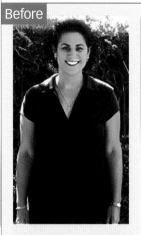

Before

"One thing I know: that when I take care of myself it's good for my family."

KELLY APISA, 35
Starting weight: 226
Lost 57 pounds

"As a single working mother, I was definitely used to putting others' needs first. Then I realized that by not taking care of myself, I wasn't being as great a mom as I could be. I had no energy, I was grumpy, and I didn't feel good about myself. I decided to make taking care of myself a commitment that's simply nonnegotiable. My workouts became no different from a doctor's appointment that I had to keep. I started getting up earlier to exercise and getting into bed earlier to get a good night's sleep. I feel 100 percent better about myself and have more energy and balance in my life than ever before. I'm a much happier person, and in so many ways it's as good for my son as it is for me."

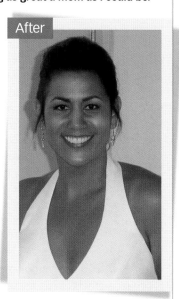

After

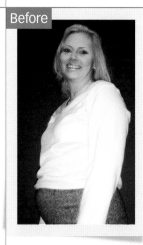

Before

"One thing I know: that the only one holding me back was me."

LYNNE HERFEL, 38
Starting weight: 184
Lost 48 pounds

"Dr. Phil talks about how baby circus elephants are attached by heavy chains to immovable steel stakes, so that by the time they weigh six tons, all that's needed to keep them in line is a little rope and a wooden stake. They don't run off even though it would be so easy, because they're conditioned to believe they can't. It made me realize that if this time was going to be different, I needed to completely reprogram myself and get rid of my self-defeating thoughts. I had to get to a place where I believed I could do it. Once I did that, everything else fell into place. That's not to say that getting up at 5:30 every morning so I have time to exercise without neglecting my family is easy! But now that I know I can succeed, changing my lifestyle isn't as daunting."

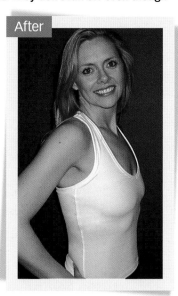

After

machines. Reengineer your surroundings in a way that pulls you in the right direction. Get all the garbage out of your house, and fill your kitchen with fruits, vegetables, whole grains, lean meats, sugar-free beverages—things you can consume until you're blue in the face without losing ground. Bring healthy snacks to work, or get in the routine of walking with your cubicle mate to buy a piece of fruit midmorning.

6. **THE BOY SCOUT MOTTO APPLIES TO CRAVINGS, TOO.** Take a close look at your day, and you'll see you've got some consistent time slots when temptation gets the best of you. It could be during an afternoon break at work, when you get home at the end of the day, or once the kids go to bed. If every morning when you get to the office you indulge in a doughnut and a hot chocolate, that can add up to nearly 30 pounds a year, even if the rest of the day you're eating spinach.

Be prepared. Successful losers identify the target time, place, activity, people, and moods that trigger the impulse to eat junk food, overeat, eat too fast, or partake in any other mindless

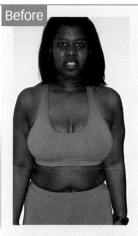

Before

"One thing I know: that mindless eating can be cured with a little attention."

JACQUETTA JACOBS, 30
Starting weight: 191
Lost 46 pounds

"**Work is stressful. I used to ease my anxiety with food. Sitting at my computer, I'd reach for Twizzlers, and before I knew it, I'd finished half the bag. Then I'd get home** from the tough day, starving and ready to unwind, and I'd eat a huge meal. I was packing on hundreds of extra calories without even noticing. Now I eat every two to three hours, choose a lot more multigrain carbs, fruits, and vegetables than I used to, and have my last meal by 7 P.M. You can't snack on junk food when it's not around. During the day, I don't carry any change on me for the vending machines. I've embraced a lifestyle that helps me cope with stress in healthy ways, and it's made all the difference."

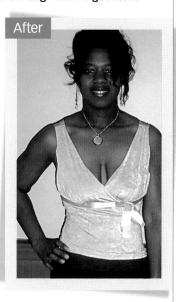

After

behavior that stands between them and their goals. Then they come up with creative and constructive ways to avoid those danger zones. Be ready for yours by planning an activity that's incompatible with eating, like exercising, playing with your kids, taking a bath, or walking the dog. It may be as simple as entering the house by a different door so you don't have to pass through the kitchen. Divert your attention and change your routine by finding new coping mechanisms that prevent you from getting derailed. When you have a strategy worked out in advance, one that is stronger than the negative pull of your past bad habits and programming, you'll be surprised by how quickly your urges will pass and your habits will change.

7. **NO ONE EVER LOST BIG WITHOUT BREAKING A SWEAT.** Weight loss winners know they don't have to run marathons but do have to get regular exercise. They learn not to be intimidated by the idea of exercise. At first it may feel forced, like any obligation. But eventually, they get to a point where they either embrace it or at the very least accept it as a necessary part of the day. They tell themselves, *I don't have to like it—I just have to do it. I just have to resolve to stop living like a lazy slug and become more active.* The physical and psychological payoffs are innumerable, and neglecting to exercise can shorten your life. You may need to experiment a bit, but find an activity you like and program it into your lifestyle so it's as much a part of your routine as showering or getting dressed.

8. **CONSTANT DEPRIVATION IS FOR MONKS.** People who succeed invariably acknowledge their efforts and progress. They've learned how and when to pat themselves on the back. When you deserve it, tell yourself, *I'm doing a great job here. I got through today well. I'm almost there.* Now, don't destroy all your hard work with precisely the kind of treat that will get you off track. Change your definition of a reward from a free-for-all with a Whitman's Sampler to getting a new haircut, buying a new outfit, or giving yourself a half hour alone to enjoy the sunset.

9. **THE BEST MOTIVATION IS YOUR OWN HAPPINESS.** When people attempt to lose weight so someone will want them or like them better, it doesn't work. Taking charge of your weight is about exercising your personal power and changing yourself from the inside out—not trying to please someone else. If you use someone else as motivation, you'll be miserable and perhaps even resentful of that person. The successful people I've worked with learned that they had to get to the point of psychological readiness where they said, *Never mind what everyone else wants; I'm doing this for me.* You would walk to hell and back again for your husband? Well, do something far less strenuous but equally loving for yourself. Challenge yourself to use your energy, your vitality toward changing your own life. This isn't about pleasing the marketing machine that tells you you're only of value if you're a size 6 or smaller. It's about feeling better every time you have to walk up a set of stairs or run to catch a bus or when you first open your eyes and feel comfortable in your own skin. **O**

Shortcut to Bliss

What lifts depression, jump-starts creativity, soothes jitters, muscles up immune systems, reignites sex lives, and zings your body with tiny arrows of pleasure? Would you believe: small—really small—amounts of regular exercise. Honestly, it's a miracle. DAVID SERVAN-SCHREIBER, MD, reports.

Jennifer Travis* was a 28-year-old student pursuing a second master's degree at the University of Wisconsin. She lived alone, rarely went out except to her classes, and constantly complained that she would never meet the man of her life. Her existence seemed empty, and she had lost hope that it would change. Her only consolation was her beloved three packs of cigarettes a day. She spent her time watching smoke waft upward in wreaths instead of concentrating on her course notes.

Jennifer wasn't surprised when the doctor at the school clinic reported that her score on a scale for depression placed her among the most affected 10 percent of the patients there. By then her depression had been going on for two years, but neither of the suggested treatments was acceptable to her. She did not want to talk to a psychologist about her mother and father or the problems of her childhood. And she refused medication because, as she said, "I may be depressed, but I'm not sick." She agreed nevertheless to take part in a research project the doctor was conducting, perhaps because it seemed like a challenge.

Jennifer was supposed to jog three times a week for 20 to 30 minutes. She could run alone or in a group—how she did it was completely up to her. At her first meeting with the jogging instructor, the reality of what she had signed up for hit her in the face. How could he possibly expect a person 20 pounds overweight who had not exercised since the age of 14 and smoked three packs a day to start running? The last time she'd gone biking, she had made it only ten minutes and thought she was going to die. "Never again," she'd sworn. And the idea that she needed an instructor to learn how to run seemed even more ridiculous.

Still, Jennifer listened to the instructor's advice, guidance that turned out to be absolutely essential to her future success.

First, he directed her to take very small steps, trotting rather than running, leaning forward very slightly, without raising her knees too much. Above all, she was told to go slowly enough to hold a conversation ("You have to be able to talk but not sing," the instructor insisted). If she got out of breath, she was ordered to slow down—if need be, to go at no more than a brisk walking pace. She must never experience pain or fatigue.

The goal at the outset was simply to cover a mile, taking as long as she liked, trying to jog as much as possible. The fact that she managed to reach this objective on the very first day was a source of satisfaction for her. After three weeks, at a rate of three weekly sessions, she was able to keep up her jogging pace for a mile and a half, then two miles without any real hardship. She had to admit that she found herself feeling a bit better—overall, she was sleeping more soundly, had more energy, and was spending less time dwelling on her problems. Then, at the end of one of her runs, she twisted her ankle—not badly enough to completely immobilize her but enough to keep her from exercising for three weeks. She was surprised at how disappointed she was not to be able to go jogging. After a week, dark thoughts came crowding in and she noticed her symptoms of depression returning.

When Jennifer's ankle healed and she was finally able to exercise again, the depression waned within a few weeks. She had never felt so well. Even her period—which was usually very painful—seemed less uncomfortable. Long after the research project ended, Jennifer was still regularly spotted running around the lake with a smile on her face.

Depression is always associated with gloomy, pessimistic, recurrent thoughts that undercut the self and others: "I'll never succeed. I'm ugly. I'm not bright enough. I have bad luck. I'm sick...." These ideas may be as excessive as they are hurtful (such as "I always disappoint everybody," which simply cannot be true). But by the time they manifest in depression, they've usually become so automatic that it is no longer obvious how abnormal they are. One of the characteristics of sustained physical effort is precisely that it puts a halt, at least temporarily, to the torrent of depressive thoughts. Most people who jog or run say that after 15 or 20 minutes, they reach a state in which they feel spontaneously positive and even creative. If negative messages pop up, which is rare, just diverting your attention to your breathing or to the sensation of your feet pressing down on the ground is usually enough to see them off.

Joggers and runners also gradually become less conscious of themselves as they go—easing the depressive inward dwelling that interferes with the ability to enjoy the simple events of life. They describe letting the rhythm of their effort lead them on—an experience some refer to as the runner's high, a kind of flow. Only those who persevere for several weeks experience it. This state, subtle as it is, often becomes addictive. After a certain amount of consistent exercise, many joggers can no longer go without their 20 minutes of running, even for a single day.

Name has been changed.

The big mistake that beginners make is to want to go too fast for too long. Truthfully, there is no magic speed or distance. What leads to a feeling of flow is persisting in an effort that you sustain at the limit of your capacities. *At* the limit, but no further. Research on states of flow has demonstrated this. For a first-timer, the distance will inevitably be short and the steps small. Later the jogger may have to go faster and longer in order to maintain flow, but probably only after he or she has already become addicted.

The project Jennifer Travis participated in was one of the early studies to show the mood-lifting power of exercise. The evidence has grown steadily more convincing ever since. In 1999 researchers at Duke University published the results of a study in which they divided depressed patients ages

France, I hardly knew anybody. Besides going to medical school, I was looking for an apartment, moving in, getting the lay of the land. Starting all over again, without parents around to tell me what to do, was fun at the beginning, but after a few months, my life seemed empty, devoid of pleasure. Without my family, my friends, my culture, my favorite hangouts, I felt as if I were slowly withering away. I remember one evening in particular, nothing seemed to matter or make sense except classical music. I listened to Schubert endlessly instead of studying. After several weeks in this stark mood, I realized that if I didn't do something, I was going to fail my exams.

I didn't know where to begin, but I knew I had to shake myself out of my stupor. I thought about squash, which I had taken up shortly before leaving Paris. Luckily, I had brought my racket with me—and it saved me.

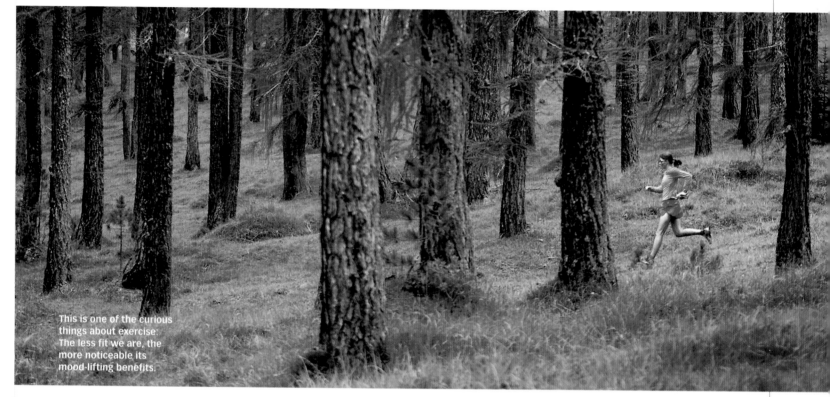

This is one of the curious things about exercise: The less fit we are, the more noticeable its mood-lifting benefits.

50 to 77 into three groups. The first did 30 minutes of jogging or brisk walking three times a week; the second took the anti-depressant Zoloft; the third did both. After four months, patients in all three groups were doing equally well, the medication offering no particular advantage over the regular practice of working out, except in relieving the symptoms a little faster. When the researchers followed up six months later, however, they found a major difference between the types of treatment. About a third of the patients who initially improved on Zoloft (alone and with exercise) had relapsed, whereas 92 percent of those benefiting from just the aerobic exercise program were still doing well. Most of the joggers and walkers had decided on their own initiative to keep exercising even after the study had ended.

I have experienced both the preventive and therapeutic value of exercise in my own life. When, at 22, I arrived in America from

During the first two weeks of playing at a local health club, nothing changed except that I finally had something to look forward to. But also, thanks to squash, I met a few people who were nice enough to invite me over for dinner. For a long time, I didn't know whether it was the exercise or my new friends that helped me most, but whatever the explanation, it didn't matter. I felt far better, and I was back in the saddle.

How can exercise change the way we feel? Deep inside our skull, we have a "brain within the brain" that is responsible for emotions. This so-called limbic region also balances heart rate, blood pressure, digestion, and all the hormones of the body. Because of such neural multitasking, when our body changes, our emotions change, too. During exercise, for example, our body releases endorphins—tiny molecules that resemble

Health

How to Save Your Own Heart

The math is simple: Cardiovascular disease is the number one killer of women. Eighty percent of it is preventable. MEHMET OZ, MD, and MICHAEL ROIZEN, MD, boil it down to the ten things we should all be doing.

1. GET AT LEAST SEVEN HOURS OF SLEEP.
That's per night, not week. And men—a needier breed—require eight. The benefit? Ask us if you still need an explanation when you wake up in the morning.

2. KNOW YOUR BLOOD PRESSURE.
What's the fastest way to age an artery? Subject it to high blood pressure, which will harden it like a garden hose that's been left out in the sun. A range of 120/80 to 130/85 mmHg is considered below the hypertension point, but it's not ideal. In fact, reducing your blood pressure from 130/85 to 115/76 can make your body up to ten years younger. There's no data to show that using drugs to lower blood pressure offers the full youth effect. So for now, you guessed it: Exercise, lose weight, reduce stress. The good news is the benefits from doing physical activity are just about instantaneous.

3. AVOID SMOKY BARS.
Don't let people puff away in your space. An hour of passive smoke can cause the same amount of aging as having two to four cigarettes. (If you're doing the smoking, we're not going to bother nagging. You know what to do.)

4. LEARN SOMETHING NEW. LOVE SOMETHING YOU DO.
Continuing to challenge the brain and being passionately engaged increases neuroplasticity, prompting the growth of extra connections. If you then have an injury like a stroke, the brain is better able to compensate for the trauma and lessen its effects.

5. WALK 30 MINUTES EVERY DAY.
One study on men suggests that for every hour of exercise, you get two extra hours of life. Rather than the "30 minutes," though, fixate on the "every day"—moving regularly is the active ingredient in exercise's powerful antiaging effect.

6. TAKE HALF AN ASPIRIN DAILY.
Yes, those big studies came out in 2005 saying low-dose aspirin does pretty much zilch to prevent heart attacks and cancer in women, but we still have little bits and pieces of the puzzle coming in—and the evidence is strong for aspirin's reducing the risk of stroke. Let's put it this way: People in the know take half an aspirin a day. If you're over 40, we recommend half a 325 milligram tablet (or two baby aspirins), with half a glass of warm water both before and after you swallow so that you're less likely to irritate your stomach. Check with your doctor to make sure you are aspirin tolerant.

7. EAT FISH THREE TIMES A WEEK.
It may not be just the omega-3s in the oil that keep the heart and arteries humming along; a number of animal studies have also indicated that fish protein provides a separate boost to cardiovascular health. Eat a variety of low-mercury fish (such as wild salmon, catfish, or tilapia). And if you're not nuts about seafood, an ounce of walnuts a day will give you a good dose of omega-3s.

8. LIVE WITHIN YOUR MEANS.
Feeling out of control financially can cost you not only sleep (see number one) but also arterial health due to chronic stress. A bankruptcy can put miles on your body's odometer.

9. FLOSS AND BRUSH.
Periodontal disease, such as gingivitis, does not affect just the gums. Any chronic infection stimulates your body to defend itself, and part of the response is to protect against bleeding with an increase in clotting tendency—a recipe for heart attack.

10. DON'T LEAVE HOME WITHOUT A STRESS-REDUCING TECHNIQUE—OR SEVERAL.
Deep breathing, meditation, yoga, running, knitting—you can't have too many ways to defuse stress. Even scrunching up your face as tightly as you can for 15 seconds and then releasing can deflect the pressure before it gets to you and starts wearing and tearing your cells. O

You Need 8 Glasses of Water a Day...and Other Rules to Blow Off

Everyone knows that sunlight will kill us, antioxidants will save us, and we should each lug around a gallon of water at all times to stay totally hydrated. Except that everyone's wrong! In an effort to help conventional wisdom catch up to the latest health findings, SARAH WILDMAN reconsiders some of the rules we live by.

Drink eight glasses of water a day. **FORGET IT!** In 2002 Dartmouth Medical School professor Heinz Valtin, MD, published an article in the *American Journal of Physiology* boldly declaring that, given all the water we get in food and various beverages, simply drinking when thirsty is more than enough for healthy adults who aren't engaging in vigorous exercise. In 2004 the nonprofit Institute of Medicine concurred, saying that the "vast majority of healthy people adequately meet their daily hydration needs by letting thirst be their guide."

Stay out of the sun. NOT ENTIRELY. Whoa—it seems that in our eagerness to avoid skin cancer, we went too far down that shady road. According to the June 2004 *Harvard Health Letter,* allowing sunlight to touch your skin (experts generally suggest ten to 15 minutes a day, twice a week) provides a number of benefits. UVB rays apparently trigger a chemical response that allows your body to produce vitamin D. Some researchers believe this chemical response may even help ward off multiple sclerosis and certain cancers. And people who suffer from seasonal affective disorder (depression caused by lack of light) find significant relief from regular sun exposure.

Antioxidant supplements prevent cancer. UH-UH. In October 2004 *The Lancet* published an analysis of 14 previous studies involving 170,000 people and found that the antioxidant supplements A, C, E, and beta-carotene did not prevent gastrointestinal cancers. More research needs to be done, but another analysis, conducted by the U.S. Preventive Services Task Force, found insufficient evidence either for or against taking A, C, E, multivitamins with folic acid or antioxidant combinations to ward off cancer or heart disease. It did conclude that beta-carotene supplements may be harmful and advised against them. There's still hope, though, that unlike vitamins alone, foods rich in antioxidants (like tomatoes and blueberries) may provide some benefit.

For the healthiest diet, follow the USDA's dietary guidelines. NOPE. In January 2005 the Department of Health and Human Services and the USDA issued revised dietary guidelines,

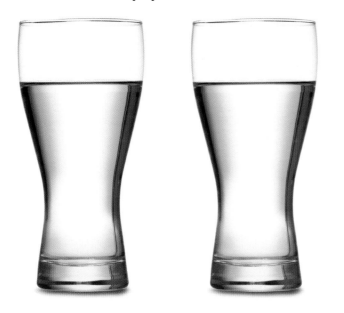

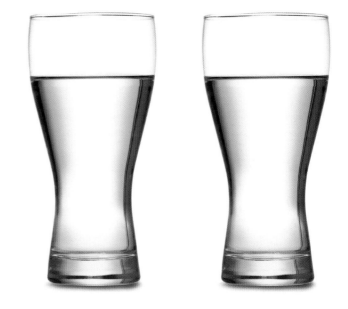

aiming to correct what Walter Willett, MD, a professor of nutrition and epidemiology at the Harvard School of Public Health, characterizes as the "faulty science" underpinning previous guidelines. While the new recommendations, which emphasize losing weight and eating fewer refined carbs, are an improvement, Willett says they've still been unduly influenced by agribusiness. For example, he says they recommend an excessive amount of dairy—as many as three servings daily. "There's no clear evidence that that amount is actually beneficial," he says. "And millions of Americans are lactose intolerant and can't consume that much dairy." (He suggests one to two servings and taking supplements, if necessary, to get 800 to 1,200 milligrams of calcium a day.) The other major problem is grouping red meat with more healthful proteins. The 2005 guidelines, like the previous ones, bear "the fingerprints of Big Beef," he says. The USDA "lumps red meat with chicken, fish, and soybeans and says, 'Consume lower-fat versions,' which doesn't make sense. Soybeans have a lot of fat, but it's good fat, while red meat"—which Willett advises us to eat sparingly—"has been linked to heart disease and colon cancer." The same day the guidelines were published, the *Journal of the American Medical Association* published a study confirming the link between red meat and colon cancer. You can find Harvard's nutritional guidelines at www.hsph.harvard.edu/nutritionsource.

Mammograms are ineffective, because by the time a tumor shows up, it has already been growing for five years. WRONG! This is a particularly dangerous canard, because currently there's no test out there that would catch cancer before mammograms do. And it presumes that all cancers grow at the same rate. They don't. Mammograms are still the most effective way of detecting—and therefore treating and beating—breast cancer as early as possible. Consider that by the time a cancer can be felt, it may have been growing for up to ten years. "Mammograms," says Susan Love, MD, author of *Dr. Susan Love's Breast Book,* "are our best tool for finding cancers. Whether *early* is the appropriate word is being questioned."

You need eight hours of sleep a night. NO, YOU DON'T. Two studies published in the journal *Sleep* in 2004 found that people who slept seven rather than eight hours lived longer than their seemingly more well-rested counterparts. That's not to say that sleep deprivation isn't real—get less than seven hours, experts say, and you may begin to lose creativity and focus.

You can rely on the FDA for independent, bottom-line health information. SORRY! "The Food and Drug Administration has become largely the captive of the industry it's supposed to be regulating," says Marcia Angell, MD, former editor in chief of *The New England Journal of Medicine* and author of *The Truth About the Drug Companies.* "Very frequently," Angell says, multiple members of the various advisory committees at the FDA "have consulting arrangements with companies whose drugs they're evaluating." Similarly, in the case of the 2004 cholesterol guidelines endorsed by the National Institutes of Health, "eight of the nine panelists reportedly were on the payroll of one or more companies that make statins." One problem, Angell explains, is that the results of the clinical trials on which those guidelines are based showed no benefit for women who don't already have heart disease. She points out that if big pharmaceutical companies "succeed in convincing doctors that the standard for cholesterol should be even lower than what's currently seen as normal, the companies have, overnight, expanded their market. Your doctor needs to be able to rely on research and recommendations by critical, unbiased scientists."

The FDA's longtime approval of now discredited arthritis drugs like Vioxx and Celebrex is also evidence of less-than-vigilant oversight. If the manufacturers knew for years about a potential for increased heart attack risk, as they allegedly did with Vioxx, why did it take so long for the drug to be pulled from the market? **O**

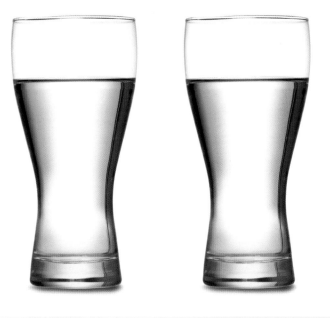

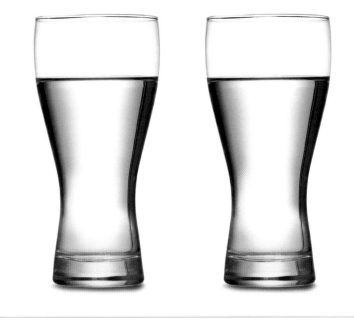

Sugar Shock: The Epidemic Hits Home

LISA KOGAN was nine weeks pregnant when she found out—almost by accident—that she had diabetes (like five million of us, she was walking around undiagnosed) and that her baby was seriously in danger. Two years later, she reflects on the one-two jab life gave her and what she's learned about living with out-of-control blood sugar.

Life can turn on a dime. One minute you're sitting in your lawyer's office discussing the possibility of adoption, the next you're standing in your bathroom staring at a little stick that—against all odds—has somehow managed to register two skinny pink lines. Anyway, that's my story. I was 41 years old, I was pregnant, I was cautiously euphoric. And then the world turned upside down.

It was September 24, 2002. Nearly three weeks after examining me, my obstetrician had sent a letter saying my glucose appeared "slightly elevated" and suggested a glucose tolerance test. Fed up with my inability to ever get her on the phone, I called a colleague's husband, a respected obstetrician-gynecologist, and read him the results of the test. There was a pause—I remember that—and then I know he said, "Uh-huh, okay, hold on a minute while I make a call." After a very long minute, he got back on the line with what struck me as an absurd question. "Are you wearing shoes?" he asked. "Yep, I'm in my sensible pregnant-girl flats," I answered. "Good," he said. "I want you to grab your bag and get into a taxi. You'll be going to 168th Street and Saint Nicholas Avenue. Take the elevator to the..." It was going way too fast. "Listen," I said, "I'm pretty beat, but maybe tomorrow." And then he cut to the chase: "You're diabetic," he said, "and this baby can't wait until tomorrow." He explained that my soon-to-be-former doctor had taken much too long to diagnose me and that my baby's organs were being formed in an environment of uncontrolled sugar. He said other things, but it was all a blur. Thirty-five minutes later, I found myself at the place that would become my second home: Columbia University's Naomi Berrie Diabetes Center in New York City.

I have endured great pain in my day. A large woman named Helga waxes my bikini line every May, and I had a roommate who once listened to Enya for nine straight hours—so believe me when I tell you I understand human suffering, and I realize that in the grand scheme of things a little finger jab or an occasional shot in the arm doesn't really hurt all that much. But needles freak me out. It's irrational, it's phobic, it's not changing anytime soon. Before I meet the doctor, I am given a hemoglobin A1C test—a simple finger stick that determines your average blood sugar for the past three months. "Not that hand; this one,"

I sob. "Wait, *this* finger. Use *this* finger. Hold it; I'm not ready," I plead as I breathe in the nauseating smell of rubbing alcohol on cotton. The little girl in the next chair rolls her eyes. A slightly more sympathetic preschooler assures me that "they're quite good here." It is not pretty when you're seated with two people under the age of 7 and the only one who wants her mommy is you. Just then I feel a hand on my shoulder. "Hi, I'm Dr. Robin Goland. We'll sit down and talk in a couple of minutes," and in a futile effort to further reassure me, she adds, "I promise you're not the first woman in history ever to be diabetic *and* pregnant." But I'm pretty sure she's wrong. "Actually, Dr. Goland, I believe I'm the first woman in history ever to be pregnant."

Holding my newly pricked finger as if I'd been bayoneted, I settle in for a chat with Dr. Goland. She is a combo platter, equal parts wry, compassionate, and no-nonsense, a slim powerhouse in her late 40s whom I imagine cheerfully defusing a midlevel nuclear device while forging a permanent peace in the Middle East and harnessing solar energy. Over time I'll find out that she has absolutely no grasp of pop culture and once forgot her child at an ice rink, but this is only our first date. Today I need her to be clear, kind, heroic—and that's exactly what she is.

She explains that there are 18 million diabetics in the United States, and nearly one-third of them are walking around undiagnosed: "The problem is that often a person with diabetes feels no different from someone with normal blood sugar. Their blood vessels could be getting damaged, but they have no idea anything's wrong. In most cases, an individual's normal blood sugar, after fasting overnight, is under 100. The symptoms people generally associate with diabetes—urinating frequently, unquenchable thirst, poor wound healing, feeling very tired—don't usually occur until the blood sugar is above 250. The slow rise in blood sugar, from out of the normal range to frank diabetes to really severe high blood sugar, can take a decade or more."

To my total shock, the result of my hemoglobin A1C test indicates that my diabetes is not gestational. Gestational diabetes usually strikes after the 20th week of pregnancy and disappears within an hour of giving birth. But at nine weeks along, it's apparent that I was diabetic before ever becoming pregnant.

YOUR PERSONAL BEST

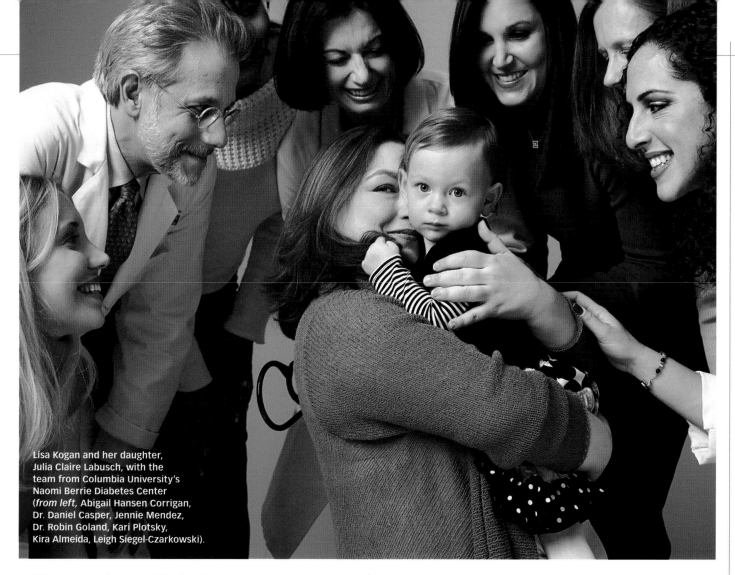

Lisa Kogan and her daughter, Julia Claire Labusch, with the team from Columbia University's Naomi Berrie Diabetes Center (*from left*, Abigail Hansen Corrigan, Dr. Daniel Casper, Jennie Mendez, Dr. Robin Goland, Kari Plotsky, Kira Almeida, Leigh Siegel-Czarkowski).

The test reveals my A1C level to be 8.4 percent. A normal count would be 6 percent, and many people are at 4 or 5 percent. Dr. Goland asks me about my family history (cancer galore). She asks me if I smoke (never). She asks me about my diet and fitness routine (used to see my trainer three times a week, currently see my refrigerator three times a night). Now it's my turn to ask the questions.

"What exactly is diabetes?"

"Well," she begins, "there's type 1 and type 2. Type 1 occurs because your own immune system attacks your insulin-producing cells. When that happens, you can't make insulin, so to survive you have to take it by injection. Type 2 is much more common. That's a disease where the pancreas makes insulin but the body doesn't respond to it normally. We call that insulin resistance. And in the end, over years, the pancreas often has trouble making insulin. The result in both of these diseases is that the blood sugar goes too high."

"Then what happens?" I ask.

"Blindness, loss of limb, kidney failure, heart attack, stroke."

With each word I shift deeper into catatonic noodle mode.

"But," she adds, brightening, "every one of these things can be delayed or prevented. Because we didn't used to know how to keep blood sugar normal and how to prevent the complications, a lot of people are under the misconception that first you get the disease, then you get the problems, and that's that. The truth is,

if you work to control it—and it *is* work—none of this is inevitable. You can be a healthy person with diabetes—you may never experience any of these complications."

My eyes scan the room as I try to take all of this in. There's a Harvard diploma hanging on the wall, pictures of three tanned tourist kids in front of some Greek ruins, a tiara-wearing teddy bear resting on the windowsill. I massage my ever expanding stomach and finally ask the million-dollar question: "Is my baby okay?"

Dr. Goland says it's too soon to tell. She wants to send me to a lab so they can run more tests, and I start a fresh round of sobbing. Directing me to the nearest box of tissues, she steps out of the room and returns followed by a band of angels. "You know what, Lisa, you don't need to get yourself to another lab. We're going to take some blood right now." Two nurses, Dr. Goland, and one vampire/medical assistant named Berenise ("She's the best") bring me into an examination room and start rolling up my sleeves in search of a good vein. It's a remarkable tribute to peer pressure and vanity that I ever allowed my ears to be pierced, and I explain how that procedure actually made me pass out. They have me lie down, and the process begins.

"So," says Dr. Goland, who seems to believe in the power of distraction, "what's Rosie really like?" Through clenched teeth, I tell her that I work for Oprah and that though I've never really said this to anyone before, "I guess the thing that makes Oprah so special to me"—they all lean forward—"is that SHE'S NEVER STABBED ME IN THE ARM WITH A SHARP NEEDLE."

Dr. Goland decides I should be hospitalized till I get the hang of everything. I beg her to let me go home. "You'll have to test your own blood tonight and give yourself a shot of insulin," she says.

"I can do that," I say, almost certain that I can't do that.

"You'll have to call me at home tonight between 10 and 11."

"Okay," I answer, "if I need you, I'll call." She scrunches her brow. "I don't think you understand—if I don't hear from you, I'll be up worrying the entire night. You have to call."

Then she presents me with a secret weapon in my brand-new war. "This is Leigh Siegel-Czarkowski—you'll be spending a lot of time together."

I recognize her from my bloodletting.

"I'll walk you through the injection and blood test now, and then we can go over it again tonight," says Leigh, a 30-something nurse practitioner and diabetes educator, as she hands me her phone number. I leave the office at around 6:30 with a glucose meter, insulin pen, test strip, needle, lancet, and splitting headache. Only later do I learn that the office closes at 5.

That night I lay everything in front of me and phone Leigh.

"I don't think I can handle this," I say, attaching the needle to the insulin pen.

"That's how I used to feel," she says, and instructs me to pinch my thigh.

"You're diabetic?"

"Since I'm 15."

"Leigh?"

"Hmm."

"Isn't there some horrible disease I can get that involves ointment?"

"Of course there is," she assures me, "but right now you've got this."

I sink the needle into flesh, push the button on the pen, force myself to count slowly to five until the drug is completely released, and pull the needle from my leg.

"Leigh?"

"I'm right here."

We listen to each other breathe for a while and finally she says, "Let's stick your finger now so you can call Dr. Goland and say goodnight."

First thing the next morning, I'm back in Leigh's office—a place I'll be hanging out in every day for hours over the next three weeks. We'll also talk at least twice daily on weekends. After conferring with Dr. Goland, it is decided that I'll prick my finger to check my blood seven times a day and control

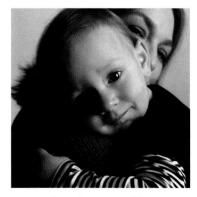

I ask the million-dollar question: "Is my baby going to be okay?"

my sugar with five injections of insulin a day. Needless to say, I am not part of the decision-making process.

I'm sent to an obstetrician a few doors down who, via sonogram, locates my baby's heartbeat and then reviews the long list of potential problems for a baby who's been marinating in sugar. Her definitive answer is that she won't know anything definitive for some time. Back at the center, I'm sent to nutritionist Kira Almeida for an eating plan tailored to my needs. I'm sent to Dr. Daniel Casper for the most thorough eye exam I've ever had. I'm sent to social worker Kari Plotsky for a head exam. Actually, Kari just wants to see if I feel like talking. I tell her I really don't, then proceed to talk for the next hour and a half.

A couple of weeks go by. I know everyone and they know me. Needles, carb counting, weighing and recording every bite of the three small meals and three small snacks that I consume at roughly the same time each day still don't come naturally, nor does willing myself to believe that I'll have a healthy baby—but I do it nonetheless. Dr. Goland checks my blood pressure, and in the peppy cheerleader style I've come to cling to pronounces me "completely amazing."

"Completely amazing people don't let themselves become diabetic," I say.

Dr. Goland shoots me the have-I-taught-you-nothing? look and pulls up a chair. "This is not your fault, Lisa."

"C'mon," I say. "I've stopped going to the gym, I've put on weight, I've—"

"Time out," she says. "Diabetes is a genetic disease. And as for being overweight, that's one of the most inheritable conditions we know of. Almost as much as having blue eyes."

"Okay," I reply, "but you've gotta admit that there's an environmental component to all this."

"Clearly, there is. But in most cases, without the genes you don't become diabetic. You could weigh 400 pounds, but if you don't have the genes, chances are your blood sugar would be normal. And," she continues, "some of the things that can trigger diabetes—age, stress, high fever, even certain medications—antagonize the effect of insulin. Someone could put you on prednisone for poison ivy and your blood sugar goes up, or you could be a really conscientious exerciser and hurt your back. It's the combination of pain and the fact that you're no longer exercising that can raise your blood sugar. I see that kind of thing once a week here. You just can't control every factor. So it's never exactly the patient's fault." She sees my doubt but plows ahead. "This is a disease where there's a huge amount of guilt and blame. Angry wives are always coming in here pointing to their husbands and saying, 'If he'd just taken care of himself, this never would've happened.' That's actually incorrect. It might not have happened at the time it happened, but it would probably happen eventually."

My lips say, "I suppose," but my eyes are glued to the scale across the tiny room.

"I think it's a little unfortunate that we believe eating is completely an issue of free will. It's not. Food intake is carefully regulated. It has to do with survival of the species. There are important circuits in the brain that are hardwired to direct how much we eat and when we feel satiated, and it's increasingly clear that there's a derangement, probably an inherited derangement, in the circuits of a person who struggles with weight."

And here I thought it was my needle phobia and constant weeping that would convince her I was deranged. "Now," she continues, "this isn't to say you couldn't go on a diet and lose weight after the baby is born—you could. It's just extremely hard to keep it off when the circuits are altered and your body is telling you you're hungry. It's also much easier for some people to gain weight. And that's their genes talking again. The thing is, if you really pay attention and you're willing to be a little hungry and exercise regularly, your genes are not your destiny."

"It's all so hard," I say.

"If it were a simple matter, nobody would be diabetic or overweight," the doctor agrees. But the good news is that I've got patients who are quite overweight—even after they take off ten or 15 pounds, they're still overweight by anybody's standard, especially their own—but through that little bit of weight loss, their blood sugar is now normal.

"They always say to me, 'What are you so excited about?' But that's what I want people to understand: For your long-term health, the difference between having a blood sugar of 100 versus 200 is enormous, and often it's those ten pounds that change everything. Diabetes is a chronic, progressive disease, but it can be staved off for years. And that's huge!"

I vow never to touch spaghetti carbonara again.

"People who struggle with diabetes still have to live in the real world. It's unrealistic to tell someone they can never have the good stuff. If there's something you love to eat, I want to make sure you can still eat it from time to time. It's impossible to always be perfect. You have to learn what your blood sugar levels are supposed to be and keep them within those limits 80 percent of the time—shoot for a solid B; the other 20 percent is a quality of life issue."

Two years later, my quality of life no longer involves shots of insulin, and I check my blood only randomly every few days. I lose weight, gain some back, and try to be kind to myself in the process. Dr. Goland tells me that my latest hemoglobin A1C is at 5.7—perfectly normal. "So does this mean I'm no longer diabetic?" I ask hopefully.

"I actually discourage my patients from thinking they're cured. The real question is, Do you have well-controlled diabetes or poorly controlled diabetes?" Mine is well under control, she tells me. And so I continue to eat a lot of vegetables, some protein, and an occasional dish of spaghetti. I walk home from the office at a fairly brisk pace two or three evenings a week, but the secret to my fitness program involves chasing after a sticky little toddler with a voracious curiosity and a mind-boggling level of energy. It took a village, but on April 26, 2003, Julia Claire Labusch was born perfect and pink, healthy and happy—the most delicious sugar substitute I've come across. ◖

Are You at Risk?

An estimated 41 million Americans between the ages of 40 and 74 are on the verge of type 2 diabetes, according to the American Diabetes Association. And because prediabetes has no symptoms, it's easy to miss. When it's caught early, however, modest weight loss and daily exercise can slow—even prevent—progression to the full-blown disease.

The trick is to get a blood glucose test every three years starting at age 45—or earlier and more frequently for anyone who's overweight and has any of these additional risk factors: high blood pressure, low HDL (good) cholesterol and/or high triglycerides, polycystic ovarian syndrome (a hormone imbalance that can cause infertility and is associated with insulin resistance), or parents or siblings with diabetes. Risk factors also include being of African-American, Hispanic, Native American, Asian, or Pacific Islander descent; having gestational diabetes or delivering an overweight baby; and not getting enough physical activity. In families with a strong history of the disease, testing should begin when overweight kids are in their teens, says endocrinologist Anne Peters, MD, a diabetes specialist and professor at the University of Southern California's Keck School of Medicine. No matter what your age, if you notice excessive thirst, frequent urination, extreme and persistent hunger, or unexplained weight loss despite overeating, get your blood glucose measured: You may already be diabetic. Other symptoms include fatigue, recurrent yeast infections, slow-healing sores, and blurry vision.

If your blood sugar indicates that you're headed for diabetes, there's a lot you can do. In a two- to five-year study, prediabetics who exercised at moderate intensity for 30 minutes five times a week and dropped, on average, 5 to 7 percent of their body weight with a low-fat, reduced-calorie diet cut their risk of the disease by 58 percent. This approach was nearly twice as effective as taking medication, which mainly helped participants who were younger than 45 and extremely obese. Eating 500 fewer calories a day should be enough to knock off the necessary weight, according to Eric Westman, MD, associate professor of medicine at Duke University.

Those already diagnosed with diabetes can also benefit from such lifestyle changes, although it's unclear how long they can control their blood sugar without medication. Typically, diabetes is treated with drugs that lower blood sugar and avert (or postpone) the need for insulin injections. "There are lots of short-term data—usually encompassing weeks to a year—showing that weight loss can ameliorate diabetes, decrease glucose levels, and reduce or even eliminate the need for medication," says David M. Nathan, MD, a professor of medicine at Harvard Medical School and chairman of the Diabetes Prevention Program, which conducted the prediabetes study. A federal trial called Look AHEAD should reveal more in the coming decades. —Jane E. Allen

For further information, call the American Diabetes Association at 800-DIABETES or go to the federal government's National Diabetes Information Clearinghouse Web site, diabetes.niddk.nih.gov.

Memory Boot Camp

How two weeks of intense training convinced 50-year-old
EMILY YOFFE that she wasn't going gaga after all.

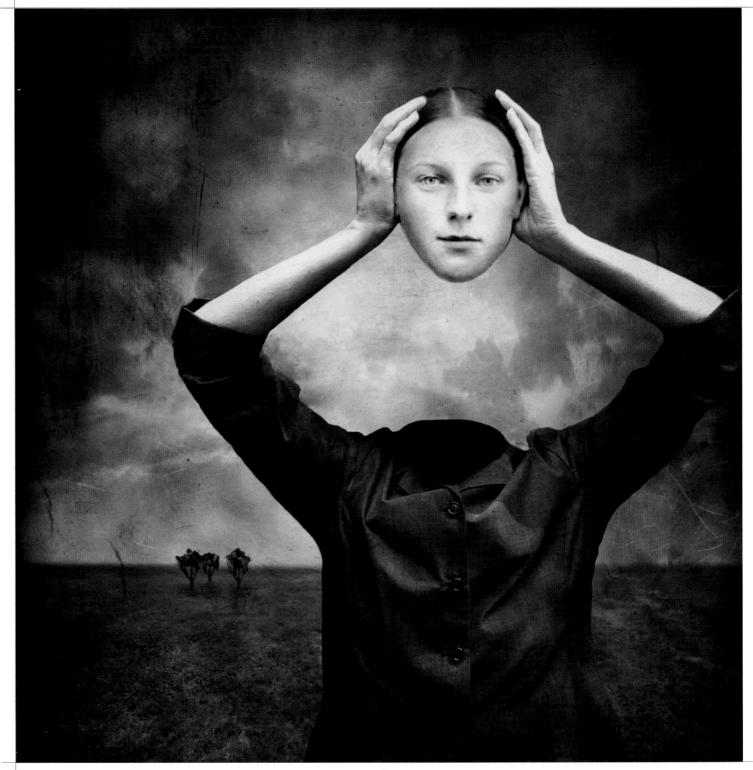

It was during my second hour of testing that I started to get concerned. I had come to the Aging and Memory Research Center at UCLA to have a baseline assessment before embarking on a two-week memory improvement program designed by the center's director, Gary Small, MD. After undergoing brain scanning in an MRI, I sat with a psychologist who gave me a list of 12 random words to memorize. Over and over, I could muster up only nine, even when the tester prompted me for the words I missed. I had been looking forward to this evaluation, thinking it would be fun. Now I realized it was fun in the same way a bikini wax or a colonoscopy is fun.

At age 50, I am well aware that my memory is not what it was 20 years ago. Occasionally, after dinner, I'll tell my 10-year-old daughter to put the leftovers "in the thing that keeps food cold." Sometimes when trying to recall who told me what, in place of the speaker, all I see is a blank face—rather like the blurred images in the Soviet newsreels of leaders who had fallen out of favor. I try to comfort myself with the fact that if you're old enough to remember Soviet newsreels, you're old enough to have these kinds of memory holes.

But what if it's possible to plug the holes, to return your brain to its former nimbleness? This is the hope offered by a study Small conducted. He took 17 healthy people, ages 35 to 69, who complained of mild but normal, age-related memory problems, and divided them into two groups. One group went on with their lives as usual. The other group followed Small's memory improvement program. At the end of two weeks, PET scans showed that those on the plan had greater efficiency in the area of the brain involved in working memory—being able to hear a new phone number and dial it shortly afterward, for example. They also performed better on tests that measured verbal fluency, like the ability to come up with words that start with the same letters.

Why not see how I measure up? I had thought. But I was getting more anxious with every test. In one exercise in which I was told to replicate designs made of colored blocks, I threw up my hands like a frustrated kindergartner and said it couldn't be done.

Following my tests, I met Dr. Small in his office. A psychiatrist and neuroscientist, he is an innovator in the early diagnosis of Alzheimer's and has written a number of popular books (the latest being *The Longevity Bible*). EVERY EIGHT SECONDS A BABY BOOMER TURNS 50 is printed on a piece of paper above his desk. Small has already entered the ranks of aging boomers; he's 54, but a wiry, youthful, cheerful 54. After I described my life and my memory complaints, he told me to pay particular attention to the stress reduction portion of his plan, which was laid out in his book *The Memory Prescription*. There was no magic formula in making the program two weeks, he explained. It's a short enough period of time that people are willing to stick with it and long enough to yield measurable results. The ultimate goal is to incorporate most of the changes into one's day-to-day life. The

"prescription" itself—based on tantalizing studies suggesting that certain behaviors might preserve memory and delay the onset of Alzheimer's—breaks down into four parts, with nothing startling to any of them (see "A Sample Day" on page 48): improved nutrition (a fruit- and vegetable-heavy, junk food–eschewing diet); physical activity (including stretching and frequent, vigorous walks); stress reduction (short relaxation and meditation breaks); and mental stimulation (a series of challenges, from doing mazes to coming up with images to associate with names, such as a frankfurter for Frank).

I was skeptical that Small's program would cause big changes in my brain, because I already have fairly healthy habits. So I was surprised when I went back home to be confronted with just how lousy many of my habits were. Take my diet: Despite being something of a food nut, I had fallen into the pattern of skipping lunch and eating part of a chocolate bar in the late afternoon as a way of not gaining weight (one of the dangers of working from home). Small told me this was particularly stressful for the brain, which needs a steady supply of glucose to keep humming.

When I started having three meals and two snacks, getting up from my desk and eating became the highlight of the day—to the point where, as feared, it was often hard to stop. But since I was also taking the doctor's advice to do more exercise, I would follow my snack (nuts and dried fruit) or lunch (a salad) by taking our beagle for a walk. Even if this plan does nothing for my memory, I thought, at least the dog will be in better shape.

It was harder to follow Small's advice on stress reduction. A natural-born procrastinator, I always find myself with too many demands to fit into too little time. Doing the program, I realized I had become addicted to stress hormones—the pumping anxiety making me feel as if I was being productive.

I learned, however, it was also fritzing out whatever brainpower I had left. Among the many studies Small cites in his book, one found that "constant stress literally shrinks a key memory center."

That was enough to inspire me to go to the bedroom for five minutes every so often and imagine myself at a beautiful beach. Sometimes it was hard not to imagine myself into a nap. But it was amazing how even a short break could clear my mind.

Then there were the brain exercises. Studies show that highly educated people or those engaged in challenging work or activities have "greater density of neuronal connections in brain areas involving complex reasoning," Small writes. What this does, supposedly, is provide a higher-functioning mental perch from which to make a descent. In practical terms, it means that people with more developed brains will still have good mental functioning at the point in life when others will notice impairment. And it means that those with denser brains who do get Alzheimer's can absorb the assault of the disease longer before it causes a loss of function.

But during my two-week brain training, an article appeared in *The Wall Street Journal* titled "Oops! Mental Training,

> Occasionally, after dinner, I'll tell my 10-year-old to put the leftovers "in the thing that keeps food cold."

Crosswords Fail to Slow Decline of Aging Brain." Oops, indeed. I called Timothy Salthouse, PhD, professor of psychology at the University of Virginia, who was quoted in the article. He explained that although practicing a specific skill—doing crossword puzzles, remembering names—can improve that ability, it doesn't mean that any other mental function will get better. "Another issue is how long the effects last," he said. "That's an open question." He also said the idea that a stimulated brain is a better-aging brain confuses cause and effect. The studies finding a link between doing crosswords and having less dementia could be due to the fact that individuals born with more complex brains are the ones drawn to challenges like puzzles—and not because people with average intelligence start doing word games at 40 or 50 to stimulate their brains.

Small agrees we don't have definitive answers but says it makes sense to apply what seems promising. And even if learning to remember names won't improve your spatial abilities, why not be better at remembering names?

Why not? One day when I saw the administrative secretary at my daughter's new school (I'd met her a half-dozen times but never remembered her name), I really looked at her—and at the nameplate on her desk—and saw that I could make a connection between her first name, Brenda, and the blonde hair she shared with my sister-in-law Brenda. For her last name, Watson, I imagined a lightbulb over her head, a reference to Thomas Edison's assistant Mr. Watson. Two days later, I was thrilled that I still knew her name. Then I realized I had totally misremembered something crucial: Thomas Edison didn't have an assistant named Mr. Watson—Alexander Graham Bell did. Oh, well, I was sticking with the lightbulb. The following week, while walking the dog (again!), I was able to break down a phone number for a missing cat and recall it when I got home a half hour later. Alas, that jolt of confidence was short-lived, too. The next morning, I was I adding an egg to my omelet. I cracked it open and put the shell in the bowl and the egg down the sink.

Back at UCLA after two weeks, I underwent a brain scan, again while trying to remember a series of words. The images revealed a 50 percent reduction in activity since the first time. This is good! It means my brain was using less fuel to do the same work.

Afterward I was put through another battery of tests with clinical psychologist Karen Miller, PhD. The differences between the two sets of results were dramatic. In the first set of tests, at one point I performed like a 60-year-old; the second time around, I scored consistently the way a 35-year-old would.

So how does it feel to have the memory of a 35-year-old again? I don't really. I am just more aware that I can get my memory to work better if I make the effort. I have techniques to remember those pesky things that plague us in modern life. I actually listen to and learn the names of new acquaintances (and I'll never forget you, Brenda Watson). All in all, I'm certainly glad I did the program. Now, if only Dr. Small would come up with a two-week regimen that would give me a 35-year-old face. **O**

Brain Training: A Sample Day

- **WAKE UP AND STRETCH:** Standing, breathe in deeply as you raise your arms out to the side and overhead; exhale as you return to starting position. Do four times.

- **MARCH IN PLACE,** lifting your knees high as you count to 20.

- **BREAKFAST:** vegetable omelet (one egg plus two egg whites) and a half cup of blueberries; green tea. (Small's diet emphasizes antioxidant-rich foods—vegetables, fruit, green tea—lean protein, and low-glycemic carbs; it's light on red meat, processed carbs, and saturated fat.)

- **MENTAL EXERCISE:** Write down two details about what the first person you see is wearing.

- **TAKE A FIVE-MINUTE OR LONGER MORNING WALK.**

- **DRINK A GLASS OF WATER.**

- **MIDMORNING SNACK:** a half cup nonfat yogurt with one tablespoon of raisins and green tea or water. (Small prescribes snacks to keep blood sugar steady and brain cells fueled; raisins and green tea are packed with antioxidants.)

- **WRITE YOUR FIRST NAME** with the hand you don't use. Now take two pencils and write your name with both hands at the same time.

- **LUNCH:** tuna sandwich on whole wheat with lettuce, tomato, and light mayo. (The omega-3s in the tuna are also key to Small's diet.) Seltzer.

- **SIT QUIETLY AND BREATHE** through your nose for two minutes. Visualize the breath as it enters and leaves your body.

- **AFTERNOON SNACK:** one cup tomato soup or juice with one to two ounces of unsalted almonds or walnuts (nuts are also high in omega-3s). Tea or water.

- **RECALL THE TWO DETAILS** you noticed this morning and compare them with what you recorded earlier.

- **DINNER:** Grilled six-ounce chicken breast with herbs, a half cup of brown rice, steamed spinach, tossed salad with oil and vinegar, and fruit sorbet. Water or a glass of wine.

- **TEN-MINUTE AFTER-DINNER WALK,** followed by a glass of water.

- **BEFORE GOING TO SLEEP,** try a brainteaser [answers on bottom of page]:
  What number follows next in this sequence? 4, 9, 16, 25, __
  John is standing behind Jim, but Jim is standing behind John. How can that be?
  Add the missing vowels and regroup the letters of this proverb: PPLW HLV NGLS SHSS SHLDNT THR WSTNS.

[Answers: 36; They're standing back to back; People who live in glass houses shouldn't throw stones.]

Women on the Rocks

It seems so civilized, so liberated: an all-girl evening gossiping, networking, sipping the cocktail du jour—and nobody's looking for Mr. Goodbar. What's wrong with this picture? RENÉ STEINKE reports.

At the Park, a lounge in downtown Manhattan with a California-like indoor patio, Jeanie Overduin and Anna Liss, both 21, sit beneath the lacy trees singing vintage Madonna songs to each other. They consider themselves moderate drinkers, at least in their age group, and they've devised a pseudoscientific system for staying out all night without getting tanked. They're on their second cocktail (on a typical night they drink anywhere from two to six), steeling themselves for a trip to a karaoke bar. Jeanie, a

event. They both cite the restorative qualities of a vodka and soda, which contains fewer calories than a lot of other cocktails—more water, too—and so they claim it's the perfect tonic for a long night. Anna says, "I think it's important to enjoy your life while you're young. When I'm older, I want to be able to say to my kids, 'Mom did that; Mom was there.'"

Women of all ages are hitting the bars more than ever. And I've been hearing reports that people who drink are putting away more alcohol than a decade ago. In fact, one out of five women

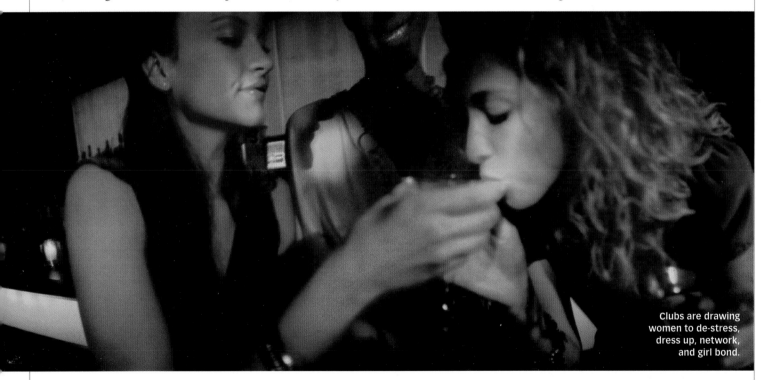

Clubs are drawing women to de-stress, dress up, network, and girl bond.

model, and Anna, an intern for a fashion designer, say they go out four times a week, often barhopping until 3 or 4 A.M. Anna still gets up to go to work by 9, even if a little bleary-eyed; Jeanie doesn't drink before a gig—"Boy, oh, boy, do I look like shit after a big night," she explains, admitting that she once skipped a casting call due to a hangover. And they talk about their partying almost as if they're in training for a sport. Anna swigs a lot of water in between alcoholic beverages. "And when I'm feeling nice and tipsy, I'll stop for a while and then pick it up again later." Jeanie does the same. Often their evening begins with a drink or two at dinner, and then they go on to a nightclub or fashion

between 18 and 44 is said to be a binger (more than three drinks per occasion)—which is particularly disturbing because health experts are finding that alcohol takes a harsher toll on women than men; even relatively small amounts can cause damage.

As a working mother who cherishes the occasional night when I share a bottle of wine with friends, I'm wondering how one navigates the line between good-hearted, harmless fun and overindulgence. Why *are* so many women gathering in pubs and clubs? How much do they really drink? How bad is it for them? The best way to find out, I decide, is to head into the New York bar scene.

On a sunny late afternoon at Joshua Tree, a postcollege pub in Manhattan's Murray Hill, 25-year-olds Monica Taylor and Erin Hamilton (who asked to use pseudonyms) are drinking sangria at an outside table. Inside the bar, a couple of guys watch a baseball game on the big-screen TVs. Monica's boyfriend didn't want her to go out again (it's Monday) because she blacked out on Saturday night. "I got completely wasted and couldn't remember getting home. The taxi could have taken me anywhere," she says, her blonde hair riffling in the city breeze. Like many New Yorkers, she is haunted by the recent killings of Imette St. Guillen and Jennifer Moore. This year, within five months of each other, both young women—Imette, a graduate student in criminal justice just shy of 25, and Jennifer, a suburban 18-year-old headed for college—went out clubbing in Manhattan. And for both, an evening of drinking ended in brutal murder. Imette's tortured body was found at a Brooklyn dumping ground, Moore's body in a New Jersey trash bin.

Though Monica is shaken by her own carelessness, she laughs it off, saying she knows people who drink a lot more than she does. And in retrospect, she understands why she drank so much

University, Nalini, a 19-year-old wearing a strappy dress, also seems oblivious to how vulnerable she really is when smashed. She admits to "pounding drinks" whenever she's out with her boyfriend and is uncomfortable or bored. Sometimes she drinks so much that she doesn't remember what she's done.

Experts are growing alarmed by the ferocity with which young women, especially teens, are drinking—in part because of new research suggesting that alcohol may be more destructive to an adolescent's developing brain than previously thought, impairing memory and learning ability. A new survey of 17- to 35-year-old women by the American Medical Association shows that 21 percent of those who went on spring break became inebriated to the point of not remembering what happened to them, 12 percent said they felt forced or pressured to have sex while drinking, and 20 percent engaged in sexual activity they regretted. The study also found that most women on spring break had or knew someone who'd had unsafe sex. And 21 percent said they had passed out from drinking.

As for older women who have outgrown their hard-partying days, many of the bargoers I talk to may be out three or four

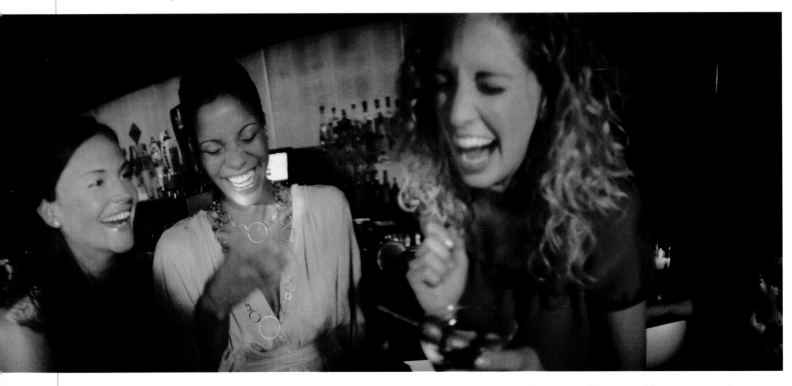

white wine that night—she felt uncomfortable at the party, where she didn't know anyone. Alcoholic excess is an unusual occurrence for Monica. But Erin has a "smart and successful" friend who often drinks until blacking out. A couple of years ago, the friend got into a cab while very inebriated, and two men pushed in the car after her and raped her. Erin widens her eyes. "That really made a lot of us wake up to what was going on with us." Despite the tragedies, though, Monica and Erin haven't necessarily slowed down—they are savvy, they say, to the city's perils, and for the most part, they insist, they know how to protect themselves.

Farther downtown at a margarita bar near New York

times a week, but they're careful to avoid hangovers so they can show up for work the next day. They could have three to six drinks each time, but they pace themselves, consuming their beer, wine, mojitos over several hours; they wouldn't do anything as inelegant as stumble or slur their words. Though these women consider their drinking habits moderate, medical experts say they are fooling themselves.

It's midnight on Saturday at Pravda, a subterranean bar in downtown Manhattan with a Soviet-era, clandestine ambience evoked by Moscow memorabilia, an entrance down a barely marked, narrow stairway, and a cocktail menu that includes caviar, a fruit-flavored concoction called the bohemian, and the specialty of the house, the Leninade (some kind of vodka–lemon juice creation). At the mirrored bar, six shiny-haired women lean together in ardent conversation. Their blouses are slinky or sheer, their eyes mascaraed and bracelets jangling, not for the men casting glances in their direction but for one another. When they go out with their boyfriends, they go to "dives," but when it's just them, they prefer a chic place where they can dress up, "so it's more of a night out." They're in their mid-20s, among them a journalist, a stock trader, an assistant producer for a television show. They're on their fourth round, laughing, gossiping, hoping no one will cut in with a silly pickup line.

I t could easily be a scene from *Sex and the City,* which seems to have transformed the ladies' night out into an *event*—an evening not only glamorous but sexy. When I track down Candace Bushnell, author of the book the series was based on, as well as *Lipstick Jungle,* she insists that groups of women have been going out together for drinks since at least the early 1980s. "*Sex and the City* was only a reflection of what women were doing, and

Champagne concoction), and eye of the tiger (rum, syrup, and three kinds of juice).

The phenomenon isn't limited to Manhattan. Like many in the bar industry, Kim Connor, owner of Big Daddy's Roadhouse in Orlando, Florida, has made a point of catering especially to women. Her ladies' room is stocked with hairspray and hand lotion, and she offers an extensive wine list. Years ago, she says, when she started in the business, women wouldn't come in by themselves. Perhaps they were deterred by the image of the seedy, sexually desperate female barfly depicted in movies like 1977's *Looking for Mr. Goodbar.* Today the stigma has vanished, and it's tempting to see the shift as a big gold star for the women's movement. "Women are definitely more independent, more in charge of their own money, more comfortable in a bar than they used to be," Connor says. A good number of us now have consuming careers, and we certainly deserve a nice vodka drink, or a few—at least as many as the man at the next table is having. And, like the old boys, why not use the bar as a place to do business? "I think women can drink better than men, don't you?" says a friendly female imbiber I meet on a Saturday night. But, in fact,

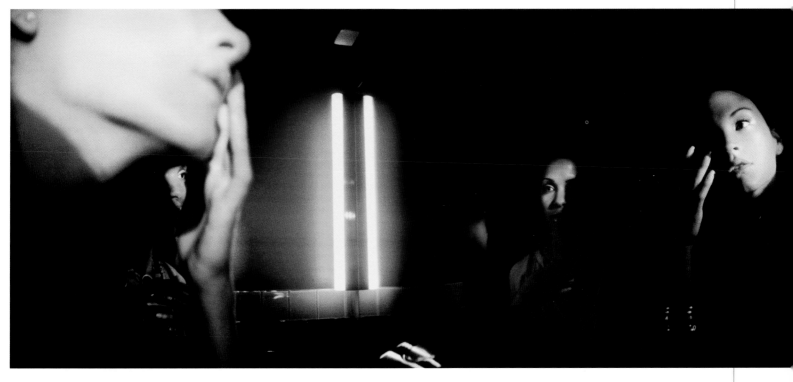

other people picked up on it," she says. Even so, Bushnell's heroine, the cocktail lounge habitué Carrie Bradshaw, obviously struck a nerve. At the bars and clubs, she is referenced countless times, and I spot several imitators, with their luxe blonde hair and high-heeled designer shoes, ordering the signature Bradshaw drink, the cosmopolitan.

The cosmo, in turn, has spawned an array of couture cocktails, helping the alcohol industry to cash in on female drinkers. In addition to the infinite variety of martinis, served in jewel-bright glasses like small works of art, there's the buckaroo (bitters, bourbon, Coke), the kir lethale (a vodka, raisin, crème de cassis,

the opposite is true—one drink for a woman, on average, is equivalent to two for a man.

"We have a lot more information on the effects of drinking on women," says Susan E. Foster, vice president and director of policy research and analysis at the National Center on Addiction and Substance Abuse at Columbia University, which recently put out a book called *Women Under the Influence.* And the news *isn't* good. Evidence suggests that compared with men, women become addicted to alcohol more quickly (see "Is Drinking a Problem For You?" page 52). It also takes lower amounts of alcohol and shorter periods of time to cause heart and liver damage

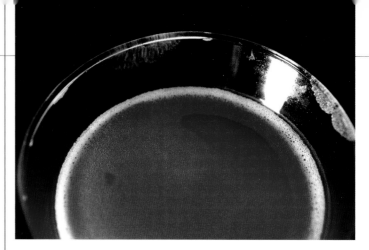

in women. Alcohol weakens our immune systems and raises our risk of breast cancer. Even our hangovers are worse than men's.

I can't help but remember when the tobacco industry cynically trumpeted the victory of women's freedom to smoke with its "You've come a long way, baby" ads. Is it really a good thing if more women find going to bars an appealing pastime?

Out in the clubs, women seem to have other things on their minds than their health, with the exception perhaps of counting cocktail calories. "I like to go out to bars because I like to get hit on," says my friend Kate Ackermann, 25. "I like to flirt, even if it doesn't go anywhere." And a surprising number of women I talk to say they met their partner out drinking. One fashion design assistant hooked up with her boyfriend at a birthday party at a lounge. "I was drunk and dancing. He just grabbed my arm." It was six months before she took his calls, though, because she couldn't remember what he looked like.

Whether or not you meet someone, "there's the sense that something might happen," says one 44-year-old. "Usually nothing happens, but it's nice to think that something could." A bar scene becomes a public spectacle where, fueled by the "liquid courage" that a drink or two confers, one can freely ogle strangers or put oneself on display. "It's all about dressing up," says Kimberley Gray, 34, who works in financial services and would never wear the silky halter she's sporting at the Park to the office. "Women describe walking into a wine bar or a bistro as though they were walking into live theater," says psychotherapist Deborah Anna Luepnitz, PhD, author of *Schopenhauer's Porcupines: Intimacy and Its Dilemmas.* "There's an air of freedom and slight unpredictability." While quick to acknowledge the dangers of club life—drunk driving, unsafe sex—Luepnitz says, "Bars and nightclubs can serve as what psychologists call potential space, a place where one experiments with identity, debating a little more forcefully, laughing louder, dancing funkier."

Some clubs play on that need to escape ordinary life by providing a fantasy environment. "There's a lot of pretending that goes on in bars," says my friend the writer Elizabeth Gilbert (*Eat, Pray, Love*). "There's something very stagey about them." As a former bartender at the Coyote Ugly Saloon in Manhattan's East Village (now famous thanks to her article that was made into a movie), Gilbert ought to know. In the 1990s, with its old-fashioned beer-swilling atmosphere, Coyote Ugly popularized an image of a cowgirl letting loose, drinking men under the table. Gilbert often saw women "come in and have one beer and suddenly be dancing on the bar!" Sometimes, she says, a woman just needs to go wild.

Most of all, true to *Sex and the City,* the women I talked to were often out knocking back drinks to be with each other, a little alcohol pushing conversations into more heated areas, encouraging them to confide something more intimate than they normally would. As my good friend Natalie Standiford, author of The Dating Game, a series of young adult novels, puts it, "Afterward I often feel as if I've come from the shrink." At the wine bar 'Inoteca, on Manhattan's Lower East Side, Tiffany Howell, 32, a music video producer, is splitting a bottle with a friend. Aside from the company, she loves the taste and smell of wine, although

Is Drinking a Problem For You?

It's not always easy to distinguish between love of a good time and a need to drink. These questions are designed to indicate alcohol dependency or abuse.

In the past year, have you...

■ ...failed to fulfill any major work, school, or home responsibilities due to drinking?

■ ...drunk alcohol in a situation that was physically dangerous, such as while driving?

■ ...been arrested for driving under the influence of alcohol or for physically hurting someone while drunk?

■ ...had ongoing relationship problems that are caused or worsened by your drinking?

If you answered yes to any of these questions, alcohol may be controlling you more than you think. Certainly, if you have any of the following four symptoms, you should try to get help: (1) a strong craving or urge to drink; (2) trouble saying no to alcohol once drinking has begun; (3) anxiety, nausea, sweating, or shakiness when you go without booze; (4) a need to drink greater amounts of alcohol in order to feel the same effects you used to.

You can call 800-662-HELP, a national hotline that will connect you with local resources.

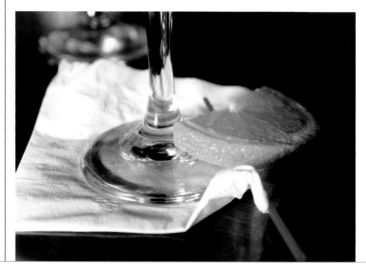

she's quick to note that she's not interested in getting drunk, just "looser," maybe. "It's amazing how a cocktail brings one back to life," says Tara Shields, a 38-year-old public relations executive, who's reviving herself over at the King Cole Bar, an old-fashioned, tweedy haunt in the St. Regis Hotel.

At certain stages in life, women say, drinking heavily requires recovery time that they don't have. "You really pay for it the next day," says Chris Maul Rice, 42, a writer and mother. But at the Rainbow Room, whose wide windows overlook Manhattan skyscrapers, I find six blonde women in their 50s and 60s sipping away the afternoon with white wine, Key lime martinis, and Grey Goose on the rocks. It turns out they're from Dallas and have been friends for 25 years, and now that they're finished with PTA meetings and their children are off to college, going out for cocktails every couple of weeks is a newfound pleasure. "Our husbands like it," says one of the women. "This way they don't have to chitchat." As they all savor their drinks, obviously enjoying one another's company, her tanned friend adds, "My daughter teases me that I still drink like a sorority girl—whatever I can get my hands on."

The reason that women can't drink like men, I discover, is not only that we tend to be physically smaller but that our bodies have more fat and less overall water content. Because water dilutes alcohol and fat retains it, a beer or martini stays in a woman's system longer than a man's. This is even more true for older women: As we age and our body composition wends its way toward more fat, less water, our tolerance for alcohol decreases. One study found that postmenopausal women on hormone replacement therapy who have just one and a half drinks a day are putting themselves at a greatly increased risk for breast cancer.

As I read up on this science, my head is spinning. Reports on alcohol are so confusing—nearly every week there seems to be a new finding that contradicts the headlines the month before. Isn't red wine good for your health? Doesn't a drink a day help ward off Alzheimer's? What about the Parisians, who have alcohol with every meal except breakfast? Denise Russo, PhD, at the National Institute on Alcohol Abuse and Alcoholism says that even if there may be some small benefits to alcohol in moderation, the risks far outweigh them, and those who don't drink shouldn't start for health reasons. Both Russo and Columbia's Foster stress that, overall, alcohol raises your odds of heart disease and breast cancer and, Russo adds, can increase your susceptibility to diseases you might otherwise fight off. Having said that, they do offer guidance on what's acceptably moderate, though they are careful to note that a lot depends on one's individual physical makeup; it's difficult to offer across-the-board standards, other than that you should have no more than one drink a day. But if you're pregnant, depressed, predisposed to alcoholism, or on certain medications, one drink is too much. For most women, Russo explains it like this: "We say in general it takes about an hour to metabolize a small drink of alcohol. You should have no more than one drink per hour, and certainly no more than two per evening." And it's not good to do it on an empty stomach.

This definition of *moderate* may be surprising to some, and the health effects of alcohol are frightening enough to make those of us who partake pay more attention to how much we're actually drinking. But if alcohol is bad for us, stress can also kill, and health experts constantly hound us to relax—which is exactly what a good night on the town can help you do. Alice Domar, PhD, executive director of the Domar Center for Complementary Healthcare just outside Boston, who is working on a book on perfectionism (*I'll Be Happy When...?*), tells me she's seen many women so driven to do everything right (diet, work, exercise) that drinking becomes the only indulgence they allow themselves, occasionally causing them to go overboard. In general, says Domar, women are under an enormous amount of pressure, and "sometimes having a glass of wine can break that cycle." The caveat is that it's "sometimes" and you don't depend on it. She goes out with her friends about once a month and speculates about why it's enjoyable to drink wine. "It just makes people talk more," she says. "They think things are funnier." And laughing is surely good for you.

I noticed when I was out at the clubs, among all those women joking with their friends, that it was hard for me to keep the moderation guidelines in mind. They seem strict and mirthless when you want to unwind. But I'm more aware now that while a little alcohol may help you warm up to a date or relax after work, drinking a lot can do the opposite, making you say something you wish you hadn't or do something that in retrospect makes you worry about yourself. Drinking offers an escape from your regular life, but for that very reason, it's the opposite of being mindful, alert to the world and its ordinary pleasures.

I still don't want to give up those occasional wine-drinking evenings with my friends, but I'm pretty alarmed by the recent health findings and concerned that so many women who think they're just out having a good time end up putting themselves in danger. Now I've formed the habit of asking myself, *Do you really want a glass of wine? Why?* The answers can be interesting. If it's because I feel stressed, I consider a bath. If it's because I'm uncomfortable at a party, I look for a friendly face. A couple of years ago, I gave up drinking entirely because I was pregnant, and I was amazed at how awake I felt in the mornings, how much reading I could do before bed, how, especially at night, I felt more attuned to music, conversation. However much I enjoy raising a glass with friends, I want to keep in mind that I'm making the choice, and that abstaining, too, brings its own clear-eyed, steady joy.

> "I got completely wasted and couldn't remember getting home. The taxi could have taken me anywhere," says Monica Taylor, 25, sipping sangria.

Beauty

Beauty and the Bitch

You know that little voice that relentlessly berates you whenever you look in the mirror, the one that makes you wince every time your appearance falls short of some impossible ideal? Enough! VALERIE MONROE cuts a tyrant down to size.

My god, you are beautiful." Has anyone ever said that to you? Yes? No? Whatever: Imagine it now. Imagine someone looking into your eyes and saying, "My God, my God, you are beautiful." What would it mean to hear that? Would it mean that you had the face of the Madonna? The body of Madonna? Would it mean that the person who was saying it was delusional? Or in love?

One morning not long ago at the *O* magazine offices, 14 of us sat around the heavy conference room table, another 12 of us in a second circle of chairs behind the first. The subject was beauty. We're a pretty vocal group, mostly outspoken and forthright, and by anyone's standards, we are also a pretty *pretty* group—even (I think) a pretty beautiful group. To wit, Beauty A: luxuriously thick, dark curls; a clear, pink complexion; deep chocolate brown eyes; delicate nose; full, generous mouth. Beauty B: a towhead; fair, poreless skin; sky blue eyes; Cupid's bow, ruby lips. Beauty C: a life-size Barbie doll, hourglass figure; huge brown eyes; ski-jump nose; perfect teeth. Beauty D...well, you get the idea. Each of these women is asked whether, in her heart, she knows she's beautiful. And beauty after beauty reveals her secret: Me, beautiful? Never! I'm plain! Even, sometimes, ugly! Don't look at me without makeup! One of the women, with creamy skin, wild dark hair, blue eyes, an athletic build, and a Jo March personality—which is to say she plunges ahead in most endeavors with great, astonishing aplomb—claps her hands smartly over her ears at the mere suggestion that she might be even the slightest, tiniest bit attractive.

And so there we all were, staring at one another, stupefied, and asking, "How can you not see how beautiful you are? Where is your critical voice coming from?"

We got an answer of downright mythical proportion from Beauty A, who long considered her luxuriously thick, dark curls the bane of her existence, a glaring, unfortunate beacon of her awkward unruliness, her inability to fit in with the prevailing ideal of womanhood. She traces her discomfort to her grandmother, a grande dame whose rigid notions about beauty were deeply entrenched in Southern tradition. There was only one way for a woman to look—discreet, well groomed, polished, ladylike. Stray from it in any way (which included wild curls) and you became a kind of pariah, judged to be unmannered, slothful,

poorly raised, and maybe loose; conforming was a way to hide anything that might threaten your station in society.

Her grandmother was a forceful woman whose notions snaked perniciously through the generations, gripping Beauty A and her sisters. It was only recently that they discovered the root of her abnegation and, consequently, their own. As a young woman, their grandmother, considered quite a beauty in her day,

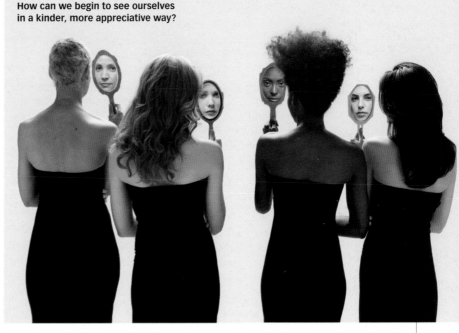

How can we begin to see ourselves in a kinder, more appreciative way?

had descended the staircase in her family home dressed and made-up for a big dance, only to be met by her own grandmother in the parlor. "Go back upstairs and fix yourself!" her grandmother had cried. "You look awful!" Bad enough. How had she transgressed? Makeup overdone? Dress too revealing? A hair out of place? She could have asked her grandmother. But how would the old woman have known? Her grandmother was *blind*. Which begs the question, What was she reacting to? What deep, unsettling fear could have inspired such an outburst? Whatever it was, the fact remains that five generations later Beauty A still struggles over her lovely mess of curls.

Shaking our heads, we asked ourselves the most important question: How can we end this deadening, compulsive self-criticism and begin to talk to ourselves about beauty in a kinder, more compassionate and appreciative, less punishing way?

If you stop to think about it—and let's do that, right now—you'll realize that most of the messages we get about the way we look have to do with denial and withholding (avoid looking older, eat less) and imperfection and loss (conceal your flaws, regain your firm complexion). Can you recall the last thing you read or heard that suggested you celebrate or even acknowledge the positive aspects of the way you look? Instead, we're bombarded with images of the young, the skinny, the oversexualized, the computer idealized. The effect on our self-image and self-esteem is even deeper than you might imagine. Psychologists call it normative discontent: It's considered normal for women to be unhappy with the way we look. Follow this line of thinking: If it's normal, then for us to fulfill our role as women, we're *supposed* to be displeased with our appearance. Does this resonate with you? Are you afraid to admit that—one day, for a few minutes, stepping out of the shower or into the bath—you actually do look okay, or maybe even (God forbid) pretty good?

From the moment we appear in the mirror in the morning, we are face-to-face with our inner critic—call her Judge Beauty—the one who presides over the viciously unforgiving Court of Egregious Imperfections. The interrogation begins: Are you thin enough? Is your complexion bright enough? Your bottom firm enough? Smile white enough? Hair shiny enough? Are your lips too thin or too full? Your eyes too small? Your nose too big? And what's your defense? Haven't been taking care of yourself? Not paying attention? Or saddest of all, were you simply *born that way?* This line of questioning is supported by a constant stream of messages nearly everywhere we look that we could be more attractive if only we wore this or drove that, ate this and not that. In ways subtle and not so subtle, culture teaches us to look cruelly upon ourselves. We're raised to pay attention to these messages—improvement being an essential element of the American dream—and to take them to heart. Ask yourself: Do you equate being pretty with being happy? Have you ever thought that if you were prettier, you might be happier?

In case you're thinking that this kind of severe self-judgment isn't all that common, here is a peek at some interesting statistics from a global study commissioned by Dove, the company that created a sensation with photographs of real women of different sizes in its Campaign for Real Beauty:

■ Only 7 percent of American women (15 to 64) have *never* been concerned about their overall physical appearance.

■ Ninety-two percent of American women (15 to 64) want to change some aspect of their physical appearance, mostly body weight and shape.

■ Almost two-thirds of American women agree that when they feel bad about themselves, it usually has to do with their looks or weight.

■ Living with beauty ideals leads almost seven in ten women globally to withdraw from important, self-actualizing activities, such as going to school or work or a job interview, *because they feel bad about their looks.*

These feelings of inadequacy, the striving for perfection, the competing, the comparing—with others or with younger versions of ourselves—is all a fool's game. No one ever wins, not even the most conventionally beautiful. As Rita Freedman, PhD, clinical psychologist and author of *Bodylove,* points out, if you think you're not pretty, you spend your life regretting that, and if you think you are, you spend your life in fear of losing your looks. Then one day, you do lose them. (You want something to cry about? We'll give you something to cry about!)

We're not supposed to be excessively concerned with the way we look; it's unseemly, prideful, immodest, vain. Vanity stems from competitiveness, says Freedman; it even suggests evil impulses (Mirror, mirror, on the wall...). But here's the rub: As women our sense of self is inextricably bound up in our appearance, and so we tread a very fine line between concern and over-concern or obsession. Freedman reports that in a classic research study, psychotherapists were asked to rate the personality traits of a healthy woman, a healthy man, and a healthy person. "Preoccupation with appearance" (vanity) was rated normal for a healthy woman but abnormal for a healthy man and for healthy people. That leaves us stuck in a damned if we do, damned if we don't dilemma, she points out: aware that we're judged by our attractiveness but ashamed to admit how deeply we value looking good, because that would mean we're...vain.

That seems like a lot of bad news. But there is a slight trend toward a more forgiving attitude: the Dove advertisements, showing robust women comfortable in their bodies; Nike ads suggesting that we focus on what our bodies can do rather than on how they look. These messages can remind us that we need to see ourselves through kinder eyes.

Maybe you've already learned how to do that, if you've been looked at kindly—by a parent, a friend, or a lover. If not, you can learn it now. A while ago I discovered a photo of a little girl at age 5 or 6, not at all a pretty child. Her demeanor is more Alfred E. Neuman than anything else. Her smile is wide and real, but what you notice most—after her seismic optimism—is that she has only one tooth on the top, one huge, white tooth, and it's taking a detour, too, a hard right when it should be going straight. Even so, she thinks she is a fine-looking child, and who (she wonders) in their right mind wouldn't agree? She's vulnerable, open, engaged with the world, a lively (if ingenuous) presence.

When I catch a glimpse of myself on a bad day, not looking the way I wish, rather than turn away from my reflection in disappointment or even disgust, I keep looking till I can see that child, that happy girl who knew that, in spite of her freckles and skinny arms and foolish, scrappy smile, she was *beautiful enough.* Can you see that innocent kid in yourself? Once you do, you will see her in everyone. Because real beauty isn't about symmetry or weight or makeup; it's about looking life right in the face and seeing all its magnificence reflected in your own. ◐

Stop Right There!

5 THINGS YOU SHOULD NEVER DO IF YOU WANT TO FEEL BEAUTIFUL

1. **DON'T USE A MAGNIFYING MIRROR, EXCEPT FOR TWEEZING YOUR BROWS.** If you've ever studied your face in one, you probably don't need an explanation as to why it's not a great idea. But Francesca Fusco, MD, assistant clinical professor of dermatology at Mt. Sinai Medical Center in New York City, offers a few good reasons. A magnifier will make you focus on things that can't be seen with the naked eye, so what's the point of knowing they're there? Also, because everything on your face looks wildly out of proportion in a magnifying mirror, you may get inappropriate ideas about what you actually need. For example, a woman focusing on the little lines above her upper lip might say "Supersize me" to the doctor holding the collagen. (And that, O Best Beloved, is how the lady got her trout lips.)

2. **DON'T USE FLUORESCENT LIGHTBULBS AROUND THE BATHROOM MIRROR.** They emit a flat, white, harsh light that makes everyone look as if she were sick. Better: halogen bulbs with a glass frost filter—MR16 are good ones, says New York City lighting designer Ira Levy, because they emit a clean, even light. In general, the prettiest, most flattering light is warm, incandescent, and dimmable.

3. **DON'T PARTICIPATE IN ANY KIND OF SKIN ANALYSIS THAT INVOLVES A MACHINE.** By using a probe on your face, these devices (often found in department stores) measure pore size, oil levels, dryness, the number and depth of wrinkles, etc., and give you a printed readout, including bar graphs, on the condition of your skin. For some reason—could it have to do with marketing?—the news is never "Nothing could possibly enhance your flawless complexion."

4. **AVOID BEING LIT FROM BELOW**—unless you want to scare the heck out of your kids. You know those little canisters of lights that sit on the floor and shine up into a room? Move away from them. Light, in nature, comes from above, and so we're accustomed to seeing the world this way, points out Stephen Dantzig, author of *Lighting Techniques for Fashion and Glamour Photography*. But light that's shining directly down on your face can be equally unflattering (which is why it's imperative to inform the paparazzi that you must not be photographed outside at high noon on a sunny day). Balanced lighting—for example, one ceiling light directly centered over the bathroom sink and one on either side—will eliminate unflattering shadows, says Levy.

5. **DON'T COMPARE YOURSELF TO WOMEN YOU SEE IN MAGAZINES OR MOVIES.** If you had 15 handlers making sure your hair and makeup were perfect, you'd look pretty glamorous, too. —*V.M.*

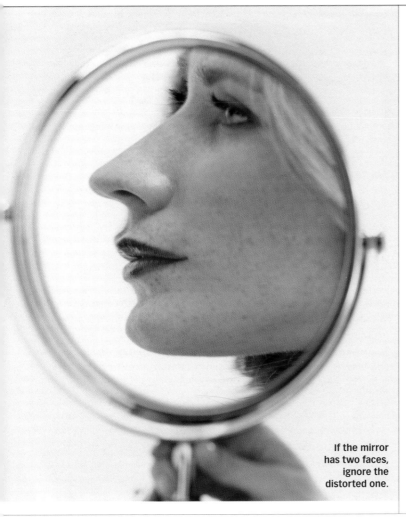

If the mirror has two faces, ignore the distorted one.

Inner Beauty: The Shining

You know it when you see it, but it's difficult to describe: inner beauty. It transcends the impression of a woman's physical traits. Feature by feature there may be nothing special about her—she may even be plain—but something about her attracts you in the most profound way. Something radiates from within. What is it?

"You're responding to empathy, compassion, an openness to others," says Matthieu Ricard, former genetic researcher, now Buddhist monk and author of *Happiness: A Guide to Developing Life's Most Important Skill*. "You see it on someone's face when she feels in harmony with our deepest nature as human beings, which is basically peaceful and loving."

But how does that harmony manifest itself physically? Through subtle expressions, says Ricard, which we pick up both consciously and unconsciously. Hundreds of almost imperceptible muscular movements constantly communicate our feelings. Think of how a classically beautiful face changes when it's transformed by contempt; less beautiful, right? Maybe even ugly? Unconditional love transforms a face, too, says Ricard. We identify with that look. It brings up in us a yearning to be loved and to be loving; and it reminds us of the best we can be, which we may have forgotten or sublimated. And so, inspired, we wind up looking out at the world through more loving eyes, passing the harmony along. That's the thing about inner beauty: Unlike physical beauty, which grabs the spotlight for itself, inner beauty shines on everyone, catching them, holding them in its embrace, making them more beautiful, too. —*V.M.*

Love Me, Love My Imperfections

They have flat chests, flabby knees, stork legs, no hips, wrinkles, age spots, bald spots, extra pounds, and scars. No wonder these five women are so darn appealing.

THE BEST MAKEUP

ANNE LAMOTT

I woke up from a nap one day years ago to find my 5-year-old son, Sam, gazing at me. He took my face into his hands, and peered at me like an old Jewish relative, and said, "I love that little face."

But I didn't love that little face yet. For too long, and despite what people told me, I had fallen for what the culture said about beauty, youth, features, heights, weights, hair textures, upper arms. Still, sometimes in certain lights I could see that I was beautiful, not in spite of but because of unusual features—funky teeth, wild hair, acne scars. My mother's nose, very English, with pinched indents at the tip, what she always called her horns—incredibly helpful, as you can imagine, to my self-esteem as a child—and which I call my proton nobulators. My father's crooked teeth. Cellulite that would make Jesus weep.

I was 40. My best friend had died two years earlier. She was 37, highly intelligent and beautiful. Until she got sick, I'd always believed that beauty protected you, surrounded you with a Guard-All shield. Her cancer kicked this belief to pieces. She was so pretty in the scarves and caps she wore to cover her bald head. Many great-looking women in Marin County, where we are in the midst of a breast cancer epidemic, have lost their hair. At the bank the other day, I ran into an old friend, the Christian Scientist mother of a classmate I had 40 years ago. She is almost 80, with great polish and style. Her hair was gone, replaced by white peach fuzz, yet she was brimming with health and joy. I said gently, "Are you just finishing up chemo?"

She said brightly, "Oh, no, this silly thing is something I go through sometimes."

I started comparing notes with her, because on top of having had impossible hair my entire life, now it is falling out. I worry that I will start looking like Richard Nixon, with dreadlocks.

"I have a fantastic doctor in Southern California who helps me with this," she said. I begged for the number, and she gave it to me and it was not until later that I asked myself, *Why would you beg for the number of a hair loss specialist from one of that doctor's bald patients?*

It was because she was so beautiful, and she knew and exuded that.

Most of us don't notice how great we look until years or decades later. I was looking at photos of myself not long ago, at various ages and weights—way before the neckular deterioration began, way before the fanny pack of menopause—and I could see how gorgeous I must have looked to everyone else. At 16, with an Afro, 20 pounds heavier than I'd been the year before, I was stunning, radiant with youth and athleticism and intelligence; only I honestly thought at the time that I resembled Marty Feldman. In my mid-20s, an anorexic hippie living in a coastal artists' community, I had a best friend who mentioned from time to time that she was the pretty one, which I would have thought went without saying. But I could see the other day, studying some old pictures, that I was the other pretty one. I looked like a waifish Renaissance fairy. Mesmerizing. Then at 33, clean and sober and healing from bulimia, 20 pounds and 20 years lighter than I am now, I'm posing in a periwinkle swimsuit, only I'm covering my thighs in shame, as if someone is photographing me in the eighth-grade gym shower instead of on a public beach. There is a rip in the photo, because I started to tear it so no one would see. Twenty pounds ago! Twenty years! Why did it take me so long to discover what a dish I was? And that my stats were not what made me beautiful?

The answer is that this culture's obsession with beauty is a crazy, sick, losing game, for both women and men, and especially for teenagers, and now, with the need to increase advertising revenues, for preadolescents, too. We're starting to see more and more anorexic 8-year-olds. That obsession is a game we cannot win: Every time we agree to play another match and step out onto the court to try again, we've already lost. The only way to win is to stay off the court. No matter how much of our time is spent in pursuit of physical beauty, even with great success, the Mirror on the Wall will always say "Snow White Lives." But this is in fact a lie—Snow White is a fairy tale. Lies cannot nourish or protect you. Only spirit and freedom can. I hate that. But it is true. There is a line I try to live by, spoken at the end of the Hindu Vedanta service, that goes, "And may the free make others free." And only freedom from fear, freedom from the lies, can make us beautiful, and keep us safe.

Although some days go better than others.

Let's start with something easy: To step into beauty, does one have to give up on losing a little weight? No, of course not. However, if you happen to be sick of suffering, you might consider it. Because if you cannot see that you're okay now, you won't be able to see it if you lose 20 pounds. It's an inside job.

I should know: I lost ten pounds last year. Someone who spent $30,000 at a supervised diet hospital told me the secret of how she lost 12 pounds there: Eat less, exercise more. Oh, and wait—this is $5,000 worth of cutting-edge advice—drink a lot of water. So I did that and in only three months lost ten pounds. I know there is not a chance anyone could sell one copy of a magazine by putting this

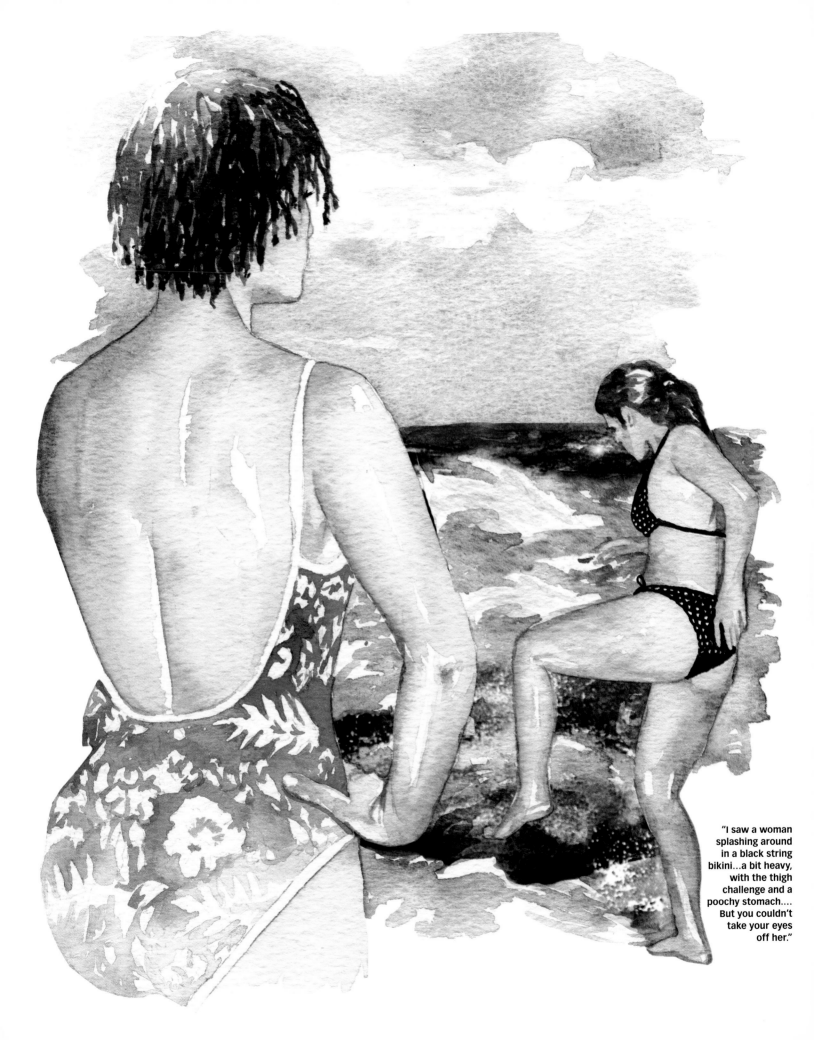

"I saw a woman splashing around in a black string bikini…a bit heavy, with the thigh challenge and a poochy stomach…. But you couldn't take your eyes off her."

on the cover: LOSE TEN POUNDS IN JUST THREE MONTHS. Oh, boy. But this is what I did, and it worked, and guess what? No one noticed, as God is my witness, except for Sam and my boyfriend and a couple of friends, whom I badgered into noticing.

Oh, and my tennis partner, who cried out joyfully, "Annie! Have you lost weight? Look how thin your neck is now!"

It's SO hopeless. What are we going to do? I don't know. But I suppose, while we are on the subject of weight, we might as well address the neck. The neckage. The situation.

The situation is deeply distressing: the wattle and the wrinkles that gather like roman shades in the back. The liver spots. The soft pouch like a frog's vocal sac—or the gular pouches of Komodo dragons—that now connects the chin to the neck. But here's the thing: It could be so much worse, as is usually the case, because at least the neck is recessed. God recessed the neck for a loving, caring reason. While the face is right out front, She set the neck back, out of the direct light, in the shadows.

Sure, you can still see that gravity is having its say, because the neck is where it all shows—it's like the thighs of the head.

But it helps to think of it as something—a pedestal, say, or a plinth—on which you'd set a work of art. A stand for the head and the face. The fact that it is not an incredibly attractive stand doesn't matter one bit. It's there to display your face, your eyes—which are where you carry who you are—your intelligence, goodness, humanity, excitement, commitment, serenity. Over time these are the things that change the whole musculature of your face, as does laughter and animation, as does especially whatever peace you can broker with the person inside.

It's furrow and pinch and judgment that make us look older—our mothers were right. They said if you made certain faces, they would stick, and they do. But our mothers forgot that faces of kindness and integrity stick, too.

I have a friend who looks like someone out of Brueghel or the Brothers Grimm, with a big pancake face and patchy brown hair. But she's lovely, and I mean this objectively, because she loves her life of friends, volunteering, and travel. She's usually in an infuriating state of wonder, of appreciating what is instead of what she wishes was.

She is radiant with spirituality and humor; she got dealt the same basic cards we all got dealt, but somehow she could see that the cards were marked, so she put them down and refused to play. You can't win with marked cards. This has left her with hands free to do what her heart secretly longs to do in this life. She puts on lipstick, a warm soft fleece vest, a matching scarf, and she's set, way ahead of the game.

Joy is the best makeup.

But a little lipstick is a close runner-up, if you ask me.

I know women from every place on the makeup continuum, some who wear none; some who wear a lot, who spackle it on, who could play Shakespeare in the park as soon as they drop the kids off. I know some who wear a lot, beautifully. I know a man who wears concealer to cover his rosacea and several 12-year-olds who doll themselves up like drag queens. I love and glom on to real drag queens; the 12-year-olds spackled in makeup make my heart ache.

But there's nothing wrong with makeup in and of itself. It only becomes a problem when you think you need to be concealed because you're unacceptable. I think we can all agree that the skin does get rattled with age, and that all those wrinkles and hectic blotches of color do not contribute to an illusion of the dewy calmness of youth. But a little makeup, while perhaps not simulating dewy youth, acts as a kind of airbrushing. It restores balance to the face. It makes you look less terminal.

Also, it distracts from the melatonin moustache.

And pretty lipstick makes you look so much less tense and mean. Left to their own devices, lips pucker with the purse strings of age, and lipstick makes them soft again.

I wear a little tinted moisturizer, powder, lipstick. They give me a face I am happier to bring into the world. I look less scary. I'm very glad to claim the crone who is coming to life within me: I just don't want her to screech so loudly that the little girl who is still around gets silenced. I don't want the crone to drown out the naughty teenager, the flirtatious middle-aged woman.

Here is my theory: I am all the ages I've ever been. You realize this at some point about your child—that even when your kid is 16, you can see all the ages in him, the baby wrapped up like a burrito in a swaddling blanket, the 1-year-old letting go of the table to take that first step, the 4-year-old sleeping, the 10-year-old on a mountain hike, climbing up an incline.

We're like Magic 8-Balls. If you ever broke one open with a hammer, you discovered that it contained a plastic geodesic dome, with answers written on every surface, floating in a cylinder of murky blue fluid. After you've asked your question, and shaken the ball, and the dome stops spinning, the blue water falls off the sides, so you can read the answer in the window. And my theory is that like our children, like every facet of the geodesic dome, every age we've ever been is who we are.

So how can I be represented by a snapshot of me during a split second at this one aging age? Isn't the truth that this me is subsumed into all the me's I've already been and will be?

Don't get me wrong: I love people who don't wear makeup. But, paradoxically, when I put on a little, it helps me feel more natural—I don't worry so much about how I look. This diminishes the destructiveness of self-consciousness.

Self-consciousness looks like the other furrows and shadows on our faces, the smudges under our eyes.

The most utterly unself-conscious woman I know is a nun named Gervais. Her hair is short and graying, with a slight curl, and she stands tall, with an economy of self-containment and abundance all at once, like bamboo. She's in touch with everything around her, but she doesn't need anything from it: The plainness and holiness of the world seem enough for her.

She has the beauty of modesty, which is a virtue the world doesn't have much truck with: one ordinary flower in a vase, as opposed to a bouquet.

When Jesus was asked about beauty, he pointed to nature, to the lilies of the field. Behold them, he said, and *behold* is a special word: It means to look upon something amazing or unexpected. Behold! It is an exhortation, not a whiny demand, like when you're talking to your child—"Behold me when I'm talking to you, sinner!" He's saying, You are freely given each moment the opportunity to see through a different pair of glasses. "Behold the lilies of the field, how they grow; they neither toil nor spin."

But that's only the minor chord. The major one follows, in his antianxiety discourse—which is the soul of this passage: that all striving after greater beauty and importance and greater greatness is foolishness. He's saying we have much to learn from lilies about giving up striving. He's saying that we could be aware of, filled with, and saved by the presence of holy beauty, rather than worshipping golden calves.

I saw a woman on the beach in Hawaii three years after my son told me that he loved my little face. I was 43, and in the early stages of seeing that I had, in fact, become a woman of beauty: I hadn't fully grown into this yet, but the truth, which bats last, was pressing through more and more of the confusion and judgment that had blinded me most of my life. The other woman, who was about my own age, was playing in the surf with her young child. She was near the shore, in water that barely reached her knees, so I could see her clearly. There was nothing physically dramatic about her. Nearby in the water and tanning on beach towels were teenage girls and young women in bikinis who were brown, lithe, smooth, and perfect, who made you want to kill yourself. But this woman looked—well—like us, like me and my friends. She was of average height, with long dark hair, a bit heavy, with the thigh challenge and a poochy stomach. The thing was, she was wearing a bikini, like all the very young women, whereas I and the other women over 30 were wearing one-piece suits made of spandex, designed for maximum suckage and disguise. But she was splashing around in a black string bikini, with both an extraordinary lack of self-consciousness and glistening confidence. You couldn't take your eyes off her. She commanded the beach.

We sneaked looks at her, as if she was a movie star. She was like the Greek goddess of Surf. And we beheld her. I thought, *That could be me someday. I could wear a bikini too....Theoretically.*

She was medicine.

Now, I knew I wasn't going to go buy a bikini any time soon. But I wondered if I could splash about like her, with abandon, my head thrown back and my arms held out to the sun. And later that day, I did. I was wearing the same old jaws-of-death swimsuit I wore that morning and a towel wrapped around my waist almost to the shore. When I dropped it, I felt shy and stricken

and jiggly. But after a minute, I straightened my shoulders, reached for my son's hand, and ran with him into the ocean, and I splashed and sploshed and ducked under the waves, and then leapt back up to the air, like Our Lady of the Tides, for all the world to see.

BODY OF EVIDENCE
BETSY CARTER

I love stories. I love when they take unpredictable turns and come alive with evocative characters. I love how the best storytellers can suggest smells or sounds, and provoke new thoughts or old memories. I thought about this the other evening after a bath when I was standing naked in front of a full-length mirror in my bedroom. Normally I avoid full-length mirrors, particularly when I'm undressed, but this night I lingered.

The first thing I noticed was my high waist. It brought me back to a night in junior high when I'd stood in the living room wearing a pair of pink shorts and a white T-shirt. I was talking on the phone with one leg bent and my foot resting on my other knee. "She looks like a stork," my father said to my mother. My mother was sitting on a rattan chair smoking a cigarette. She turned so I wouldn't see her laugh, but the steady bursts of smoke plumes over her head gave her away. I got off the phone and whined: "Daaaad, quit it." Oh yeah, I was a real whiner. Still, it was nice visiting with my folks in that old living room, even for those few seconds. And Dad was right: I am built like a stork.

I looked at the crescent-shaped memento on my knee. When I was 10, I picked up a bottle of Clorox to wash my Patrol Girl belt and accidentally banged the bleach against the wall. The bottle broke, gashing my knee. My father scooped me up, threw me into the bathtub, and ran the water. I'd forgotten the frightened look on his face and how the house smelled of Clorox for weeks.

And so it went. Everywhere I looked, I saw a story: the breast cancer saga, writ large; the freckles on my shoulders that evoked my mother's voice ("With skin like yours, you'll burn to a crisp"); the birthmark on my hip that is a duplicate of my father's and his father before him.

Over the years, as the stories accrued, I became more self-conscious about my body. I miss being unself-conscious about my nakedness. You know the kind of naked I mean: ripping off your clothes for a skinny-dip; being undressed with someone because he's cute and you can; walking around the gym towel-less after a hot shower. Then I look at my very imperfect body and see its patches of history, like stamps on my passport. Those stamps aren't the kind of thing that would make me throw off my towel at the gym or be the first to jump naked into a lake. But like a good story, they remind me of where I've been, and of the annoying and endearing people I've met along the way.

SAVED BY THE CITY

ELIZABETH BERN

When I was growing up in the Midwest, the gold standard for beauty was embodied by Farrah Fawcett-then-Majors: blonde, tan, curvaceous. I was none of these things and used to joke that with my dark hair (on which the ubiquitous Sun-In was useless) and pale skin, I looked like a photo negative of who I should have been. I was also skinny enough to be banished to the boys' department for jeans; I can still remember the heat of the shame that swept through me when an unkind salesgirl crowed, "You have no hips!"

At 21, I arrived in New York by train, hopped in a cab, and asked the driver to take me to "downtown Greenwich Village." Like so many midwestern girls who flock to the city each June, I was clueless, bedazzled, thrilled. Dropped off at Washington Square Park, I realized that, for the first time in my life, I fit in— because there was simply no way not to, no sole way to be or to look in this simmering cauldron of beauty and defiant style.

The dark/pale coloring that had once inspired the meaner girls to call me "witch" was viewed here as striking; "too skinny,"

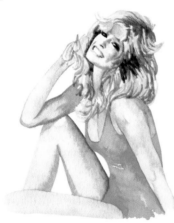

I learned, scarcely exists in Manhattan's lexicon. Voilà: I looked better! I can't say that overnight I stopped wanting to resemble someone else (or that I never do so now), but I understood on a visceral level how deeply subjective beauty is, how wholly dependent on context, how mutable, how wide.

PADDING MY RÉSUMÉ

CATHLEEN MEDWICK

As a teenager in the early 1960s, I had a small waist, slim legs, breasts as pointy as ballistic missiles. Or at least my bra made them look that way. Like my mother, I was flat-chested. Unlike her, I didn't care. When I went to college and became a hippie, I casually trashed my padded bras. Years later, while my friends were cramming themselves into devices engineered to hoist their bosoms back up to sea level, I wore a soft scrap of lingerie designed for 13-year-olds.

It was only curiosity that made me volunteer, in 1994, at the women's magazine where I then worked, to test-drive a hot new product called the Wonderbra. The solid construction made me feel ridiculously top-heavy; my sexiest inclination was to claw at my now-itchy breasts. When I ventured outside, though,

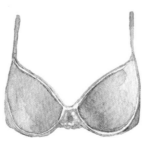

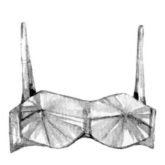

I heard a couple of guys say, "Wow, big ones!" and I thought, *Okay, this is why women love being busty.* Of course, when I turned, I saw the men loading two enormous paintings into a truck. I went back to the office, dropped off the Wonderbra, and said goodbye to the sexpot I'd never be.

But one day not long ago, in a rare burst of midlife daring, I bought a lightly padded bra. I put it on and something remarkable happened. I felt uplifted! I felt womanly. When I entered a room, I led with my chest, as if I were the bearer of something precious. People ogled my sweater, even though they'd seen it often before. I became a magnet for hugs.

Would I have been more glamorous all these years if I'd had a working relationship with cleavage? I'll never know. Lately I seem to have two identities, womanly and gender neutral, and I find that I'm comfortable with both. Bra or no bra, wonders never cease.

CUTE...OR SMART?

MADELEINE CHESTNUT

In my mother's view, to be gorgeous was to be brainless. And to be brainless was to commit the sins she'd never forgiven herself for: promiscuity and educational poverty. The "fast girl" who'd gotten pregnant out of wedlock twice before age 20, Mom sought a strange kind of redemption: She may not have kept her skirt down and her grades up, but she would certainly raise girls who did.

Which is why, when she caught 12-year-old me experimenting with lipstick, she pounced: "Do you think you're cute?" she spat, hurling the lipstick into the garbage. "Now go start on your algebra."

I was nearly 30 the first time someone—a boyfriend I loved—told me I was beautiful. "Me?" I said. Chatty, yes. Witty, maybe. But my mother had spent 20 years and hundreds of dollars on SAT prep to make sure I put *smart* into the slot where other girls put *pretty.* "Can't you see yourself?" my boyfriend quizzed. I couldn't.

Then, two summers later, I found a photo I'd never seen before: my mother at 19, Rockette legs emerging from teensy hot pants, nipples at full salute, Afro stretching toward the sky, a bootylicious hottie babe modeling a stunning figure I can only dream of, yet bearing a face almost exactly like my own. *Can't you see yourself?* No—but now I could see the woman in the photo. And I could see that whatever erroneous notions Mom might have given me, she gave them along with her intelligence, her courage, her imagination, and, yes, her beauty. **O**

The Plain Truth About the Beautiful People

SIMON DOONAN grew up worshipping the BP—Countess This or Princess That—and only when he became a New York style czar himself did he recognize true glitz when he saw it.

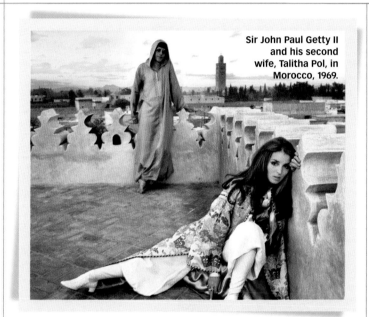

Sir John Paul Getty II and his second wife, Talitha Pol, in Morocco, 1969.

No detail of their fancy-schmancy lives was too trivial for our consideration: We simply had to know everything about their hairdressers, their palazzi, their caftans (the Beautiful People always seemed to be photographed wearing caftans), their eating habits, or lack thereof, and the unguents they slapped on their gorgeous faces.

What were the qualifications needed to become one of the BP? Were there membership dues? Nobody seemed to know. It was all very mysterious. There were certain obvious common denominators: Most Beautiful People had loads of disposable cash, loads of thick hair, and tons of fake lashes. Having a closet full of Valentino couture seemed like it might speed up the approval process. And, yes, they were undeniably beautiful. All the Beautiful People—at least the chicks—had cheekbones on which you could easily land a private jet.

And what possible function, you are no doubt wondering, did they serve? The truth is a little sad: Simply put, the BP were invented to fill up magazine pages and to remind us ordinary mortals that we can never be too rich or too thin.

In other words, they existed in order to depress the living hell out of the rest of us.

Once upon a time, long before Angelina and Lindsay and Blahniks and bling, there lived a long-lost tribe called the Beautiful People. We earthlings worshipped at their altar, and we called them the BP for short.

Back in the 1960s, the BP were big news: Every magazine was crammed with fascinating drivel about these glamour-pusses. Some names, like Princess Grace and Jackie O, were familiar to us commoners; most were not. Many BP had fake-sounding aristocratic titles like Countess Consuelo Crespi and Princess Ira von Fürstenberg. Several BP were married to the moguls of the day: There were Guinnesses and Gettys, as well as an Agnelli or two.

Where did they live? It wasn't the Bronx, that's for sure. The Beautiful People were totally Euro-fabulous: For them it was all about Rome and Monte Carlo and Saint-Tropez in the summer and Gstaad in the winter.

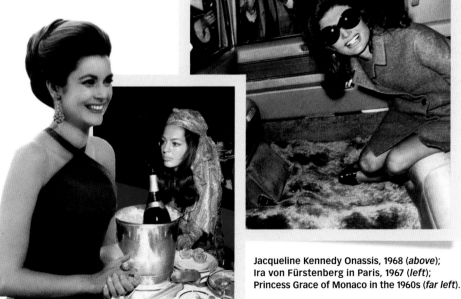

Jacqueline Kennedy Onassis, 1968 (*above*); Ira von Fürstenberg in Paris, 1967 (*left*); Princess Grace of Monaco in the 1960s (*far left*).

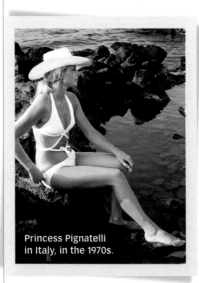

Princess Pignatelli in Italy, in the 1970s.

As a fashion-obsessed teen growing up in a gritty industrial town, it was inevitable that I would fall under the spell of the Beautiful People. And fall I did, one rainy Saturday in 1968. There I was rummaging petulantly through my mother's pile of fashion mags while plotting how to escape the family home and move to swinging London, when I chanced upon a copy of a now extinct magazine called *Nova*. On the cover was a portrait of a haughty blonde woman lying on a leopard bedspread. PRINCESS PIGNATELLI PLUCKS EACH HAIR OFF HER LEGS WITH TWEEZERS read the provocative headline. *Good for her!* I thought and flicked to the relevant page.

Luciana Pignatelli, I quickly found out, was the self-appointed queen of the Beautiful People. She wrote *The Beautiful People's Diet Book* and *The Beautiful People's Beauty Book.* She was the conduit between us lowly mortals down here on earth and the BP high up there on Mount Olympus. A missionary of sorts, she aimed to share their fashion tips and beauty secrets with us so that we might become just a tad more beautiful, or at least less unbeautiful.

Most of her suggestions had limited application to my working-class life. Finding out how to take care of my minks and sables was interesting but utterly useless since my winter coat was a food-stained duffle with a missing toggle.

As I contemplated the glamorous *principessa,* it was impossible for me not to make comparisons with my mother, Betty Doonan. Here was everything my mother could have been. Like the *principessa,* Betty Doonan dyed her hair blonde and never appeared in public without high heels and a full face of maquillage, but there the resemblance ended. Though she would happily have spent her days pulling each hair out of her legs with tweezers, fate had not dealt my mother that kind of hand.

While the Beautiful People's glamour seemed ethereal and goddesslike, Betty Doonan's was a lot more down-to-earth—think Lana Turner with a dash of Robert Mitchum thrown in. A tough, working-class broad, she had left school at the age of 13 to train as a pork butcher. In the Second World War, Betty joined the air force and became a spitfire electrician. Nobody messed with Betty Doonan.

During my childhood, Betty always worked at least two jobs. When she wasn't working, she was dealing with our demanding live-in relatives and lodgers. These included, but were not limited to, my schizophrenic uncle, Ken; my grandmother (postlobotomy); and my blind aunt, Phyllis. Yes, Betty was a schlepper and a trouper. When she wasn't riding her bike up the hill with a basketful of groceries, she was cutting up Aunt Phyllis's food into bite-size chunks.

Like all teenagers, I was idiotically ashamed of my folks. All I could think about was escaping to the fashionable excitement of the big (Emerald) city where the Beautiful People were waiting, or so I thought, to welcome me into their bracelet-encrusted arms.

God punished me for my superficial aspirations. When I got

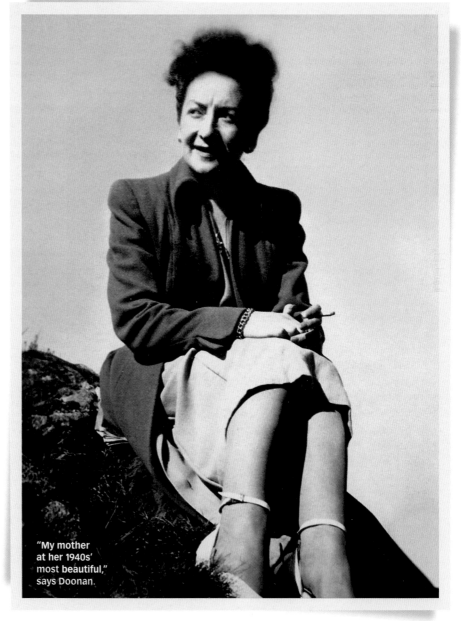

"My mother at her 1940s' most beautiful," says Doonan.

to the big city, there were no caftans or tiaras or palazzi. There was just a seething mass of people like me, all trying to pay the rent and extract a few chuckles from their daily grind.

Luckily for me, I had inherited Betty's work ethic, her optimism, and her love of a well-cut skirt. Slowly but surely, I began to claw my way into the world of fashion and style and soon found myself rubbing shoulders with many Beautiful People. It wasn't long before I realized that good-looking, glamorous people were no different from the rest of us. Some were geniuses; some were idiots. Some were jolly and perky, and some were suicidal. There was one noteworthy difference: Many of these folk, especially the really rich, really good-looking ones, had never felt the need to develop a sense of humor. None of them were as much fun as Betty or Aunt Phyllis.

I decided to chronicle, and ridicule, my pursuit of the Beautiful People in a book called *Nasty: My Family and Other Glamorous Varmints*. I set about charting my starry-eyed progress down the Yellow Brick Road. Before I was even halfway through, I realized that the Beautiful People—surprise, surprise!—were the ones I had struggled to leave behind.

Just call me Dorothy.

My promotional book tour was something of a revelation. Many of the people I met had a hard time grasping this basic concept. Despite the universality of my message—"There's no place like home!"—many of the journalists and book-signing attendees would yes me to death, laugh obligingly at my family anecdotes, and then, without fail, they would say something like "Okay, that's all great, but who is more beautiful, Angelina Jolie or Nicole Kidman?"

Oy vey!

We, with our Brads and Beyoncés and Katie-and-Toms and our rampant celebrity culture, are still hypnotized by the idea of the Beautiful People. The situation is, if anything, worse than it was in the early 1960s. Contemporary media is slavishly devoted to putting beautiful people on Mount Olympus so that we can worship them. And the only way we can get close to our gods—and feel good about ourselves—is to subject ourselves to humiliating makeovers and brutal surgical procedures à la *The Swan, Extreme Makeover, I Want a Famous Face*, and so on.

Is there any hope for us? Or are we all headed straight to BP hell?

Here's an optimistic thought: Now that surface beauty has become a commodity that can be acquired by anybody with enough shekels to hire the right stylist and the perfect plastic surgeon, maybe, just maybe, it will lose some of its mystery and power. If you can buy beauty at the shopping mall, maybe it's not so special after all. With the loss of its mystique, might we now have the perfect opportunity to give beauty a much broader definition, something that reaches way beyond the purely physical?

Any new definition of beauty should obviously include stuff like courage and accomplishment and selflessness, but let's not forget humor. Let's celebrate those individuals who have retained the ability to be childlike and silly.

Various beautiful people in my day-to-day life spring to mind: I'm thinking of one particular colleague who made me laugh so hard recently that I bit on a fork and chipped my front tooth. And what about the salon receptionist who wears a different wig every week and pretends it's her real hair? Surely my doorman would qualify. He once saw me leaving my apartment building on Halloween dressed as the queen of England, and ten years later, he curtsies and calls me "your majesty" every time he hands me my mail.

Any definition of the really beautiful people needs to encompass people like my courageous blind aunt, Phyllis, who always rose cheerfully above her handicap, with (or in spite of) Lassie, her Seeing Eye dog. I'll never forget the time Aunt Phyllis returned from a friend's funeral with her knees grazed and grass in her hair.

"What the hell happened?" asked my mum, dabbing disinfectant on Phyllis's wounds.

"Lassie led me into the open grave," Aunt Phyllis replied and collapsed on the floor laughing.

Now that's what I call beautiful. 🅞

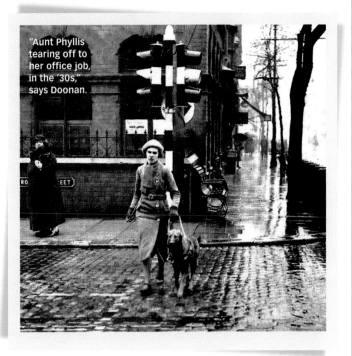

"Aunt Phyllis tearing off to her office job, in the '30s," says Doonan.

"Me, in the late 1960s," says Doonan.

All I could think about was escaping to the big city.

Balance

Overhelpers Anonymous

If you're always lending a hand, a shoulder, an ear, even a buck or two to people who can perfectly well solve their own problems, MARTHA BECK wants you to get over your rescuing addiction and start taking care of yourself.

Michelle and I met for coffee not long after her youngest child headed off to college. She said she'd been roaming around her empty nest, assembling care packages for her kids, ironing her husband's socks. I clucked sympathetically and reached for my iced coffee when Michelle beat me to it. She reached across the table, grabbed my glass, lifted it a couple of inches, and handed it to me. A few minutes later, she did it again. Then again. After the third time, I said, "Um, Michelle, could you not do that?"

"Oh, I'm so sorry," she said—and reached across the table to hand me my glass again. Then the two of us laughed, as friends will when one of them appears to be possessed, because we both knew what was happening. Michelle had entered a zone we call overhelping. I know that I do the same thing when I'm stressed-out or upset. Maybe you do, too. We get stuck in help mode, draining our own energy, annoying friends, creating weakness and dependency in family members. If this complex sounds all too familiar to you, the following information may be, uh, helpful.

RECOGNIZING WHEN IT'S TIME TO STOP

I love the cartoon house cat named Eek!, whose motto is "It never hurts to help!" In every episode of his television show, Eek! rushes to assist someone, invariably creating disasters that make World War II look like a Tupperware party. Resisting our inner Eek!, knowing when it does hurt to help, is key to loving well. Let's start with a quiz:

1. T F **I'm often exhausted by caring for others.**

2. T F **I do things for people without waiting to be asked, then feel hurt if they aren't grateful.**

3. T F **The thought of not caring for anyone makes me nervous.**

4. T F **I frequently complain about the stress of caring for others.**

5. T F **I feel yearning or envy when the people I help realize their dreams.**

6. T F **I'm feeling smaller and more invisible as I help others grow and achieve.**

7. T F **It would be scary to pursue my deepest hopes without anyone helping me.**

8. T F **I've given up on my own dreams; I just want my loved ones to be happy.**

9. T F **I feel I'm the only person who can do things right.**

10. T F **I'm trying to solve a thousand problems, none of them my own.**

11. T F **I'm exhausted by having to fix countless needy or incompetent people.**

12. T F **The people I help couldn't function without me.**

If you answered *true* to even one question, your intentions are good but the result is likely bad. You're pouring energy into doing things for others that you subconsciously know they should do for themselves. While healthy help is based on a desire to improve others' lives, overhelping is actually about the helper's emotional needs. Recognizing what's really going on—and dealing with your own wants in new ways—is essential to breaking dysfunctional patterns.

VARIANT #1: HORMONAL HELPFULNESS

My friend Michelle began ironing socks and treating me like a toddler because taking care of other people, while taxing, eased her anxiety like a hit of opium. Literally.

When my first baby was born, I knew my body would start secreting oxytocin, which stimulates lactation. This seemed weird but logical. What I hadn't expected was the number oxytocin would do on my emotions. I was desperate to feed, pat, carry, diaper, caress, and rock anything that seemed to need help—my baby, certainly, but also my hamster, my local TV news anchorperson, and my broken toaster. When I wasn't doing something helpful, I'd get almost frantic.

These reactions probably evolved so that mothers would care for their babies even at risk to themselves. But all women, not just mothers, secrete oxytocin under pressure. For decades, the famous fight-or-flight response (mediated by hormones like adrenaline) was primarily studied in men. Only in recent years have researchers found that in women the fight-or-flight response is tempered by a rush of oxytocin, the "tend and befriend" hormone. When things go wrong, we may fight or flee, but also feel strong urges to support and comfort others.

When we actually can help, by rocking the baby, cheering a friend, fixing the ailing toaster, we get a hit of "endogenous opioids," internally produced chemicals that affect our brains like opium.

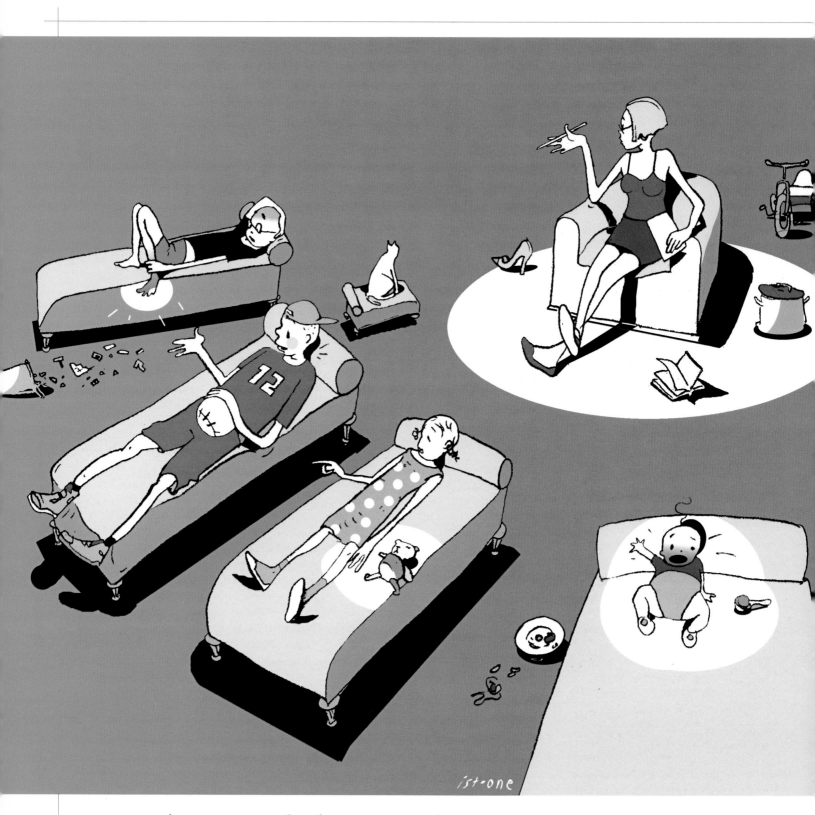

I was desperate to feed, pat, carry, diaper, caress, and rock anything that seemed to need my help—my baby, certainly, but also my hamster, my local TV news anchorperson, and my broken toaster.

These create a fine, floaty, glowy feeling, one of the main reasons I enjoy being a girl. It's also why I do life coaching (I get paid to get high!), and why Michelle couldn't stop picking up my 12-ounce glass of coffee. Both of us like to self-medicate with the helper hormone.

To see if you do the same thing, go back to the quiz and check your answers to questions 1 through 4. If you answered *true* to any of these, part of your helpfulness is meant to allay your own anxiety. Instead I would encourage you to use the following strategies:

THE FIX: Turning Helper Hormones on Yourself

Therapists and self-help books constantly advise us to get manicures, pedicures, massages, and spa treatments. This advice has a solid biological basis. Any nurturing we direct toward ourselves, especially if it involves physical touch, triggers the same endogenous-opioid surge we get from doing things for others. If you're a hormonal overhelper, schedule a foot rub from a reflexologist, lure your mate into bed, pet the cat until it purrs in your lap. Get touched.

Be especially diligent about this in times of stress. Overhelpers may offer assistance to get a "fix" when they themselves need comfort. This is a quick trip to exhaustion and resentment. The next time you're upset, instead of focusing on trying to help others, pat your own hand and tell yourself kind things ("It's okay, sweetie, the hamster doesn't hate you. He bit you only because he didn't need you to diaper him"). The more you place your full attention on giving yourself comfort, the less you'll help others who don't want it.

VARIANT #2: AVOIDANCE ASSISTANCE

"I'm dying to start my own business," says Susan, a 30-something homemaker, "but I'm too busy pitching in with my sister's and my husband's lives. I never get a minute to myself." This makes Susan's loved ones grind their teeth to the gums. They experience her constant support as intrusive and frustrating. "I don't need Susan's advice," her sister tells me, "but she spends hours giving it to me. Please, Susan, get a life!"

Susan concentrates on other people's problems to avoid the scary prospect of following personal dreams. Author Julia Cameron uses the term "shadow artist" to refer to someone who lurks on the fringes of achievement, helping others attain the rewards they really want for themselves. Take a look at questions 5 through 8 on the quiz. One or more *true* responses means you may be shadowing when you might want to stand in the limelight.

THE FIX: Connect with Anger

Avoidance assisters rarely admit to being angry—just worn-out and disappointed. But anger is a healthy response to overhelping at the cost of your own dreams, so give your frustration a voice. Fill in the blanks below with any words that come to mind.

"I'm so tired of helping [name]_____. If I never had to worry about him/her again, I'd have time to_____
_____."

Now take half an hour off from assisting others, and spend those 30 minutes working on the thing you supposedly never have time for. If you're an avoidance assister, this may feel terrifying. Get used to it. Taking your own risks and creating your best destiny is always scary, but both you and others will benefit if you pour your helpful energy into your own life.

VARIANT #3: MESSIAH MADNESS

Every night, Ivan gives his girlfriend the same speech. "I practically have to run that whole office by myself," he complains. "Today I had to work with Jim on a brief, then check all the correspondence, because that new paralegal can't spell. And Brenda needed advice on her new case—I mean, how much can one man do?"

Ivan's girlfriend, bloodstream brimming with oxytocin, responds by feeding and petting him, all the time thinking, *So who died and made you God?* She knows that Ivan has a messiah complex. When she suggests delegating work, he ignores her. The son of two alcoholics, Ivan learned young that service justified his existence. Cleaning up his dad's empties, calling in excuses to his mom's boss, and caring for his younger brother, Ivan formed a belief he still unconsciously holds: The moment he stops helping is the moment he stops mattering.

The only problem is that this assistance comes off as arrogance. To ensure that he'll always be needed, Ivan criticizes his coworkers mercilessly. Their work is never good enough until he's "fixed" it. He thinks they depend on him. Actually, they sort of wish they could set him on fire. If you answered *true* to questions 9 through 12 on the overhelper quiz, it's time to climb down off your cross and offer less aid to those you think are helpless.

THE FIX: Give Support, Not Help

There's a big difference between help and support. Help tells the recipient, "You're needy and weak—I'm needed and strong." It forces others into a supplicant's position, while the helper gets to play savior. If you really want to serve others, stop doing things you resent (resentment is a sign of overhelping) and say something like this:

"You know, Bob, I'm positive you'll figure out a way to solve your problem. You can do it! I'm right here, cheering!"

Say this to yourself, right now, and you'll feel that even as self-talk, it's empowering. Offer that same encouragement to others.

If the bad news is that you're an overhelper, the good news is that you can stop right now. Nurture yourself, support others without assuming responsibility you resent, and feel your energy switch from "Eek!" to "Aah!" You'll become a contented, self-contained source of personal well-being, a model who shows others how they can achieve the same state. And that's the kind of help that really never hurts. ◻

The Rule of 10-10-10

By asking herself three easy—and utterly profound—questions,
SUZY WELCH has managed to solve just about every personal and professional
quandary in her life. An amazing, spectacularly snappy guide to decision-making.

Back in my 20s, when I was still trying to figure out how to do it all—the perfect mommy/good wife/successful career woman/happy homemaker thing—I happened to be seated next to a kindly older gentleman at a dinner party. In the course of small talk, he mentioned that he came from a family with 11 children. At the time, I had one toddler and was hanging on by my fingernails.

"How, how, *how*," I practically cried, "did your mother do it?"

The man's eyes crinkled up; he'd heard the question before.

"Well, my dear, those were simpler days," he said gently. "After my mother finished the breakfast dishes, she started making lunch."

"*Oh, come on!*" I wanted to scream, "*Give me the magic formula!*"

As if he'd heard my thoughts, the man added, "Don't worry. Everything will sort itself out eventually."

How old-fashioned he seemed. How wise he turned out to be.

Which is not to say I've cracked the do-it-all problem at the ripe old age of 46. There is no foolproof way to manage something as untidy as life, and I still have days when I feel as if I am juggling eggs on a roller coaster. But I have—over a decade of tinkering and practice—devised a method, for lack of a better word, to help me balance my multiple life roles and navigate the daily dilemmas of an overstuffed existence.

I call it 10-10-10.

Here's how it works. Every time I find myself in a situation where there appears to be no solution that will make everyone happy, I ask myself three questions:

What are the consequences of my decision in 10 minutes?
In 10 months?
And in 10 years?

The answers usually tell me what I need to know not only to make the most reasoned move but to explain my choice to the family members, friends, or coworkers who will feel its impact.

I've used 10-10-10 to make some of the most meaningful decisions in my life—my divorce, for one. But the effectiveness of 10-10-10 crept up on me when I started using it on a much smaller scale.

The first time was a typical weekday. Dropping the kids off at school on the way to work, I promised that I would definitely, absolutely see them at dinner so we could do homework together and watch our favorite TV show. I also promised our babysitter the evening off.

At 5 P.M., of course, a crisis erupted at the office. During this period, I was hoping for a promotion, so walking out the door with my boss's hands wrapped around my ankle seemed particularly ill-advised. I called home to test the waters. The babysitter nearly burst into tears when I mentioned staying late. Two of the kids were fighting, and one was sulking for an unknown reason. (The other was still at swimming practice, thank God.) My daughter grabbed the phone and put in her two cents: "You love work more than us."

My gut was all over the place—go, stay, go—and that's when 10-10-10 was officially born. I slowed my thought process down and systematically began to pick it apart. *What exactly,* I asked myself, *were the immediate repercussions of staying at work versus rushing home?*

If I stayed, my boss would jot it down in her little book of good deeds, and my children and babysitter would turn purple. If I rushed home, my boss would get someone else to help her, and my triumphant arrival at the front door would be greeted with the usual grunts and sighs, and probably a demand for the latest video game or some exciting new shampoo.

In 10 months? Assuming I didn't make staying late a daily feature of our lives (which I knew I wouldn't), the kids would be fine. As for the babysitter, she would be back at school, and I would be but a distant memory. At work, though, if I left, my boss might start to question my commitment and my availability, not the impression I was eager to encourage.

In 10 years, the fact that I worked late (or not) would be irrelevant. My career would be someplace I couldn't foresee. The babysitter would be working on Wall Street. And my kids would love or hate me for reasons much bigger than one late night at the office.

And so I stayed without flinching. I got my gold star at work, and the home-front grumbles faded as anticipated.

The second time I used 10-10-10, the ante was higher. I'd been asked to run a Saturday meeting for the company's executives—a big deal in terms of exposure. Unfortunately, the meeting fell on the same day my son went for his junior black belt in karate, a test that was four grueling years in the making.

Again, I ran through the time frames.

In 10 minutes, both choices stank. My son would be devastated. I could picture his sweet face all screwed up and turning pink as he fought back tears; he was the kind of kid who got sad, not mad. My boss obviously wouldn't cry, but her disappointment would surely be palpable.

In 10 months, I figured, the pain would be buried. Why? Because I would shovel frantically to make it so. If I attended the off-site, I would love my son extravagantly in the months that followed, spoil him with my attention, and apologize until he could stand it no more. If I didn't go, I would pull the same kind of performance at work, with my boss at the receiving end.

But 10 years...there was the problem. My kids would be gone and my career at full-throttle, whether I had gotten one promotion or not. But on some visceral level, my son would still know that I had chosen to miss one of the seminal events of his life for my own advancement.

That was damage I could never undo.

So I skipped the off-site. And late that Saturday afternoon, I cheered as my son received his black belt, his face pink as he tried to hold back tears.

About a year later, 10-10-10 changed my life.

Like many marriages, mine took a long time to come apart. The stakes of doing something—that is, ending it for real—seemed unbearably high: the children, the friends, the house, the backyard barbecues. And so we waited, and waited, for something to unfreeze us—a decision, one way or another.

One spring morning, I stole away from work and family, and hiked to the top of a mountain about an hour north of Boston. I needed the time and silence to work this tangled problem through. The 10-minute question came first, and it was painfully easy to answer—divorce meant chaos and despair all around. In 10 months, the mess would surely be worse, what with the

upheaval, and lawyers, too. All I could think was, *Awful, awful, awfulness—not just in 10 months, in 20, and maybe more.* In 10 years, though—in 10 wonderful years—we would have our lives back, of that I was certain. Different lives, but honest ones, free of unhappiness, uncertainty, and pretending.

That night, after a long talk about how things would unfold over the coming days, months, and years, my husband and I agreed we'd found a shared reason—and a road map—to say goodbye.

Using 10-10-10 in a divorce situation is at the extreme end of the spectrum, but over the past few years, my friends and family have borrowed it to wrestle with dilemmas of all sizes.

A woman I know, for instance, used 10-10-10 to help her resolve a difficult situation with an old friend. Lori and Sarah (let's call them) roomed together in college and, soon after, married men who got along so well that the couples came to spend many Saturdays together. Eventually, however, Sarah divorced and remarried a man that Lori and her husband found unbearably sarcastic.

A year of awkwardness ensued, as Lori made every kind of excuse to avoid get-togethers. When Sarah finally stopped calling, Lori wondered if it was time to let the relationship go. She turned to 10-10-10 to determine what to do next.

Lori predicted that the 10-minute and 10-month consequences of ending the relationship would feel something like the death of a friend who had been very ill. There would be sorrow—but also a mitigating portion of relief. In 10 years, though, those feelings would be gone, replaced by regret. That was an outcome she couldn't accept. The only option, then, was to tell Sarah the truth and ask her to consider returning to the one-on-one friendship of their college days.

She knew that the immediate consequences of that conversation could be irreparable harm: no more friendship and an ugly wound, too. But if they could survive one tough talk, Lori figured, they had decades of good times ahead of them.

The conversation was not easy, but the friendship's history carried them through it. Today, Lori says, "We both feel grateful that we didn't lose it all."

Another friend of mine finds herself using 10-10-10 to get through the patches of second-guessing that occasionally interrupt a life she loves but never planned on. Fifteen years ago, she was a sales representative for a pharmaceutical company. She loved the job, and the job loved her. The first in her family to attend college, she was looking forward to a long and successful corporate career.

Then came marriage and two children. My friend tried to keep working, but one day, when she returned from a week on the road, the nanny put her son in her arms, and he didn't recognize her. She quit, telling herself she would go back the minute she could.

That minute never came. She has three children now, the youngest a baby.

> My gut was all over the place—go, stay, go—and that's when 10-10-10 was officially born.

"The other day, I was cleaning the refrigerator and Sammy was crying his head off, and inside I was screaming, *What have I done?*" she told me recently. "10-10-10 reminded me."

Both the 10-minute and 10-year scenarios made her shudder. "Short term, I'm looking at a lot of diapers and spit up," she said, "and long term, I'm seeing a big black hole. Kids gone, but so is my career."

But, she says, "for me it's all about the time in between. When Sammy catches a ball, and Emma has her first flute recital, and Alex starts to shave, I'll be there. I gave up one dream, but I got a reality I couldn't walk away from."

> "I was cleaning the fridge, the baby was crying his head off, and I was thinking, *What have I done?*" a friend said. "10-10-10 reminded me."

Incidentally, this friend introduced her sister to 10-10-10, and she recently wrote me about her own twist to the method. It's important, she said, to make sure you're not basing too many decisions on any particular time frame. "If I'm responding to the 10-minute consequences, I'm probably living too impulsively," she explained.

A graduate student who heard me speak about 10-10-10 at Harvard not long ago questioned how much the process could help her. "I think your method works," she said, "only if you already know what you want from life." She said that 10-10-10 helped me realize I should go to my son's karate test because I valued being a good mother more than career success.

I told her that knowing your priorities may help you with the 10-10-10 process, but it can also help you discover them. Using 10-10-10 to sort out my divorce, for example, helped me learn that I valued living authentically more than living the "perfect picture" for all to see.

Speaking of pictures, I recently came across one of myself in an old photo album, taken just about the time of my conversation with that kindly man at the dinner party. Baby on hip, phone to ear—I look distracted, to say the least.

My face is different now. It's aged more than a little, that's for sure. But the anxiety is gone. Without a doubt, there are a couple of good reasons for that (no more babies on hips, for one). Still, I know that the three questions of 10-10-10 played a large part over the years. They had the uncanny ability to help me slow my life down and make it my own. Today, at least most of the time, my face wears a look of, well, I guess it is a happy calm. It's a look, in fact, that might even say something old-fashioned like "Don't worry. Everything will sort itself out in the end." ▣

Five Ways to Get a Life

Quick fixes that can rebalance your day
BY JULIE MORGENSTERN

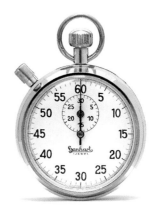

1 Shorten your workday by 30 minutes.
I promise you'll get more done than if you put in your usual nine to ten hours. That's because committing to leaving earlier gives you a deadline and forces you to eliminate the little time wasters (silly interruptions, procrastination, perfectionism) that eat up your day.

2 Avoid multitasking.
Recent studies show that it can take the brain twice as long to process each thing it's working on when switching back and forth between activities. By learning to focus fully on one project at a time, you can regain the extra hour or two you crave. Just don't squander it on mundane chores!

3 Break the habit of total self-reliance.
Insisting on doing everything yourself burdens you and prevents others from feeling valuable and needed. Delegate more at home and at work, and free your time for things you love and excel at.

4 Capture all your to-dos in one place.
People who haphazardly write lists on stray notepads, Post-its, and backs of envelopes waste time wondering what to do next and worrying that they're forgetting something. Choose only one tool (planner, Palm, notebook) to track everything you need to do, and prioritize from the top down. Start every morning with the most important item, not the many small, easy tasks. You can always squeeze the little things into the gaps. Conquering the big to-dos gives meaning to your day.

5 Schedule one purely joyful activity each week.
Think of an activity—dancing, reading, playing guitar—that you haven't done for a long time and that brings you instant happiness. Put it in your datebook as a nonnegotiable appointment with yourself, and watch the quality of your life transform. ▣

Nora Ephron's Aha! Moment

At a crowded, chaotic screening, the *Bewitched* director learned a bit of magic.

This Aha! moment is probably going to seem like no big deal. And there are probably all sorts of Aha! moments I should be writing about instead.

Like the Aha! moment when I realized that life is too short to break up with your friends.

Or the Aha! moment when I realized I should eat more cheese.

(The "eat more cheese" Aha! moment took place on an airplane about ten years ago. It was right before New Year's, and I'd been thinking about my resolutions for the next year and trying to come up with something I would actually be able to stick to, as opposed to my annual vow to exercise every single day. Suddenly, almost out of nowhere, I was served a plate of cheese.

both children and half a brain, I watched in mounting frustration. Finally, I couldn't stand it another second. I turned to Bob and I said, "It's really very simple. Someone should go get some folding chairs and set them up in the aisles."

Bob looked at me. "Nora," he said. *"We can't do everything."*

What an epiphany! What a shimmering moment! Had we been outdoors, I would now remember whether the day was hot or cold, and where the light was coming from, that's how amazing it was; but since we were in a dark, crowded screening room that was becoming more crowded by the second, all I can remember is that my brain cleared in an amazing way. We can't do everything. I was overcome.

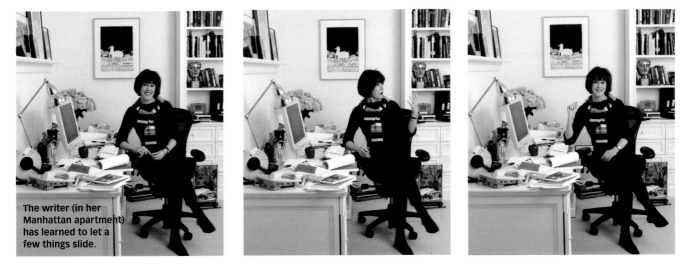

The writer (in her Manhattan apartment) has learned to let a few things slide.

It was delicious. It reminded me of how much I loved cheese. So I resolved, at that moment, to eat more of it, and I pretty much have. Presumably this is not a true Aha! moment, yet it was a blinding insight about something that would improve my life, and it has.)

Anyway, here is the moment I truly think of as my own favorite Aha! But before I tell it, a little background. I'm very bossy. What's more, I'm good at solving problems, and when I see a problem that isn't being solved, I'm only too happy to step in. But all that changed one night about 15 years ago when I went to a small screening for a movie. I was sitting in my seat before the movie began, and as the room filled up, it became clear that there were not going to be enough seats. People were bunching up in the aisles and looking around helplessly. I was sitting next to my friend Bob Gottlieb, watching all this. The director of the movie decided to solve the problem by asking all the children to share seats. This was a ludicrous suggestion, as anyone with children (or half a brain) could tell, and since I was in possession of

> "I'm good at solving problems, and when I see a problem that isn't being solved, I'm only too happy to step in."

I had been given the secret of life.

Now I am not going to tell you that from that day forth I never again interfered, or bossed anyone around, or stepped in with a solution that was not remotely necessary. But every year there are truly dozens of times that I watch things go wrong, things I could solve by simply raising my hand or my voice, and I say to myself, "Nora, we can't do everything." You would be amazed at how often things sort themselves out without any help from me whatsoever. ◘

We Interrupt This Book...

Phones ring. E-mails beep. Colleagues step in to chat. Now, where were you? Oh, yes, having your time blown into a thousand unproductive little shards. JULIE MORGENSTERN helps you take back your day.

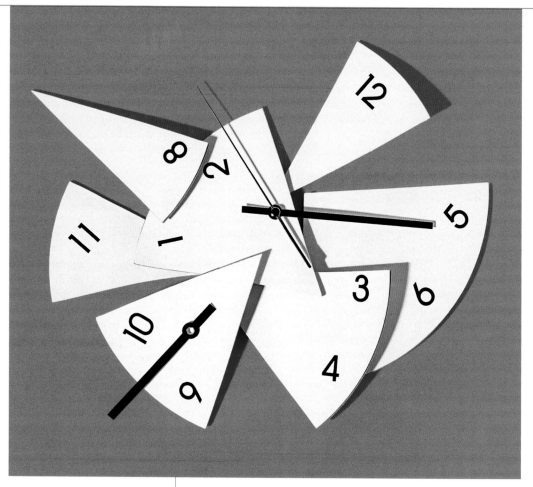

I know a woman who's an incurable optimist: She shows up for work actually believing she'll get through her to-do list. Slipping into her desk chair, bagel in one hand, latte in the other, she decides to check her e-mail before diving into the presentation she has to write, and whoosh...she's sucked into a ton of annoying little requests. She sends brief answers and 40 minutes later gets started on her presentation. Just as inspiration starts to flow, the phone rings. Then heads start popping in: "Got a minute?" "Can we have a quick meeting?" "Can I run something by you?"

Reluctant to say no to anyone, she responds to all the interruptions as they come. Her stress level escalates as her grip on her day loosens. She'd hoped to meet a friend after work for a movie but ends up staying past 8 again, when the office is finally quiet enough for her to focus on her own agenda.

Most of us spend our days in environments that make us feel scattered.

If you're an office worker, you're interrupted every three minutes on average, according to researchers at the School of Information and Computer Science at UC–Irvine. A related study showed that it can take 25 minutes to regain your concentration after each interruption, which means that brilliant train of thought you were riding might get permanently derailed. Preliminary research published by Hewlett-Packard Labs showed that in 41 percent of all cases, we never return to our original activity.

Caught off guard, we drop everything to solve problems other people not only could but should handle. One quick question leads to another and another, and soon the day is shot.

WHY CAN'T YOU JUST SAY NO?

Most people claim they give in to sudden requests because they hate letting others down. I say it's more about not disappointing ourselves: We're hooked on feeling needed. If we take a hard look at ourselves, we might see that we unwittingly encourage people to come to us for every little thing. Interruptions can also be a welcome distraction. Faced with an unpleasant task, we're more than happy to turn our attention elsewhere. Finally, we often don't say no because of simple disorganization. In a choppy and shapeless day, we handle disruption immediately because we figure, if not now, when?

While it's important to be reasonably accessible to the people you live and work with, you don't want to spend most of your waking hours in helper mode at the expense of completing your own critical tasks. Even if you're in crisis management or, for that matter, if you're a stay-at-home mom, you need to prioritize requests. Otherwise you get trapped in a whirlwind of multitasking where you start many things and finish nothing.

KEEP A LOG

The first step in taking back control is to know exactly what you're up against. Track yourself for a week. For each interruption, note the time and the way it came about (via e-mail, telephone, or drop-by visitor). Include the interruptions you visited on yourself with incessant checking of e-mail, walks to the watercooler, and klatching with friends. Write down how long you spent on each, and grade it:

A = critical and urgent
B = important, not urgent
C = unnecessary

Add up the total minutes spent on A-level interruptions, and divide by five to get your daily average. That's the amount of time each day you must leave open for the inevitable crises that must be handled immediately.

You'll likely have two or three people who can break in anytime (your boss, one or two key colleagues, and perhaps your spouse or child). Postpone dealing with as many of the others as you can. Many issues are important (B level), but, as you'll see from your log, they can wait. The delay has a payoff: It allows you to prepare to respond in a more focused, efficient way.

Breaking an ingrained habit is a tall order, but I want to get you off autopilot and have you weigh each interruption. You're more in charge than you think.

GET RID OF PESKY DISTRACTIONS

Some interruptions are simply a waste of time, so your next step is to cut way down on them:

■ **REARRANGE YOUR SPACE.** If your office feels like Grand Central, make it less inviting. Close your door just enough to avoid eye contact with people passing by. In a cubicle, move your chair or position a plant for a blocking effect.

■ **BREAK THE E-ADDICTION.** Turn off your e-mail alert, and let voice mail pick up when you really need to concentrate. I highly recommend the radical concept of not checking e-mail for the first hour of the day. Instead, spend that time on your most imperative task. The sense of accomplishment you feel from knocking off that big to-do fuels you with energy all day long and lets you meet the demands of others less resentfully. In all but a few work situations, there's nothing wrong with letting e-mail wait until 10 A.M.

■ **IF YOU'RE SUPERVISING PEOPLE,** empower them to make decisions so you're not constantly inundated with tiny questions and concerns. Be clear on the destination, but let people be creative on the path. Tell subordinates exactly which decisions they can make without you. If someone comes to you with a problem she could handle on her own, turn it back around. ("Can you make that call? I won't be able to get to it for two days" or "Come up with a few solutions, then let's meet.")

PUT DISRUPTIONS ON YOUR OWN TIMETABLE

Third, although it might sound like an oxymoron, you can schedule interruptions:

■ **ESTABLISH SEVERAL "OPEN" TIMES** throughout the day when anyone can stop by—at your convenience. Try alternating one hour closed door, one hour open. In most situations, people are fine with waiting as long as they know when they will be heard.

■ **BEGIN THE CONVERSATION WITH** "What can I do for you?" rather than "How are you?" The latter is an invitation to chat. You want to get straight to the point.

■ **ASK HOW LONG EACH PERSON WILL NEED.** Fifteen minutes? A half hour? You can choose between setting up the meeting for later or saying something like "Let's talk now; I've got a conference call in 20 minutes." This approach forces people to stick to the amount of time they've requested.

■ **REHEARSE A FEW COMFORTABLE EXIT LINES** in case someone gets you at a bad moment. For example, "I'm in the middle of finishing a project; can we talk this afternoon?" or "I'd love to help you out, but this week is impossible."

■ **EVEN FOR PEOPLE WHOSE INTERRUPTIONS** you take anytime, there's no offense in asking when they need the request filled. Within the hour? The day? You'll be surprised how often there's no rush.

> If you're an office worker, you're interrupted every three minutes on average.

RECOVER QUICKLY

Whenever you stop in the middle of completing a task, take a moment to jot down exactly what you'd planned to do next and how long it will take. For example, "Write closing paragraph: 30 minutes." If you're working on a document, put a bright-colored Post-it on the exact spot where you left off. This will make it easier to get reoriented.

Finally, don't respond to any interruption without first asking yourself the million dollar questions: Whom will you let down by saying yes? Did you also make a promise to someone else? Whose disappointed face can you tolerate least—the person's in front of you or your boss's? As for my friend, the former office night owl, she learned that sometimes the answer is herself, and her friend with the movie tickets. 〇

Happiness

What I Know for Sure: Oprah

"Your base level of pleasure is determined by how you view your whole life"

I take my pleasures seriously. I work hard and pleasure well; I believe in the yin and yang of life. It doesn't take a lot to make me happy because I take pleasure from everything I do. Some pleasures are higher rated than others, of course. And because I try to practice what I preach—living in the moment—I am consciously attuned most of the time to how much pleasure I am receiving.

Just last night, I was laughing so hard on the phone with my friend Gayle that my head started to hurt. She was confronting me about a bad hair day and wanted to make sure I was aware that the "do" wasn't doing it for me. Mid-howl I thought, *Isn't this a gift—after 20-odd years of nightly phone calls, to have someone who tells me the truth and to laugh this loudly about it?* I call that five-star pleasure.

Being aware of and creating four- and five-star experiences makes you blessed. For me just waking up "clothed in my right mind," being able to put my feet on the floor, walk to the bathroom, and do what needs to be done there is a five-starrer. I think of all the stories I've done about people who aren't healthy enough to do that.

Then I move on to the little pleasures. A strong cup of coffee with the perfect hazelnut creamer: four stars. Going for a walk through the woods with all five dogs unleashed: five stars. (Picking up their poop: a half star for solid; no stars for diarrhea!) Working out: one star, still. Sitting under my oaks, reading the Sunday papers: four stars. A great book: five. Hanging out at Quincy Jones's kitchen table, talking about

everything and nuthin': five stars. Being able to do good things for other people: five plus. The enjoyment comes from knowing the receiver understands the spirit of the gift. I make an effort to do something good for somebody every day, whether I know that person or not.

What I know for sure is that pleasure is energy reciprocated: What you put out comes back. Your base level of pleasure is determined by how you view your whole life.

More important than 20/20 eyesight is your internal vision, your own sweet spirit whispering through your life with guidance and grace—now, that's pleasure. **O**

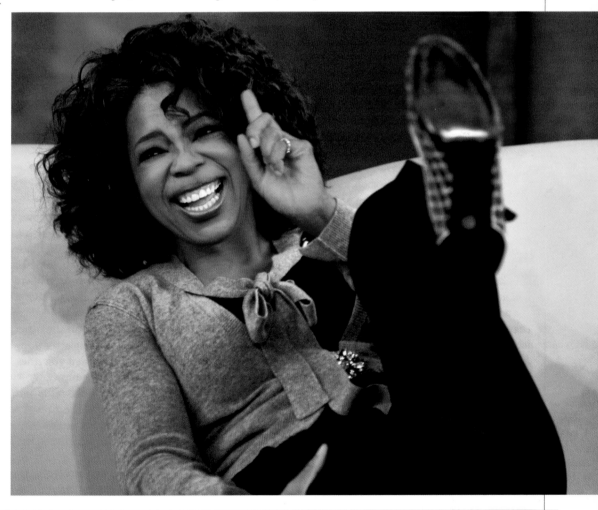

Getting Through It

Lynn Sherr's Aha! Moment

Her husband was gone, and she couldn't get on with life.
Then, as the cameras rolled, she found her way.

For nearly six years, I'd been holding my breath.

My husband, Larry, a captivating hunk, was under siege from lymphoma, the cancer that was killing him. Our lives had become a series of lowered expectations: one more vacation, one more weekend, one more day, one more hour.

The clock ran out one February morning in 1992. At home, surrounded by his family, Larry died.

Without him, I was lost. He was my best friend, my deepest love, my soul mate, my pal. Larry was part of every single thing I did, my first kiss in the morning, my last stop at night, and dozens of moments in between. I had to learn to exhale in a world I'd now inhabit alone.

But I couldn't. I wore his clothes, slept on his side of the bed, took secret comfort in leaving his sunglasses on the hall table, his book by the bedside. I told myself I was coping, but when my office was relocated half a block away, I panicked. *Oh God,* I thought, *I can't change offices; Larry won't know where to find me.*

A friend suggested, from her own experience, "Don't touch the closets, don't remove anything. It's nice to have him there for a while. Gradually, you'll start impinging on his territory, and one of these days you'll just say, 'I need more space.'" She was right, but when I finally gathered the hangers, seeing his outline in every shirt and jacket, I wept giant tears as I imagined Larry saying, hurt and confused, "You gave away all my clothes. I have nothing to wear."

Later came another improvisation: When we couldn't decide where to spread Larry's ashes, I tucked the box with his earthly remains into my lingerie drawer. I thought that might make him happy.

Something told me I wasn't doing any of this right. All the books, and some of my well-intentioned but clueless friends, talked about moving on, about getting by, about—what does it mean, anyway?—closure. But I couldn't even say the words out loud: *My husband died.*

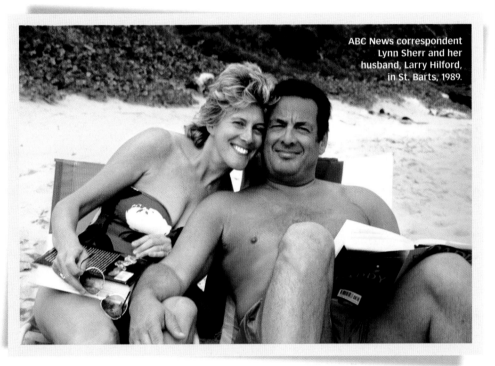

ABC News correspondent Lynn Sherr and her husband, Larry Hilford, in St. Barts, 1989.

Well-intentioned but clueless friends talked about moving on.

What I could do was describe the waves of grief, massive swells of sadness that washed through me without warning and pinned me to the pain of my broken heart.

"It doesn't wait; it just comes to get you," said my very supportive therapist. "You're functioning on two levels. And the grief is always there. Set aside more time to cry, to emote. Let some of it out, and you'll be stronger."

She understood that my moods bounced crazily, that I wanted constantly to rewrite the story, to fix the ending so that magically Larry would see another doctor and be cured. And she said I might next feel guilty because Larry was not on my mind all the time.

I started to get it, but my sorrow still lingered. I couldn't put it behind me.

The breakthrough came several years later, during a story I was doing for *20/20* about the agony of loss. I was interviewing Jimmie Holland, a pioneering psychiatrist at New York's Memorial Sloan-Kettering Cancer Center and a recognized authority on bereavement. I'd met her during Larry's last living days, but somehow the distance my job gave me—as a professional asking the questions for everyone, rather than a patient seeking solace for herself—brought new clarity to the issue.

I remember the scene perfectly: We were sitting in her vacation home in Eastern Maryland. The room was country quiet, and I could hear the water lapping against the shore outside. I asked my questions as a reporter, but her answers drilled into my soul. In a calm, reassuring voice, Holland rejected the popular formula that grief is a finite process ending after we pass through a series of such predictable stages as denial, anger, and then acceptance.

"We saw people in the medical world accepting those stages and putting people into boxes and trying to move them along and being very rigid about it," she told me. "And if you didn't go through stage one, two, three, four, five, you were abnormal in some way. We have put pressure on people to say, 'You have a certain amount of time to grieve and get on with it. We don't want to hear any more about your grief.' Well, wrong! You can't do this to people. Your pattern of grief is as unique as your pattern of love."

Bingo! I didn't have to follow anyone's pattern. I didn't have to stop being sad. Not only was sadness okay, it was necessary. Nobody can tell you how to mourn. And it's not self-indulgence; it's not wallowing; it's hanging on to something important. We should not avoid bereavement. We should embrace it, welcoming our moments of sorrow as a time to reconnect with the person we've lost.

Her words washed over me in a flood of warmth. I nodded slightly, the way one does during a television interview, acknowledging the truth of her statements. I was still in reporter mode, so I couldn't exult. I didn't want to break the spell, so I just quietly digested her wisdom as the cameras continued to roll.

It was only later that day, as I headed home, that I reran her words in my head and allowed myself to appreciate their impact. She was talking about me! She had freed me to mourn.

It was a stunning revelation. Grief was not something I'd recover from but an ongoing process, one that lasts—thank goodness—forever. I could breathe again.

Today the waves of pain are less frequent but no less intense. I cry unexpectedly and then feel better. I've learned to live without Larry but not to forget him; to honor the memory of what was, while functioning in the world that is. To welcome the sadness that keeps us connected. And every time I open my lingerie drawer, I realize that his ashes are fine exactly where they are. **O**

Saving Nico

She was waddling home to an empty house, hugely pregnant, her brain already on maternity leave, when the mugger pounced. Broke her wrist. Tied her up. What would you have done? LISA WOLFE surprised even herself.

As a married woman who wanted a child, I should have been thrilled to be pregnant. Which I was. The first six weeks. Then I began to inflate. And inflate. You had to see it to believe it, or at least that's what those who saw it said. Never mind my belly, which you would expect to take on new dimensions, but my thighs, underarms, and cheeks seemed to be growing little ones in them, too.

Even worse than losing my body, I proceeded to lose my mind. I had treasured my mind. The only daughter and granddaughter of two very frustrated women, I saw it as the vehicle for making sure I took advantage of the sorts of personal and professional opportunities they never had. But suddenly, it would focus on only three things: when I might sleep, when I might eat, and why even if I didn't eat everything I was thinking of eating, I was slapping on the pounds as if I did.

Most upsetting of all, I lost my ambition. I had a job I loved at *60 Minutes* in London. It was a chance to travel, meet interesting people, put stories on the air that could make a difference—and all I wanted to do was sleep. After years of promising to be a powerful new breed of woman, I felt I was betraying my deepest values. My guilt grew to rival my weight.

Luckily, my boss let me work from home as many days as possible. One of those days, when I was seven months pregnant, I ran out of milk. I waddled to the store to get some. I waddled home. I put my key in the door and heard a voice ask, "Excuse me, do you know Tony Roberts?" I turned around to see who was speaking, and I saw a giant man coming at me, his massive hands grabbing for my neck. He pushed me inside the house, onto the floor, and beat me as I screamed for help. "I'm pregnant!" I shouted. He hit me on the head. I fell forward. He twisted my wrist. I heard it crack like a bite into a carrot.

This was the moment I realized this was life, not a movie: I was in danger and so was my baby. I stopped screaming. Got really silent. An almost eerie calm came over me.

The man blindfolded me and tied my hands behind my back. He pulled me off the floor, threw me against the wall, and said,

> I stopped screaming. Got really silent. An almost eerie calm came over me.

"Take me to the jewelry. And I mean the good stuff. You show me junk and there's going to be trouble."

I thought of the best thing we had: my engagement ring. It hadn't fit me since my sixth week, so I was keeping it in a drawer. "Up in the bedroom," I said.

"Show me," the guy commanded, yanking me forward and grabbing the knot of hands behind my back. My husband and I were renting a tiny mews house whose staircase was so narrow that I could feel the guy's body rubbing on the walls as I led him up. "To the right," I said when we got to the top.

He pushed me into the bedroom and onto the floor. He kicked me in the thigh, hard, but it didn't hurt. Nothing hurt. "If you look in the back of the top dresser drawer, you'll find my engagement ring," I said. "Take it. Take everything. I don't care. All I care is that you don't hurt my baby. He's my first baby, the first grandchild on both sides of the family, and we know he's a boy."

He didn't speak or hit me, which I took to mean I was on the right track. "We're going to call him Nico," I said. I heard drawers open, feet shuffle, grunts. "My husband has a good watch," I said. "I'm not sure where, but we'll find it. Go to the other room on this floor, and you'll see a desk. Look in the top drawer."

I felt him leave the room. I felt him come back. He untied my hands and retied them with something firmer. "What's that?" I asked.

"Computer cable. In case you get any ideas. And I cut the phone line."

"It never occurred to me to use the phone," I answered truthfully. "And I don't know if you're interested in silver, but we have some downstairs that we got for our wedding."

And on this went for nearly two hours, the guy ransacking our home and me responding more calmly than I typically do to missing the subway. At one point, I even began to do the deep breathing exercises I had learned in prenatal class, which may not be much help in labor but can sure boost your confidence if you're getting mugged. "I'm not going to call the police," I actually heard myself say.

"You're not?"

"No. That's about revenge. I'm not interested in revenge. I'm only interested in one thing—that you don't hurt my baby."

"I didn't come here to hurt your baby!" the guy blurted. "I didn't come here to hurt your baby! I came here because some of us weren't born with silver spoons in our mouths."

I had done it. I had unraveled him. Relief poured into my body like liquid.

"Where's the cash?" he asked.

"We don't have any cash."

"Everyone keeps cash in the house."

"Well, we don't," I said. "We were worried about it getting stolen."

"Then where's your bank card?

I had to think. My bank card was in my wallet, which I had brought to the store. Only then did I realize that I was still wearing my coat. No wonder sweat was pouring from my chest like a waterfall. "It's here in my pocket," I said.

The guy dug through my pockets with strange but unmistakable

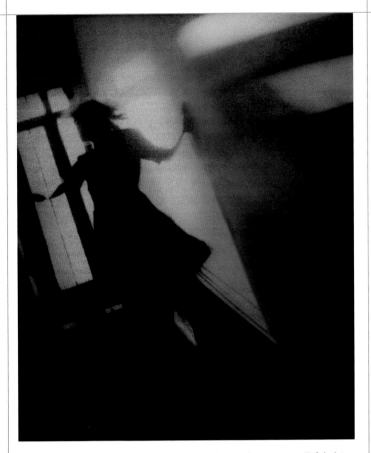

determination not to touch my body through my coat. I felt him pull out my wallet. "What's your PIN number?" he asked.

"9999," I said.

"That better be true."

"You think I would lie?" I asked, actually almost offended.

"I'm going to the cash machine. You stay here. If this PIN is wrong, I'm coming back and there will be trouble."

I felt him leave the room. I felt him come back. "And another thing," he said.

"Yeah?"

"Good luck with your baby."

And he was gone. My mind, of course, was not working as sharply as my instinct. I sat in place a ridiculously long time before I realized he wasn't coming back. I pushed my blindfold up with my knees. I ran down the stairs and used my chin to unlatch the front door, my elbow to hail a taxi to the police station.

Joy was a strange thing to feel as the police whizzed me to the hospital, my wrist broken, my teeth loose, my belly bloated as an elephant's. But joy was unmistakably what it was. My baby had been in danger, and I had served him well. The police said so themselves. They said that by humanizing myself and my unborn child, I had probably avoided further injury. How did you know what to do, they kept asking? The answer was, I just did. I have had a harder time knowing which salad dressing to choose from the thousands on the grocery shelf than what to do that wretched day. The very force I had been cursing the previous seven months for making me so fat and stupid and lazy gave me directions, and I simply followed. Pregnancy had not, after all, stolen my power, but enabled me to tap a whole new source of it. ⬤

Let the Sun Shine In

Shadowed by memories of a lost husband and father, this room (like its owner) needed an infusion of joy. How to brighten the mood without painting over the past? That's where the brilliant and intuitive Nate Berkus—who has transformed so many rooms on TV for Oprah—comes in. BY LISA KOGAN

Not a lot of living goes on in Hilary Offenberg's midtown Manhattan living room. A palette of chocolate and charcoal is punctuated with only a trace of taupe in the sisal rug. Three sedate watercolors hang above an overstuffed L-shaped sofa; a Rothko print in tangerine and Pepto-Bismol pink provides a small, if incongruous, bright spot. The one true wild card comes from Hilary's 2-year-old daughter, Carly, whose stuffed animals lounge comfortably in front of the flat-screen TV. The space is sophisticated, beautiful, and just a little bit dark—very much like Hilary herself.

Enter Nate Berkus, the young designer with a spectacular talent for transforming his clients' houses into reflections of who they are and who they hope to become. Having made over more than his share of decorating disasters, he is slightly baffled by why he's been asked to redo this particular room. "Hilary," he says, "the place looks pretty good. Tell me what bothers you." She nods in semi-agreement. "The thing is," she answers slowly, "this lighting is abominable, and these end tables are from my old apartment. So is that," she says, pointing to a wobbly silver desk lamp on a small pine trunk. "I bought the cowhide on 33rd Street to throw over the table there...." Her voice trails off,

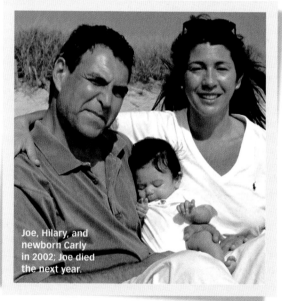

Joe, Hilary, and newborn Carly in 2002; Joe died the next year.

but Nate doesn't jump in to fill the silence. Instead he sits quietly waiting for her to collect her thoughts. She smooths the glossy brown hair away from her eyes, picks at an imaginary thread on her sweater, takes a deep breath, and continues: "This is the room where my husband, Joe, fought dying for 22 months. All he could do was watch TV and feel lousy. For a long time, I couldn't even bear to sit in this room. Being in here still fills me with sadness."

"Talk to me about Joe," Nate says. Hilary reaches for one of the many photographs resting on the built-in cabinetry. "This is Joe. He was really cute and really, *really* nice"—she waits a beat—"and nobody has any idea how I landed him." She looks at Nate to see if she's broken the tension; he smiles, and she goes on. "Joe and I got married in 2000. He was diagnosed with cancer in 2001.

Two days later, I found out I was pregnant. Carly was born in 2002." She stares at the shot of a crinkly newborn Carly wrapped in her husband's still-strong arms. "He died in 2003, three weeks and three days after Carly's first birthday."

Late-afternoon light bounces shadows across the dove white walls. Finally Nate speaks. "What did you guys like to do?" he asks. She walks Nate over to the trunk, takes off the wobbly lamp, and together they kneel down and lift its lid. "We loved the beach—that's where we took all our vacations," she says. "We eloped to St. Thomas. Joe saved the newspaper from our wedding day." As she hands him the January 20, 2000, edition of the *Virgin Islands Independent,* something falls from its pages. "Oh, it's Joey's passport," she whispers, pressing it to her for a second. Next she pulls out a random valentine, a Mother's Day card for "a great mother to be," a Christmas note from 1999 inscribed with Joe's fat, loopy cursive, "Here's to our life together." "It's still a shock to see his handwriting," she murmurs, picking up a small container of beach glass and pouring the emerald, aqua, and milky gray shards into Nate's open palm. "You know what kind of cancer he had? It was called a carcinoma of unknown origin. I mean, who ever heard of that? He was still in his 40s, for God's sake."

Nate puts down the beach glass and guides Hilary back to the sofa. "We need to breathe a little fresh air into this place," he says. "I want you to feel happy to be home."

"But I don't want to erase him," she answers quickly.

"I know you don't. My challenge will be to help you and Carly find a new beginning while still honoring Joe's memory." Hilary gets that Nate gets it, and she visibly relaxes.

"Is there anything else I should know?" Nate asks.

"Um, I've always kind of wanted a pool boy," she says with a perfectly straight face. "Hilary," Nate replies with great solemnity, "you don't have a pool."

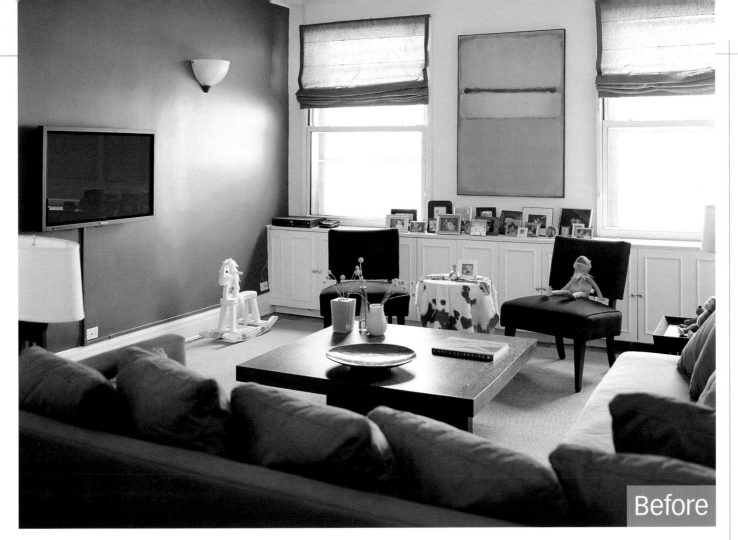

Before

"I know," she says, laughing, "but I've still always wanted a..." Now Nate is laughing, too. "C'mon," he says, attempting professionalism, "what else?"

"What else, what else?" Hilary repeats. "Well, I love brown. I like it with baby blue, yellow. I'm not normally a pink person," she adds, glancing at the Rothko. "And I don't know anything about technology—I mean, I'm practically still churning my own butter—but it would be great if I could somehow check my work e-mail." Hilary fingers Joe's wedding ring, which hangs from a chain around her neck. "And," she says, "there's the feather thing." The feather thing? "I know this sounds a little crazy, but ever since Joe died I keep finding feathers. Not dirty pigeon feathers—pristine white feathers in really unexpected places. Like I found this one right at my front door." She points to a slender white feather on the coffee table. "I always think it's Joe, checking in...keeping an eye on us."

As if on cue, the front door opens and in bursts Carly, her grandma Doris in tow.

"Hi, Carly; my name is Nate." Carly looks into the sky blue eyes of the man who regularly receives marriage proposals from women the world over, removes her pacifier, and emits the sort of blood-curdling shriek seldom heard outside of Freddy Krueger films. She runs to her room, Doris trailing close behind. The guy who's made *People's* Sexiest Man Alive list has at last met a female who finds him less than enchanting. "Okay, so that went pretty well," he deadpans. ▶

WE'VE SEEN WORSE...

Tasteful and urbane, Hilary's living room has a few inspired flourishes, like the cowhide table cover. But the lighting is dingy, the palette is too subdued, and the flat-screen TV is too dominant. More troubling still, the room is filled with painful reminders. Nate's challenge, he says, is to help Hilary and Carly "find a new beginning while still honoring Joe's memory."

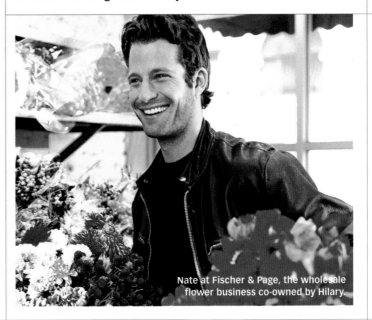

Nate at Fischer & Page, the wholesale flower business co-owned by Hilary.

HERE COMES THE SUN

To brighten the room, Nate brings the outside in—painting the walls the color of sunshine, adding numerous lamps and sconces, and enlivening the space with flowers and trees (for someone in the flower business, Hilary had strikingly little plant life).

A A Drexel Heritage credenza, which Nate paints black, provides what he calls "an extra spot to stash Carly's zoo." It also anchors the TV, de-emphasizing it so the space is less of a screening room and more of a conversation pit. The TV is now hooked up to Microsoft's MSN TV 2 Internet service—and look, no wires!

B Nate reupholsters two black slipper chairs in a chic cream-and-chocolate Lulu DK fabric, then adds brown felt bolsters.

C In one of many gestures of tender genius, Nate mounts and frames a perfect white feather—feathers have been mysteriously floating into Hilary's life like silent messages from her late husband.

D Hilary and Joe loved the beach, so Nate finds a terrarium lamp from Roost, fills it with sand, and in the sand places keepsakes from their Caribbean honeymoon. Next to the lamp is a photo album titled "Hilary, Joe, and Carly: Our Life in Pictures." The album replaces a busy collection of framed snapshots that had cluttered the windowsill.

DETAILS *Clockwise from center left:* Drexel Heritage credenza. Williams-Sonoma Home crystal lamp. Linens 'n Things wooden frames. Boston Head Light wall sconce. Arteriors Home nickel floor lamp. Design Within Reach Arco Floor lamp. Williams-Sonoma Home leather chair, pewter-rimmed hurricanes, and chrome-plated stools. Mark Snider hand-beaded pillow. Carini Lang Purple Peonies rug.

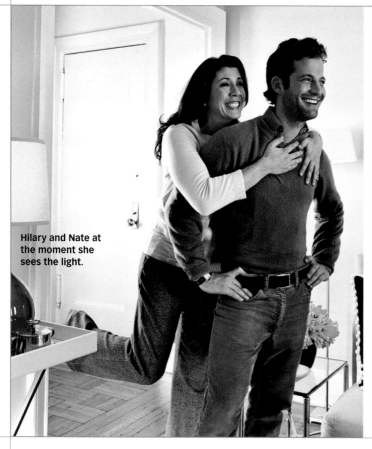

Hilary and Nate at the moment she sees the light.

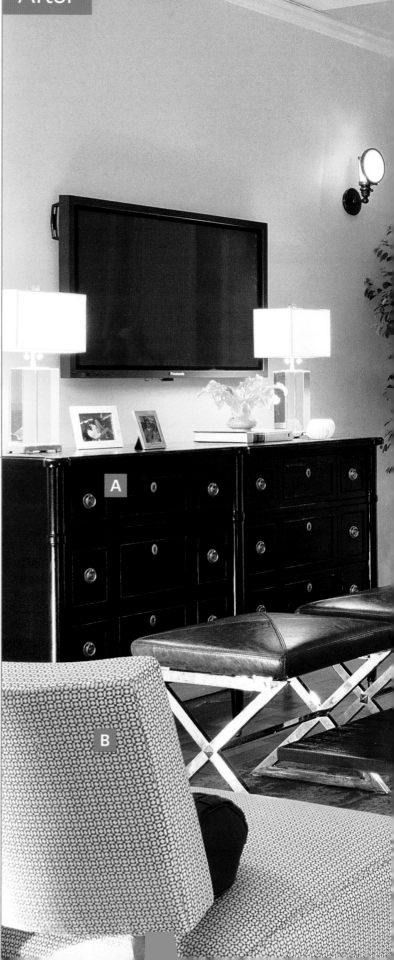

After

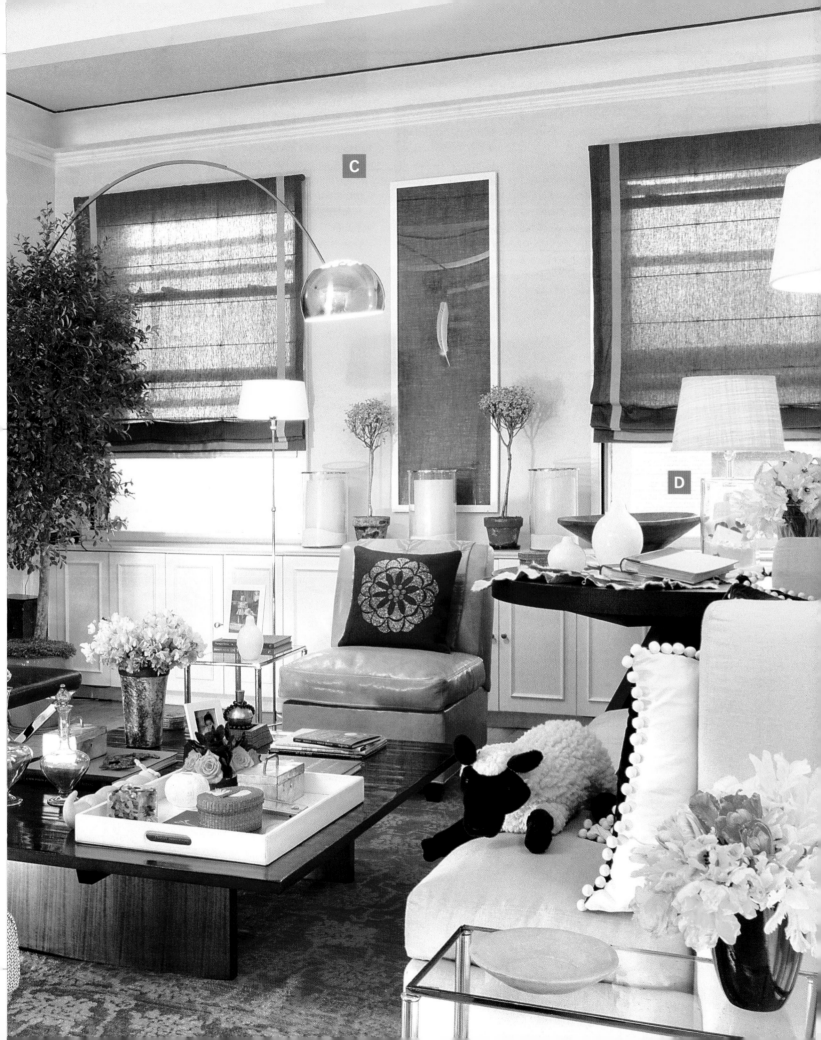

Cry Me a River

From her vantage point in Harlem, New Orleanian SARAH BROOM talks
about the days after Katrina—the waiting, the anguish over her two missing
brothers (was that Carl on TV? Michael?), the uplift of family, and how
she'll remember her jazzy, brassy, beautiful, like-no-other city.

When you are from a huge, wild New Orleans family and realize that your city is underneath so much water it can't breathe, and when the other thing you know is that your two hard-headed brothers are somewhere in all of that mess, you simply try to get your legs to carry you through the way they did before: easy and glide-like. In your day-to-day, you neglect the serious consideration of any newspaper or broadcast except to scan for names and faces of the missing—Broom, Michael, Carl, my brothers.

It has been three full days since Hurricane Katrina hit and I am in Harlem, where there is nothing to do but feel helpless. Tonight all the windows of my duplex are wide open to let the outside sounds come in. I am being particular about this because my loud-mouthed, dancing-on-narrow-sidewalk neighbors remind me of home. I sit cross-legged before the television set and watch CNN on mute. I am entirely uninterested in what the reporters have to say, am on a private manhunt for two faces I know well.

Right before my eyes is a brown-skinned man with chicken legs being lifted from a roof. He's wearing white boxer shorts and he's barefoot. He twines his legs around the rescuer's bulk to get lifted into the sky where a helicopter awaits him. "It's Carl," I exclaim. "I know it!" "That doesn't look anything like your brother," my friend says. But I had faith in that lanky man in boxers until the next day when there was no call. I would spend the next night watching again for a skinny man who maybe had a dog with him. Imagine this being all you can do. It is as paltry as it sounds.

The day before the storm came, my mother, my sister Karen, her two teenagers, and my brother Troy packed a bag apiece and drove to Hattiesburg, Mississippi. In the rush, my nephew forgot his eyeglasses. As they were leaving town, I sat in a New York park listening to jazz. While I was tapping my foot, my brother Carl gathered up his family to go to a shelter. He had his green motorized boat with him in the back of his pickup. At the shelter, Carl told them to go on in. "I'll be all right," he said. He turned around and went back home to wait for the hurricane.

Something you need to know about growing up in New Orleans: During the months of hurricane season, you might evacuate three or four times for naught. You'd pack up your most important possessions and drive as far as gas money would carry you. When you've lived this way for most of your life—every

single summer thinking, *Is it the big one?*—you forget the wrath of Hurricane Betsy. You get careless.

When I called my chef brother, Michael, to make sure he was leaving, he claimed he was crossing the Texas border at that very moment. "I'm out of there, baby," he said. This, it turns out, was the lie you tell your nosy younger sister who you know would come right through the phone and strangle you if you said the truth. This is all I knew about my mother, Ivory, and the four of my 11 siblings who called New Orleans home.

Carl and Michael swam for their lives in Hurricane Betsy, the 1965 storm that was sweet compared to Katrina. But Carl, who loves fishing—especially at night—never demonized the Mississippi the way I did. I never trusted it. It was and still is a mean, ugly river that only pretends calm; growing up near it made me dislike big bodies of water, made me terrified of waves.

I think about the stories we like to tell about Hurricane Betsy, especially at Christmas when we are all together, that go like this: Everyone was asleep when someone yelled, "Get out of bed." My oldest sister, Deborah, placed her feet on the floor and felt water. My mom yelled, "Get the baby." Everyone remembers charcoal blackness and the rush of water into the house. They swam through live wires and snakes to get to higher ground. The dogs swam, too, go the stories.

My mother calls from Hattiesburg on Monday—the day Katrina hits—and says, "Water is coming into the house. We're calling for help." The phone goes out right as she's talking, so that's all I have to go on for three days. Those two lines keep replaying in my head—during half-sleep, at dinners where I appear to have it together, at every moment of quiet.

Still no word from the boys, but it is early on and phone lines are out. When your mobile phone rings, you sprint from wherever you are to answer, and when it's a friend "just checking in," you are mightily disappointed.

On the Wednesday after Katrina, my mom calls and says she's safe. The water had buried her car, but she and her group were okay. By Friday, they are all in Dallas. On Saturday, they fly to Vacaville, California, where my brother Byron lives. This is the first time my brother Troy has flown, so we have to talk him into it.

I leave New York for Vacaville, where Byron has turned his gym and two home offices into sleeping spaces. On the first night,

Catching the spirit: Tuba Fats and band making sweet music on the old stone streets.

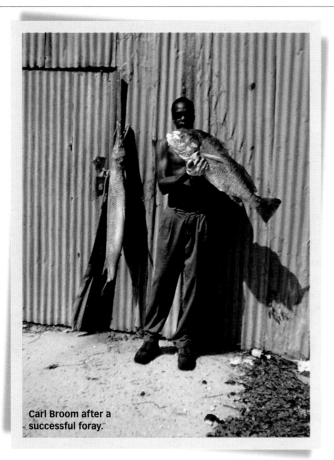

Carl Broom after a
successful foray.

Herman, who lived next door to where we grew up, has a nightmare that wakes the house.

He is 34 years old, still dehydrated, and can barely walk on his swollen feet. During the storm, he sat one whole day on the roof of our childhood home until it split in two under him and he had to swim to higher ground. Herman swears he saw Carl in a boat helping people near the Superdome. This sounds like exactly the kind of thing Carl would be doing, so most everyone believes him, except for me. I keep saying, "I need to hear from him." Whenever Herman repeats his Carl-the-rescuer story, I look at him angrily.

Neighbors have brought over piles of used clothes, and so my family, whom I have never seen ask for anything, slowly look for things they like, though it is mostly about need now. They are prideful people, but when you have one pair of pants to your name, that is no longer a trait you can rightfully claim. My mom was going around in a pair of uncomfortable gold shoes. When I asked her why, my mom, in her soft voice, said, "My good ones got messed up in all that water." Those good ones were brown

suede, her favorites. So there are these moments that remind you of what little your family has now—so suddenly! And that leads you to think of your two brothers you haven't yet heard from. You hope that the Mississippi has not had its way with them.

There are ten of us in this house. When your displaced family is not stocking up on underwear or telling each other stories meant to reassure or help you forget, you are all watching the news and yelling things at the TV. Attitude helps you get through. Or you eat red beans and rice with smoked sausage, and that feels like home. I imagine that for Troy, who until now has never left New Orleans for more than a day or two, this blue California sky must be strange. I notice, too, that my niece and nephew have the knowing eyes of grown people now.

Exactly one week after Hurricane Katrina hit, we hear from Michael. He's in San Antonio with 15 other people, some of them his girlfriend's family. He calls New Orleans after Hurricane Katrina "a disgrace to humanity." Says he will never go back, and this hurts my heart because, of all people, Michael has always loved the city with all his might. He was the one to show it off to me, the one who helped me fall so deeply in love with it. But I believe him because I do not hear any play in his voice.

Two days later I am driving my mother to the grocery store, where we have come looking for coffee and chicory, when, like a good rhythm, Carl calls. I yell incomprehensibly, saying his name in a drawn-out bayou drawl. I am sappy and my words have run off without me.

Carl starts talking nonstop: "I fell asleep, and when I woke up water was coming through the doors so quick. The front yard looked like a river. I got up into the attic with a meat cleaver and knocked out a hole in the roof big enough to get my shoulders through at an angle. The dogs beat me out.

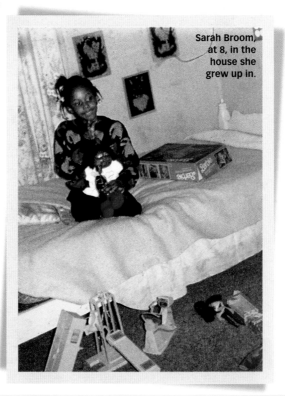

Sarah Broom,
at 8, in the
house she
grew up in.

"I was on the roof for three days with three gallons of water—I'd pour some on my head when it got too hot. You couldn't stay in the attic. It felt like 200 degrees in there. Mostly I was sitting on tar paper. When people saw that water, their eyes started getting big, they started sucking on five, six cigarettes in a row. People didn't think that thing was gonna do what it did. Nobody had a chance."

Carl remembered the life jacket in his boat, but that was underwater with a shed on top of it. He dove down twice for the jacket and then used its reflectors to signal a rescuer. Which is how he got off the roof of the house with his two Pekingese dogs, Mindie and Tiger. Later, from the convention center, he and "some dude" struck out on their own in a paddleboat, heading toward the interstate. But the paddleboat only got them so far because of the downed trees. They had to swim 30 yards through a mess of debris and dead bodies until they got picked up and taken to the airport. "There was so much despair in that place," Carl said. I'd never heard him say *despair* before. He left and walked a few miles to a distant cousin's house in Kenner, Louisiana, where he slept for three days straight.

When all of your 11 siblings are accounted for—and no second earlier than that—you let yourself mourn the city of your birth. Those feelings tried to surface earlier, but I rebuked them.

But now I am free to remember.

I was in New Orleans two days before the storm hit. I sent bragging, languorous e-mails to friends: "I am at an outdoor café drinking café au lait. A brass band has just gone by me."

Even when you have left New Orleans for better things, the city does not let go of you, so when you're back it feels as though you are returning to an old lover, the one who always takes you in no matter how far you've wandered.

I wish I could help you understand what it means to feel homesick now. I do not yet have the kind of imagination I need to understand this violation, all the world watching as my city drowned. I have known New Orleans in the same way I've known my name. I have loved it hard, the hardest of any one thing outside of family—and fanatically. I couldn't help it. My grandmother Beulah was a tough Creole woman who spoke French. My father, Simon, played the banjo and the trumpet in a brass band. You learn to move around the world in a certain, wide-eyed way when you are born into all of this richness of spirit.

In quiet moments, you think about those street musicians you came to know with their voices of gold. Theirs was an audience of passersby, and you paid by dropping a dollar or two in a hat. I am remembering one trombonist who had the eyes of my brother Carl. He looked like a hard man, looked as though he could fight for his life. But for those eyes and for all that he put into his horn, I gave him $5.

> I have known New Orleans in the same way I've known my name. I have loved it hard, the hardest of any one thing outside of family—and fanatically.

And the man in the wheelchair who, when there was a citywide blackout and you were stranded together on the sidewalk, took out his lighter, pretended it was a flashlight, and sang the blues to calm your nerves. You hope he made it out.

I wish you could hear the sounds our brass bands make, I wish you could know the kind of drumbeat that sends you dancing exuberant midstreet, sends you strutting and second-line dancing

so hard, you start to believe your life depends on movement. And perhaps it does.

I have only two immediate family members in Louisiana now, 25 days after the storm: Carl and Eddie. They are a half hour's drive from New Orleans. I called the other day, and they were in the backyard having a seafood boil. I wish I could write the sound of deep sadness in the voice of grown men you've known all your life. Carl can't get to his home yet; the water's too high. He was

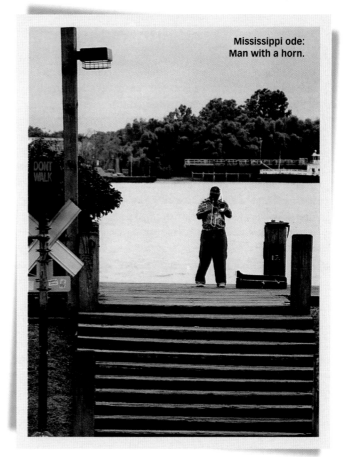

Mississippi ode: Man with a horn.

lamenting the loss of his good clothes and his toothbrush to get the two of us laughing again. Michael is still in Texas, where he's signed a one-year lease and has a cooking job. He tells me it is "a much better life." The California group is still out there. The teenagers are in new schools trying to fit in, but my niece is asking when they will go back. Another sister, Valeria, is in Alabama starting anew.

There is no neat ending to a story like this; that would not feel right anyway.

The Broom clan may be a displaced people now with far fewer possessions than before, but wherever there is ground, there can be dancing. We don't even need a drum; we've got our hands for that. And a wild, big New Orleans family spread out around the country is a dangerous and wonder-working thing to behold—like our city itself. New Orleans will resurrect, it will, just as all mighty things do, but it will take its own sweet, slow-moving time. That is the kind of rapturous idea that gets your legs moving again, gets your heart burning with joy the moment you think it. ◖

Dreaming Big

What I Know for Sure: Oprah
"Every sunrise is like a new page, a chance to receive each day in all its glory"

I remember being 15 years old, standing in the drugstore three corners from my house, waiting for the September issue of *Seventeen* to arrive. I was a faithful reader all through my teens, until I turned 18. But the back-to-school issue was the most anticipated, and I couldn't risk having it sell out.

I never had enough money at one time to buy a subscription, but I would sacrifice two school lunches a month for the 50 cents to buy the magazine filled with spectacular fashion, ideas, and dreams. It gave me hope that one day I could live like the girls in those pages.

The September issue heralded the beginning of a new school year—a chance to grow, make fresh impressions, and move forward. I loved everything about going back to school, including shopping for supplies, like a new notebook filled with crisp sheets of paper. I liked to have lots of paper and lots of pencils. I would fill my book satchel with them before school and come home empty-handed after sharing with all the kids who forgot their own. My stepmother soon started rationing—only 20 sheets a day and one pencil—to stop me from giving everything

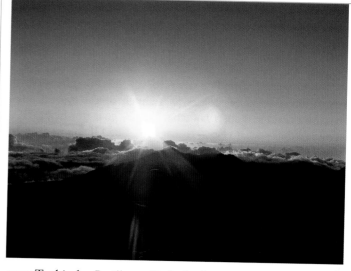

away. To this day, I still get a little thrill when I see stacks of clean white paper. To me each page represents a fresh start.

What I know for sure is that every sunrise is like a new page, a chance to right ourselves and receive each day in all its glory.

Each day is a wonder. I forget it sometimes when I'm caught up in my own stuff—deadlines, obligations, expectations. But the summer of 2006, I was able to strike a fine balance between work and renewal. Not only did I see the USA in a Chevrolet (on a road trip with my friend Gayle), but I also traveled to South Africa to oversee the Leadership Academy for Girls I was building there.

In July I sat on my porch in Hawaii and took pictures of the sunset each evening. Every day I would hike the hills in back of my house with my three rambunctious white retrievers. At 4:30 one morning, Stedman and I drove to the top of the Haleakala Crater and watched the sun rise. That's on the list of things to do before you die. You get to watch the day slowly unfold above the clouds. The sun casts a pink haze over the sky long before you see its rays, and the ridge below the cloud begins to glow. It's so still up there, you can hear life whispering to you. I could feel the depth and potential of my own existence.

No matter what our troubles, when the earth turns on its axis one more time and we see what appears to be the sun rising, I feel it's the universe calling for a change in ourselves. You have one more day. Rise with it! **O**

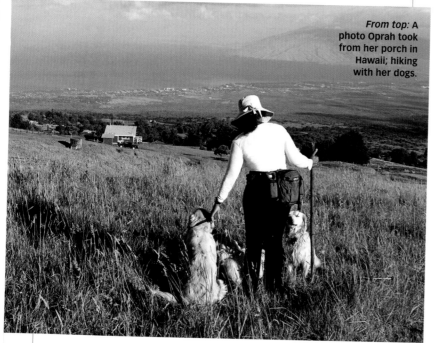

From top: A photo Oprah took from her porch in Hawaii; hiking with her dogs.

Spirituality

Are You Waiting for Your Life to Begin?

SHARON SALZBERG mulls over the downsides, upsides, priceless lessons, and incredibly productive uses of that stretch of time between Now and When.

Walking down the street in New York City one day, I ran into two friends who were so blissful, they could have lit up the street with their smiles. They were well into the process of adopting a second daughter from China, and a few hours before our meeting, they had gone to the agency to pick up her photo. She was so beautiful! We stood on the sidewalk, mesmerized by her little face, with people swirling around us, unconscious of the scene playing out before them: the vitality and tenderness and vulnerability of falling intensely in love. Every single detail of that photo was important. As horns honked and dogs walked by and folks went about their day, we could only stand there and admire her.

Then came the waiting.

It went on for longer than usual and was very hard. This was at the time of SARS, and for months, all adoptions from that area of China were postponed. My friends and many others who'd memorized their girls' photos were left waiting, and wondering: What if their daughters were hungry or sick? What if additional time in the orphanage stamped fear deep into the little girls' bones? That kind of waiting can be nearly unbearable, laced through with helplessness about not being able to do anything or not knowing how to react. However we wait, whether in openness or in pain, we find ourselves in the place between the known and the unknown, where we have let go of what is apparent and familiar and have yet to discover what is coming next.

Most often we wait because we are not in control of the unfolding of events. Our conviction about what should be resolved by tomorrow doesn't always make it so. Our sense of timeliness and the correct pace for change isn't automatically the one the airlines follow, or the U.S. government, or the Chinese government, or a friend who, we believe, owes us an apology. Our grief, our fear, the lag between a biopsy and the report, or a plain old monotonous day doesn't inevitably speed up because we would have it be that way. Like it or not, for good or ill, we have to wait.

But sometimes we wait because it has become a habit, a way to hold life in abeyance, a means to cocoon ourselves against change and elect numbness. We may become accustomed to not fully engaging, to not trying, to not risking our hearts. In my early meditation practice, I went to a retreat center in India where I received instruction in making a mental note of my physical and

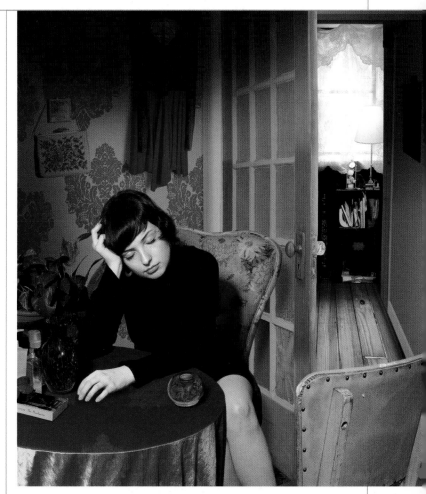

emotional experiences throughout the day. Whether I was sitting, standing, walking, lying down, eating, or taking a shower, a part of my mind was witnessing the predominant activity and silently noting it. Strangely, I found that the single most common mental note I made was *waiting*. Finally, I said to myself, *What are you waiting for?* I realized I was waiting for something exciting enough or important enough or distinctive enough for me to make note of it. I was approaching life as though I were a tape recorder with the pause button on. I was waiting for life to happen, for a better experience to happen, for a sense of connection to happen…later.

We might wait full of hope for a better day, or calmly, or distractedly, or with a certainty born merely from our thoughts that the terrible mental picture scaring us is bound to come true. This last can be like watching a door slowly swing open in a horror movie, sure nothing good is on the other side of it, powerless to race over and shut it tight against the intrusion. That's an awful kind of waiting.

And sometimes waiting can be a blessing. It might be a respite, a pause within which we allow healing to have its own rhythm, or things to take their time, or nature to follow its course. It can be a time when we relinquish our efforts to be in control and instead empty ourselves of demands and expectations and constraints.

In the best-case scenario, the landscape of waiting is a delicate one: an unbounded, translucent stretch of time before reality returns to ground and reshape our sense of what will be possible for us. We can mentally perform any act of boldness, imagine a novel feeling of contentment, or envision a magical turn in our lives. Waiting is a world in between worlds, where anything might yet happen, where everything is still to be made manifest, and where, for a while, there are no limits.

Sometimes in that in-between space we connect to a larger truth that moves us without our will or contrivance. As I was writing this, I got a call that a friend had died. I asked if his son had arrived from across the country in time to see him alive. My caller responded, "His son got here an hour before the death—it

> Waiting is a world in between worlds, where anything might yet happen, where everything is still to be made manifest, and where, for a while, there are no limits.

was almost as though the father was waiting for him." I know so many stories like that: "It was uncanny—she held on until she knew her son wouldn't be reneging on any responsibilities, then she died." Obviously, we don't make conscious decisions dictating when to die a natural death. But somehow, in the process of letting go, we seem to know intuitively when it is time to welcome change or to say goodbye.

Perhaps the lesson is that when we find ourselves waiting, whether through force of circumstance or lingering habit, we should listen deeply. When the delay is grueling, as it was for my friends who had to postpone their trip to China, we need to do everything we can to minimize our own or someone else's suffering, and not confuse waiting with being inert or defeated. Whatever the particulars, we should feel the ground beneath us and observe the space around us. And remember to breathe. We can learn to pervade the terrain of waiting with our awareness, to make it vital and connected and fully alive. ◑

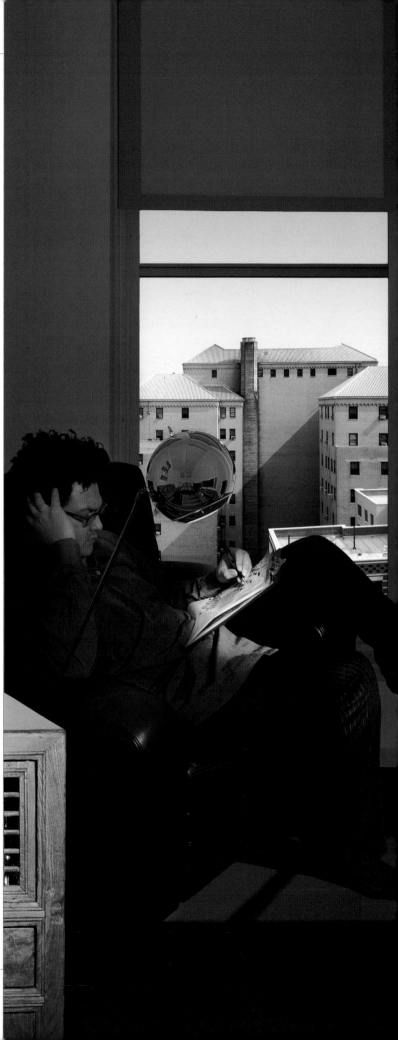

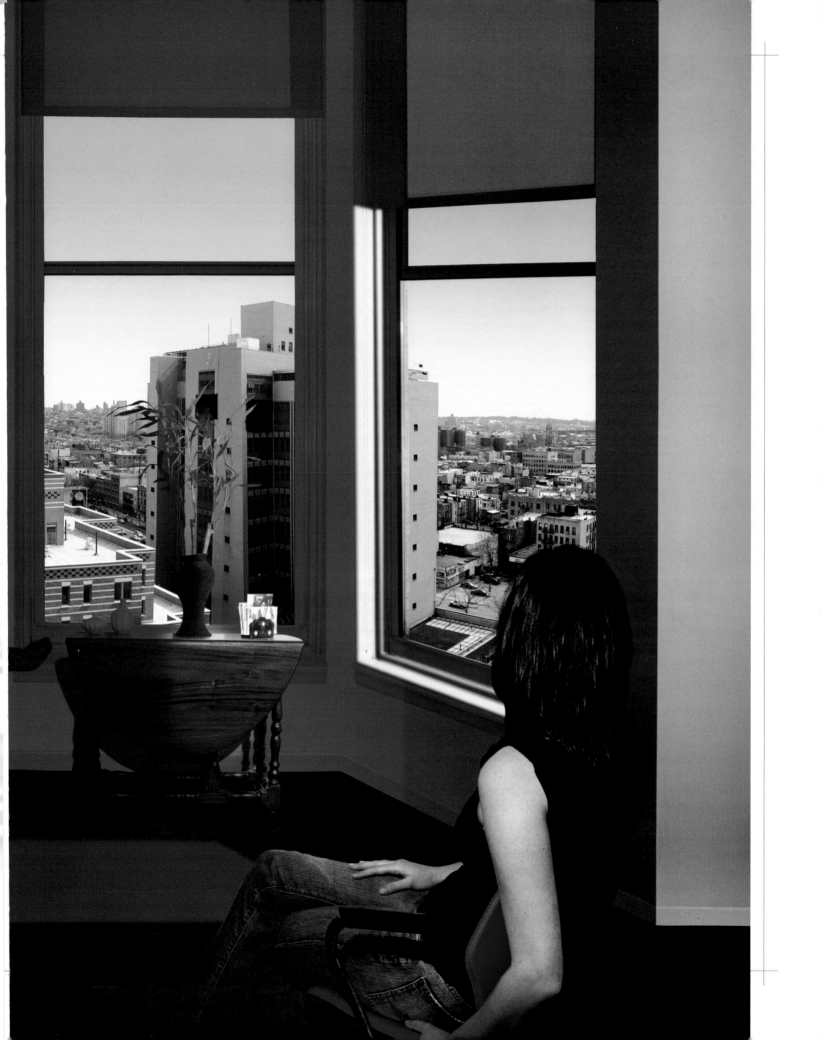

Going Solo

Single Saturday

How loneliness made VALERIE MONROE feel a little less alone.

I had spent the summer Saturday by myself, meandering through a part of the city I was still, after 30 years here, unfamiliar with, and it had yielded up a banquet of pleasure. A small, old, redbrick church, and next to it, protected by a black wrought-iron fence, a pristine lawn dotted with pale, deep-set gravestones, tilting one way and another in the dappled late-afternoon sunlight. A hidden lane, bright green moss sprouting thickly between its cobblestones, leading down toward the riverbank and a series of playful bronze sculptures of baby animals tumbling in the grass.

Around suppertime I realized that I wasn't far from one of my favorite restaurants. I rarely go there, because it's expensive and always packed, but I thought I might be able to sit at the bar and have a dozen of their tasty oysters and a glass of wine. After all the meandering, I was very hungry. I could see from the street that there was one seat left at the bar, already crowded with people who seemed to have recently napped and showered and spent some time figuring out what to wear and who now looked especially fine and happy to see one another. I was feeling a little bit like Pigpen, in my dusty sandals and shift. But I wanted those oysters. (And that glass of Chablis.) So I went in, navigated the crowd, *excuse me'd* over to the empty seat, and sat down, a bit self-consciously. I was a middle-aged woman alone at a bar among strangers. Where were my friends? Didn't I have any? My own personal bugaboo settled over me like a soggy towel, seriously dampening my pleasure: Was this experience my first step on the path that leads inexorably to rubber-soled flats, loose, tentlike garments, and an obsessive interest in public television?

I sighed aloud. If that was my future, I might as well enjoy myself getting there. I asked the bartender to recommend a wine. He offered me a taste of something delicious. The first dozen oysters were so astoundingly good, I had to have a second. As I was savoring them—deeply savoring them—I became aware

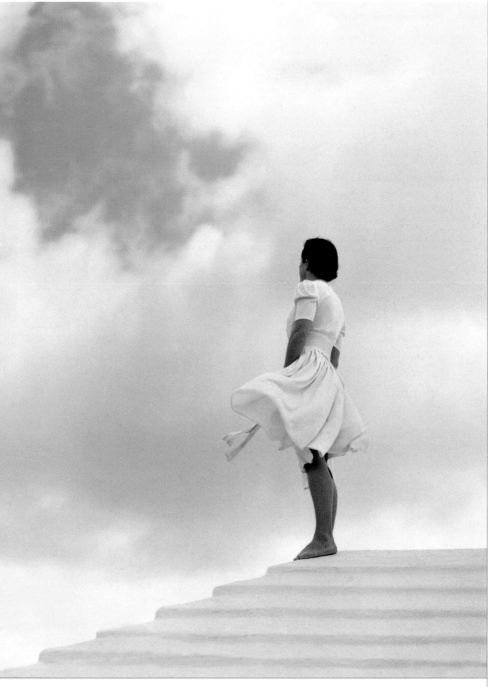

of the couple sitting next to me. He was chattering animatedly while she, half-listening, watched my every slurp and sip. Finally, she interrupted him: "I have to have what she's having," she said, pointing at my plate.

I was completely happy. Why had I felt a need to judge or label myself? (Middle-aged woman eating and drinking alone, no friends, crazy lady.) I've been running away from being alone all my life, even though I often enjoy it. I've avoided it because Loneliness, Being Alone's ugly stepsister, is uncomfortable, sometimes painful. It's the pain that sociologist Robert S. Weiss, PhD, describes as "separation distress without an object": You're longing for connection but don't know with what or whom. Which—in me, anyway—leads to a kind of emotional chaos. Not long after my date with the oysters, I began to wonder what would happen if I could tolerate that distress without reaching out to anchor myself with a phone call or an e-mail, a book, the television, a plate of shellfish. If I could just *be* with the loneliness without trying to fix it. To do that, I'd have to let go of the judgments I'd attached to being alone—that it's a problem, a punishment for not being good enough in some way.

One night alone in my apartment, I felt restless and sad. The water on the river outside my window was unusually dark,

> I'd have to let go of the judgments I'd attached to being alone—that it's a problem, a punishment for not being good enough in some way.

opal-black, smooth as glass. A barge sat parked just a little upriver; a string of twinkling white lights hung festively along its deck. It was too early to go to sleep—I wasn't tired anyway—but too late to go out. I didn't feel like reading. I thought about making a phone call; didn't really feel like that, either. I missed my husband. I missed my son. I even missed my mother. What to do with myself? I was staring out my window at that beautiful barge with nothing to do, no one to speak to. Just a person, staring out the window. Can you understand what I mean when I say that as I allowed the feeling of loneliness to arise in me I felt a heartbreaking compassion, recognizing that every person everywhere throughout history has been subject to the very same loneliness I was feeling in that moment? I started to weep, with sadness and awe and grief and joy. I felt connected to the world in a new, different way, admiring the capability of the heart to hold all those feelings at once. Such strong feelings! And of course because it *was* my heart, too, how full I felt, and complete.

This profound loneliness was, in fact, exactly the opposite of what I'd always been afraid of. I had, I realized, once again meandered into a place that I was, after many years, still unfamiliar with. And once again, it had yielded up a banquet of pleasure, unexpected and glorious. O

You Time

We're here to say you have the right to a moment—many moments—all to yourself.

THE VOYAGE IN
FRANCINE PROSE

There's a deep and utterly unique pleasure that comes—when you're traveling alone—the minute the train pulls out of the station. It's unlike the exhilaration and the vague anxiety of a plane's takeoff, unlike the wary alertness of leaving the driveway. Is it the comfort of the plush seats? The old-fashioned charm of the fact that the conductor still says "All aboard!"? I think it has more to do with a kind of promise. For the next few hours, you will be out of time, free and (especially if you ride in one of the cell-phone-free "quiet cars") at peace; nothing will interfere with your enjoyment of your own company. It's a bit like a long nap, except you remain awake, soothed and rocked by the rumble of the wheels on the track, reading or daydreaming, entertained by the spectacle of the world streaming smoothly by—a delightful reverie from which you will emerge having arrived at your destination.

THE EMPTY APARTMENT
AMY GROSS

I was 26 the first time I ever lived alone, and I was so lonely that on the way home—from the store, from work—my steps would slow as I neared my building. On the street was life and the possibility of bumping into someone, having a conversation, a little social moment. Up in the apartment was...nothing. Emptiness. Stillness. Solitary confinement—being cut off from the herd. Years later my marriage went bad, but I was afraid to let go, to be on my own. I can't live alone, I said to a friend. Why not? she asked. Because I went crazy the last time I lived alone, I said. You were 26, she said. And that set me free. When the 26-year-old me got back to her apartment and closed the door behind her, there was no one home. Here's the great, unexpected thing about growing up: Now when I'm alone, there's somebody there—me.

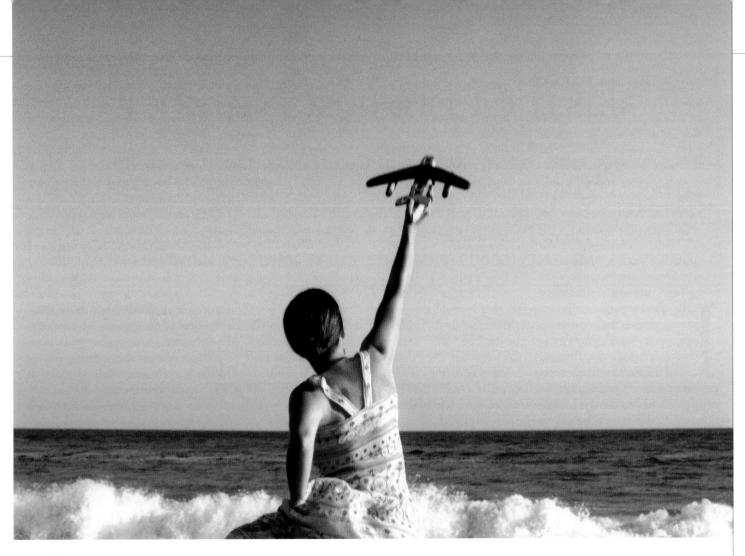

FINDING MY PLACE

CATHLEEN MEDWICK

I rest my ankle boyishly on one knee—exactly the way my mother taught me not to—and ease the book onto my lap. I drop my eyes, and already I am resting; my hard-bitten fingers turn the pages, turning and smoothing until I find my place. Then, quietly, I go in. I pay attention, but I don't have to speak. This is like meditation: disappearing and being all here.

MY OWN PRIVATE MOVIE THEATER

LILA KEARY

I sing to a standing-room-only amphitheater with Roberta Flack's voice. I accept the Oscar for best original screenplay as every nasty seventh-grade girl I ever met looks on in awe.

I meander through Paris and picnic by the Seine. I lie quietly in a metal tube hoping the MRI I am having will determine that the tumor on the bone that cradles my brain is shrinking according to schedule. Actually, I'm tone-deaf, my screenplay is an aborted paragraph on a lost legal pad, and I never liked Paris, but that last one is true.

There are people who panic when they have to be still for an MRI—people who'd have a nervous breakdown if they had to be alone for the better part of an hour in a metallic barrel. But I've lived through this too many times to be nervous. So I imagine music, make a tremendously touching I'd-like-to-thank-God-and-my-agent speech, and float along a French river. For a brief moment in time, everything stops and I get to be whomever I want to be, doing just as I please. If that's as good as it gets...well, that's pretty damn good.

PRIVATE DANCER

GAYLE KING

This is best done in the privacy of your own home, with you scantily clad and the music cranked up LOUD! A microphone is a nice touch, but if you don't have one handy (and most of us don't), a hairbrush or candle serves the purpose. The music varies depending on my mood. When I'm exceptionally happy, Josh Groban is perfection—everything he sings makes me smile—and a BeBe Winans song is always soothing. The other day I was dancing around the family room all by myself to Tina Turner. She was so loud the walls were shaking—that was exhilarating. And when I'm feeling really frisky, rapper 50 Cent is the best to make a 50-year-old feel like a teenager—appropriate since my dance moves still resemble those I was doing in seventh grade. But, hey, I don't even get embarrassed about that because I'm all alone, and in those moments, me with my music as high as it will go, I am, as Tina sings, feeling simply the best. I call it a party of one. ◖

them was John Cacioppo, PhD, currently a professor at the University of Chicago's department of psychology. "When I became interested in the topic in 1994, loneliness was thought to be a gnawing, chronic disease with no redeeming qualities," says Cacioppo, quoting Weiss on the subject. "As a neuroscientist, that didn't make sense to me. Everything has evolved for a purpose, or it doesn't stick around."

The way Cacioppo sees it, loneliness is what propelled the solitary Neolithic hunter-gatherer back into the fold, where the group shares its meager supplies and survives, while his impervious buddy carries on only to die high in the Italian Alps and be discovered as a subzero mummy by 20th-century hikers. The implication of this theory is that loneliness is handed down, and with the help of the Netherlands Twin Register Study, Cacioppo estimates that, unlike eye color (100 percent inheritable), loneliness is only 48 percent inheritable. Cacioppo likens it to a pain threshold: If you're born with a low social-pain threshold but raised in a caring and supportive environment and taught techniques for managing your discomfort, you might never become lonely. Alternatively, if you're continually bruised throughout your formative years, no matter what your genetic setting, you might plunge into lonely episodes repeatedly.

Cacioppo knew epidemiologic evidence showed that social isolation is comparable to sedentary lifestyles, poor diet, and high blood pressure as a cause of morbidity and mortality, but he didn't know why. In the past 12 years, he's done a number of studies on physiological differences between the lonely and nonlonely, paying close attention to two groups—college students and 50- to 68-year-old Chicago adults. His team's findings on stress and perceived stress pointed out some interesting differences between the socially isolated and the socially connected.

For example, lonely and nonlonely young adults were faced with approximately the same number of negative and positive life events, but the nonlonely group coped better with stressors. (In the older group, the lonely had slightly more negative life experiences.) To the lonely, the same irritation felt like a bigger hassle than it did to the nonlonely, while a happy coincidence wouldn't lift their spirits as much as it would the nonlonely. Cacioppo's team also did a brain-imaging study with the young adults, and the preliminary results suggest physiological reasons

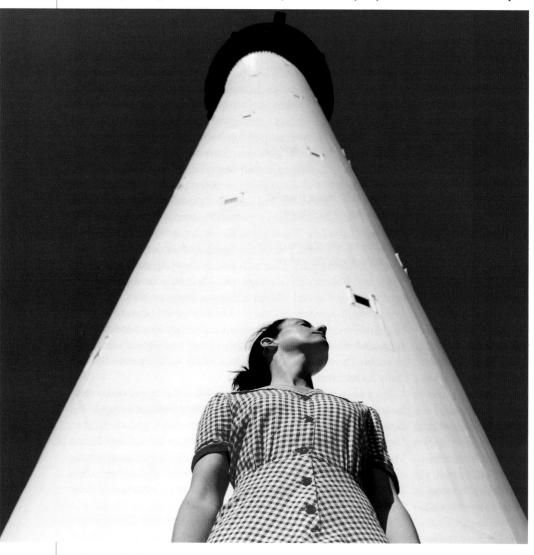

for the different outlooks. Researchers scanned lonely and nonlonely people while certain images flashed before them. When the nonlonely looked at positive pictures of people (happy, smiling folk), they showed greater activation in the reward center of the brain than when viewing an equally positive photo of an object (a cake). A lonely person, however, showed no difference in that part of the brain, suggesting that he intuitively associates connecting with others as a less rewarding experience than the nonlonely do.

Faced with negative pictures, the nonlonely person didn't react differently to an object (a dirty toilet) and a person (a battered woman). But the lonely did; they showed a much stronger response in the threat surveillance part of the brain to the negative picture of a person than to the object. The finding indicates that when a lonely person has a negative interaction, or even sees a negative interaction, he'll feel more threatened than the average person.

"Lonely individuals want to connect with other people," Cacioppo theorizes, "but they also expect to be ultimately rejected or negatively evaluated. So they engage in self-protective behavior." That preemptive defensiveness can elicit the very responses they fear most: Studies out of the University of Minnesota, in which people were given information about a stranger they were about to meet,

involved wit
themselves
adjustments
negative vis
wired to cor
tail party in
social functi
base, a mid-

Before lo
a social gatl
see what ex
ner? Are th
they new m
can tell ther

To meet
these slots,
mends joir
insists the
project—nc
series—bec
gives partic
talk about.
thing they
associate cl
at Harvar
they'll need
carry them
awkward ea

"People
can be," say
Life with
Webster. "F
She's not sa
something
problem of
19th. "Basi
says Olds.
sufficient,
lean on peo
do our own
of connecti
we don't b
because we
favor, Olds
and it's in t
eventually
was missing

Olds ack
getting inv
"They're so
bit welcom
says. "One
come off a
says. We all
the ever pe

demonstrated that our assumptions affect our interactions. For instance, if the subjects were told the stranger was aggressive—even if he wasn't—they would pick up on certain cues, ignoring others, and their behavior would unknowingly evoke aggressive behavior from the stranger, reinforcing their initial suppositions.

Along with this defensive sensitivity, the lonely tend to remember more social cues about encounters, according to studies at Northwestern University. This could be a vestige of being alone on a Neolithic plain, where a solitary person would be ever vigilant for danger. But today this capacity for hyperobservation coupled with their tendency to negatively interpret information guarantees that the lonely retain more "proof" of others' retreat, which not only confirms their view of being alone in an unfriendly world but informs their future behavior, further transforming them into the tense and anxious people Weiss first observed some 30 years ago.

"We're much more social architects of our world than we realize," says Cacioppo. "This fear of being rejected means the lonely don't open up. They also tend to select relationships badly. They're looking for the quick fix. With anybody." But easy friendships aren't always the most satisfying. The lonely stay in these substandard relationships to protect themselves from complete isolation. They find themselves at offices or cocktail parties, over-40 softball games or continuing ed courses, and because there are people in their lives, they often don't ever realize that the lack of intimate connection in their relationships reinforces a sense of not being understood or cared for in a significant way.

This kind of disconnection is, not surprisingly, often inescapably bound up with depression and results in a terrible feedback loop—the lonelier people feel, the more morose they become, leading to less and less social effort, which calls down more unhappiness on their head. But as intertwined as loneliness and depression are, researchers have discovered that they are not the same thing. As Russell explains it, "Depressed people are dissatisfied with everything in their life; lonely people are dissatisfied with their relationships." Loneliness is a distinct condition—unfortunately, a condition that has been found to be a huge causal factor of depression. Cacioppo's research has shown that a lonely woman has an eight times greater likelihood of becoming depressed than one who's not. For men, the incidence is even more striking: 13 to one.

It's enough to make a person sick—and loneliness does. In the 1980s and '90s, Janice Kiecolt-Glaser, PhD, professor at Ohio State University College of Medicine, demonstrated that lonely individuals had poorer immune function than the nonlonely. In 1995 Cacioppo and his team started examining the effects of social isolation on an individual's circulatory system. Among the college students, both the lonely and nonlonely had similar blood pressure levels. But when Cacioppo and his researchers looked closer, they discovered that the measure of

> A lonely woman has an eight times greater likelihood of becoming depressed than one who's not.

the constriction of the blood vessels, the total peripheral resistance (TPR), differed in the two groups. Whenever Cacioppo tested them, the lonely college students had higher TPR, a sign of stress.

Both groups were young, which means their physiological resilience tended to be pretty high—the heart is working fine and the body's many systems are compensating for the increased TPR in the lonely. But in older adults, increased TPR contributes to high blood pressure. "That led us to hypothesize that as the students grew older, we'd see higher blood pressure," says Cacioppo.

Cacioppo has not done a longitudinal study with those 20-somethings, but his older group, part of a five-year Chicago Health, Aging, and Social Relations Study (CHASRS), has reached the typical age for arterial stiffening. He and his team have discovered an association between loneliness and high blood pressure. Normal systolic blood pressure is less than 120 mmHg (millimeters of mercury, the standard unit of measurement). Looking at the CHASRS participants, Cacioppo says, "we found that as they get older, there's approximately a .7 mmHg increase a year per what's called standard deviation of loneliness." That doesn't sound like much, but let's assume at age 20 you have normal blood pressure. If you're chronically lonely, by the time you're 50, using Cacioppo's rate of increase, you could be hypertensive. And by the time you're 65, you could be seriously hypertensive, with an even greater risk of heart attack and stroke.

Cacioppo's team thinks one of the reasons for increased TPR might have to do with something they'd noticed while studying the restorative process of sleep among college students in the '90s. "We found that lonely people sleep less efficiently and complain about more daytime dysfunction and sleepiness," says Cacioppo. "We found it in the young adults and in the older adults. So this process that detoxifies isn't there."

As in the other studies, his team has taken into account age, gender, ethnicity, income, education, marital status, family history, level of physical activity, depressive symptomatology, social support—and this association of poor restorative process and increased TPR appears only in the lonely. In the older adults, Cacioppo found a link between poor restorative process and high blood pressure. It will take more years of study to prove that loneliness is the cause, but the association is compelling. Richard Suzman, PhD, of the National Institute on Aging, a government agency that has helped fund Cacioppo's research, wrote in an e-mail that the findings "suggest that we will pay more attention to the experience in the future, including testing whether interventions to reduce the experience of loneliness also reduce blood pressure in a cost-effective manner."

Cacioppo, Russell, Weiss, and Suzman are not aware of anyone specifically looking into how to lower blood pressure by reducing loneliness. Part of the difficulty, Cacioppo notes, is that since the increase in blood pressure is so incredibly subtle, it takes decades to see the results of chronic loneliness in hypertensive blood

What Never to Say to a Single Woman Over 35

LISA KOGAN gives a well-meaning world fair warning.

Allow me to introduce myself. I am a gainfully employed, God-fearing, law-abiding citizen, and I come in peace. I don't bet on baseball, I take excellent care of my gums, I keep my tray table locked and upright from takeoff to landing. Oh, and there's one more thing: I am what is commonly referred to in polite society as "an unmarried woman." Truth be told, I now have a boyfriend and a baby girl—it's all very modern—but much of my 30s involved ostensibly concerned bystanders averting their eyes, asking how many cats I own, and sharing their private theories on where it all went so hideously wrong for me. Ah, yes, I remember it well. And when I start to forget, I still have plenty of single girlfriends in various states of angst to remind me of the grotesque fix-ups, the ham-handed remarks, and the brutal Thanksgiving dinners. For those valiant, traumatized souls, I present my list of the ten things one must never say, think, or do when dealing with a single woman over the age of 35.

1. **HEY, COUSIN CHRISTY,** how 'bout we break with tradition and dispense with that bridal bouquet toss? Believe it or not, it's actually a touch degrading to be shoved front and center next to your spinster aunt Mitzi from Winnipeg as a roomful of revelers hopped up on Champagne and jumbo shrimp chant, "You're next, you're next."

2. **THE WORD** *PICKY*—as in "the reason you refuse to meet my podiatrist's brother-in-law for a night of miniature golf is that you're too picky"—is not only offensive, it's inaccurate. Hell, I'd have dated Ted Bundy if he were willing to meet in a well-lit, public place. No, I suspect it was your description of his "slight comb-over" and "profound desire to one day shake Dick Cheney's hand" that made me release that "catch" back into the wilds of New Jersey.

3. **DON'T CONFUSE BEING UNMARRIED WITH BEING 11.** My love of SpongeBob-shaped macaroni and cheese notwithstanding, I never wanted to sit at the children's table. Nor did I want to ride in the backseat with your darling toddler, his pet tarantula, his Spider-Man glitter glue, and his melting Fudgsicle.

4. **KINDLY STOP FILLING EVERY CONVERSATIONAL LULL** by announcing how much you love *Will & Grace.* Being single is not the same thing as being gay, just as being married is not proof of being straight...but I'll cover that concept more fully in my upcoming "Uncle Barry's Very Special Surprise" article.

5. **HAS ANYBODY OUT THERE NOTICED** that the institution of matrimony is falling apart faster than Courtney Love on a can of Red Bull? Now, I honestly don't care if your marriage is so gothic in its dysfunction that it makes the couple from *Who's Afraid of Virginia Woolf?* look like Will and Jada—I'm not here to judge. All I ask is that you quit judging me. Perhaps we're not suffering a fear of intimacy as much as a fear of being trapped in a crummy marriage.

6. **REMEMBER THAT LITTLE FACTOID** you used to bandy about—you know, the one where 40-year-old women have a greater chance of being shot by terrorists than of making it to the altar? Then you may also recall that Susan Faludi refuted that myth 14 years ago. So, okay, Ms. Faludi is probably rethinking that (thanks a lot, Osama!), but you don't have to rub it in.

7. **ENOUGH WITH THE "CONSTRUCTIVE" CRITICISM ALREADY.** We live in a world of stunning technological advancement, but it remains physically impossible to wear your heart on your sleeve *and* be emotionally distant, dress like a slut *and* a librarian, try much too hard *and* not make any real effort.

8. **NEW RULE:** You may discuss everything from the fall of the Roman Empire to the rise of Rem Koolhaas with your single friend. But her uterus, ovaries, entire reproductive system are off-limits. Sending clippings about a 74-year-old Ukrainian woman who just gave birth to triplets along with a peppy little "Keep hope alive!" Post-it note will do irreparable damage to your relationship and—if the woman is particularly resourceful—may even get your tires slashed.

9. **HERE'S A PHRASE THAT MUST NEVER,** *EVER* **CROSS YOUR LIPS:** "Let me tell you why a terrific gal like you is still single...." Because that terrific gal is then likely to explain in dark and visceral detail what happened to the last gentleman who uttered those very words—and, trust me, you really don't want to know.

10. **I'VE LOOKED AT SINGLE LIFE** from both sides now, and here's what I think: Single women are not Sarah Jessica Parker in *Sex and the City* any more than they're Glenn Close in *Fatal Attraction.* For one thing, very few have Manolo Blahniks in their closets. For another, very few have sex with Michael Douglas in their kitchens. They sometimes get lonely, frustrated, they sometimes get flat-out goofy. They are human beings—tickle them and they laugh, prick them and they bleed, offer them chocolate and they eat.... In other words, they're pretty much like all the married women I know. **O**

"Alone time is when I distance myself from the voices of the world so I can hear my own"

I used to fear being alone. I understood why after John Bradshaw, who pioneered the concept of the inner child, appeared on my show 14 years ago. John took my audience and me through a profound exercise. He asked us to close our eyes and go back to the home we grew up in, to visualize the house.... *Come closer, look inside the window and find yourself inside. What do you see? And more important, what do you feel?* For me it was an overwhelmingly sad yet powerful exercise. What I felt at almost every stage of my development was alone. Not lonely—because there were always people around—but I knew that my soul's survival depended on me. I felt I would have to fend for myself. I now think that the sense of being apart from others is what led me to trust so firmly in something bigger than I could articulate and feel a connection to God.

As a girl, I used to love when company would come to my grandmother's house after church. When they left, I dreaded being alone with my senile grandfather and my grandmother, who was often exhausted and impatient and had no time for me.

I was the only child for miles around, so I had to learn to play, entertain, and be with myself. I invented new ways to be solitary. I had books and homemade dolls and chores and farm animals I often named and talked to out loud. I'm sure that all that time alone was critical in defining the adult I would become.

Looking back through John Bradshaw's window into my life, I was sad that the people closest to me didn't seem to realize what a sweet-spirited little girl I was. But I also felt strengthened, seeing it for myself.

These days I'm often surrounded by other people. I have to interact constantly, so when I get to spend time with just me, I delight in every moment. Alone time is when I recharge and go back to my center, distancing myself from the voices of the world so I can hear my own with clarity. It's when I consciously count my blessings, take a deep breath, and try to absorb the wonder and glory of all my experiences.

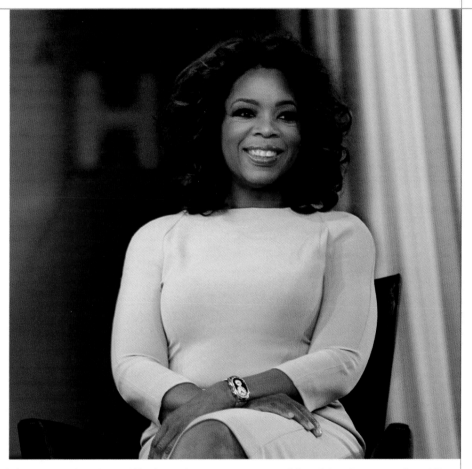

I'll admit that my 30s were a blur. After I appeared in *The Color Purple,* when I was 31 years old, my show went into national syndication and my world went on hyperspeed. At one point I visited 21 cities in 20 days. I would do speaking engagements at night after taping my show. I was trying to fulfill the responsibilities of a blossoming career and hadn't yet learned the art of saying no.

That was the unhealthiest period of my life. I was so out of balance. Fat and disconnected. Always doing, always going. I thought that if I stopped, I would surely fail. Now I know for sure that if you don't replenish your well, it runs dry. And things around you falter.

So on any given Sunday, you will find me alone. Filling myself up. Cherishing life and loving every solitary moment. **O**

Working

The Little Chill

A glance at her watch, a roll of the eye, a quick doodle: The almost imperceptible gestures researchers call microinequities can have a huge impact on the way your day, job—life—is going. LISE FUNDERBURG reports.

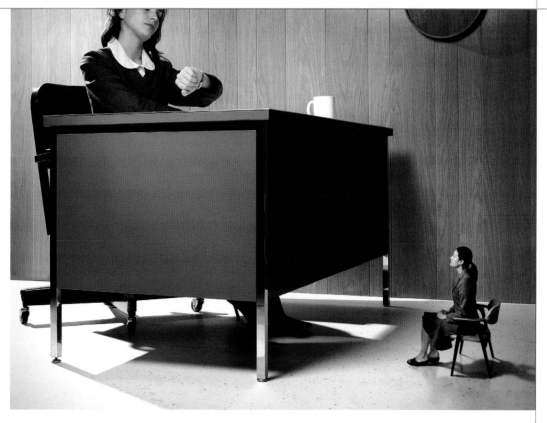

Being left off a group memo, in the grand scheme of things, can't compare to, say, being fired. Watching your bank teller's eyes drift off as you ask for your account balance isn't the same as being turned down for a mortgage—just as earning a big grin of confidence from your boss as you wow a client isn't winning the lottery. But for most of us, life is defined by the daily collection of small-scale slings and arrows or pats on the back. No one argues the importance of the small scale better than Stephen Young, president of Insight Education Systems, a management consulting firm in Montclair, New Jersey, and author of *Micromessaging: Why Great Leadership Goes Beyond Words.* He calls these make-or-break communications micromessages.

The 2,000 to 4,000 subtle signals we send each other every day are as automatic as breathing and often as invisible as air. They crop up in almost every human interaction. They're largely nonverbal, mostly communicated through nods, eye contact, head turns, and gestures such as glancing at your watch when another person is talking. They can be positive (microadvantages) or negative (microinequities). You can be micropraised, microadored, and microsupported. Or microinsulted, microignored, microjudged, microgoaded, and microdismissed.

If you were to look at microinequities through a *Law & Order* lens, people would fall into one of two camps: microperps and

> "Words play a very small role in telling others our true opinions of them."

microvictims. Microperps, often unwittingly, exploit the power of their positions with weapons that would pass any security checkpoint: They're the bosses who read e-mails while you're explaining a problem you're having; the doctors who ignore you, the patient, and speak to your spouse instead; the clerk who says, "May I help you?" and "Thank you" but never looks you in the eye; and the friend who starts apologies with, "If that hurt your feelings...."

A microvic is simply the person on the receiving end. He's the student who never gets called on and eventually stops raising his hand; the junior executive whose ideas are consistently met with "That won't work," "We've tried that before," or, worse, the complete flyover, "Anyone else?" until she stops making suggestions; and the black woman who opens the door to her large suburban home only to have the workman on the threshold look past her and ask, "Is the lady of the house here?"

Since these messages often travel on a below-the-radar frequency, they're near impossible for most of us to identify, let alone harness for good or safely disarm. Until Steve Young gets ahold of them.

Young runs a seminar called "Microinequities: The Power of Small." It's part communication theory and part street theater, and combines academic research with Young's decades of experience in the corporate world, including five years as senior vice president of global diversity for JPMorgan Chase. He's learned how to hold an audience's attention. Today, for instance, he's in Princeton, and he's got a group of about 50 school administrators from New Jersey in the palm of his hand.

"Most of us believe words convey the essence of what we mean," he says. "But words play a very small role in telling others our true opinions of them." Micromessages make our expectations and feelings crystal clear. Young asks one principal if she'd be willing to help him with an exercise; she agrees and waits for instruction.

"Hi there," Young says brightly from across the room, with a friendly wave of recognition. The principal smiles and waves back. Then Young's body melts into an oleaginous slither as he turns his torso away but keeps his eyes trained on her, looking her up and down and appraising her with a heavy-lidded leer. The principal giggles at first, then squirms in her seat.

"Ooh, that's good!" she says, realizing her discomfort is the desired outcome. When he doesn't immediately cease, she wags a chastising finger at him. "Cut that out," she orders, ever the principal. The room breaks into laughter.

"What did I say?" he asks the crowd.

"Nothing," many call out, realizing that their answer makes his point.

After a short break, Young tells the principals that to understand why people perpetrate microinequities, they have to look at the roots of micromessages: the assumptions we make about our place in the world, other people's position in the social hierarchy, or our beliefs about certain individuals and groups. Young describes a 1960s study in which Harvard social psychologist Robert Rosenthal asked a group of students to document differences between two strains of rats, one bright and one less so. The students came up with reams of evidence supporting distinctions between the two, only to find out afterward that these rats were from the same genetic line.

This phenomenon of getting the outcome you expect has come to be known as the Pygmalion effect, the way the eye of the beholder determines whether someone is a Cockney flower girl or cultured princess of mysterious provenance. Young explains that preconceived notions—about race, class, ethnicity, and gender—are essentially filters. If someone believes, for instance, that old

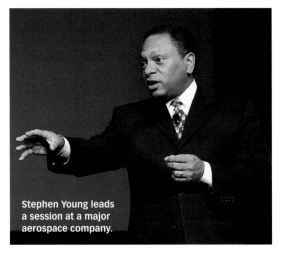

Stephen Young leads a session at a major aerospace company.

"The point," says Young, "is how clearly your performance was affected by how you were being listened to."

people can't learn anything new, he'll tend to notice events that confirm that opinion—and not register an older employee picking up a new skill. These "confirmed" assumptions, in turn, affect the micromessages he sends to the employee. Over time, micromessages conveying lack of confidence or impatience will hurt the worker's performance, further reinforcing the original belief.

"When I assume you are a bright rat or a dull rat," Young says, "my filters go into place and distort the rat's [actual performance]." For the principals, all of whom struggle to close the insidious, widely reported achievement gap between white and non-white students, Young links this last point to the education system. "Most students learn by second or third grade whether they're seen as a bright rat or a dull rat," he says. "And rats perceived to be dull begin to meet that expectation." The principals, who had been laughing a minute earlier, are now absolutely silent, many nodding in agreement.

To show how people can be influenced by someone else's behavior, Young asks the principals to pair off. One person is told to give generic job interview information—current position, responsibilities, challenges—while the other listens. The listener is instructed to give her full attention: She looks the speaker in the eye, nods, smiles encouragingly, and never interrupts. Then, on a predetermined cue, the speaker describes his last job, and the listener switches into fidget mode. She looks around, checks her cell phone, BlackBerry, calendar—anything she can come up with to appear disinterested or bored while the speaker keeps talking.

"Be creative," Young advises the listeners. "Anything short of leaving the room."

At the experiment's end, Young canvasses the speakers. How was your performance in the first half of the experiment, he asks, on a scale of one to five? "Five," most people answer. And in the second half? "Zero," some say. Others pipe up with "One" and "Negative five." The speakers report that they grew angry, lost their train of thought, and started rambling when the listeners turned inattentive. "I was bored," marvels one speaker about the second portion of the experiment, "and I was talking about my own stuff!"

Young mentions that he once paired up to do the exercise with the CEO of a Fortune 500 company who said he wanted to punch Young when he started to get antsy. "I can see what this would do in an interview situation," says one administrator. "If someone isn't listening, the candidate might start babbling and seem like an idiot. And that person may have been someone of value."

The amazing thing about this exercise, Young reminds them, is that the participants know what's going on—they're not being duped about rat smarts—and still they end up faltering. "The point here," Young tells the group, "is how clearly your performance was affected by how you were being listened to." Skill had nothing to do with race, gender, age, or sexual orientation—simply the quality of someone else's attention.

The term *microinequities* was coined in 1973 by Mary Rowe, PhD, currently the ombudsperson and adjunct professor of management at Massachusetts Institute of Technology. She arrived at MIT expecting to address policy-level problems of racial and gender exclusion. She found that one essential problem that kept people of color and women from coming into the institution and thriving was what happened to them in the halls and by the watercooler.

"In my first week at MIT," Rowe remembers, "an African-American woman came to my office and said, 'Everybody's polite to me, but the place is still so cold.' " Rowe asked the woman to keep a diary, which they'd then review. When the woman returned after several weeks, the diary's pages were blank.

"She said, 'No one has spoken to me,' " Rowe says. "The problem wasn't that anyone was rude or mean or unpleasant; it was that she felt invisible. It was just awful for her." Rowe kept happening on similar experiences, and a pattern emerged linking positive small-scale interactions to productivity and success in recruitment. At MIT, Rowe saw one white department head make his department ranks swell with women and minorities. He did it through the tiniest of steps: striking up conversations on planes when he was seated next to a person of color, seeking out women at conferences and asking them about their work, and giving new employees close and constant attention.

This professor, Rowe explains, intuitively conferred micro-affirmations, the discreet behaviors that offer encouragement, bring out the best in people, make them strive to do better, and elicit their loyalty and trust.

What struck Young about Rowe's theories was how tangible they were, and how widely applicable. Over the years, Young has seen plenty of diversity training programs come and go. Most suffer from well-intentioned but hard-to-apply core themes—"Everyone is of value" or "In diversity lies strength." Young has embraced and built upon Rowe's work, in part because it addresses the ways in which people continue to be discriminated against. Although our country has made great strides in terms of legislating equal access—women can vote and anyone can drink from any water fountain—the interpersonal acts of discrimination have been much harder to tackle. "We've done a great job of managing the elephants while the ants walk by," he says. The labeling of microinequities gives people the means to identify and then address these lingering prejudices.

But what also excites Young about Rowe's theories is how they encompass the insensitivities that result from an imbalance of power between two people—and who on this planet hasn't been on both sides of that equation? A boss can interrupt an underling, and the underling can't retaliate. A nanny has to deal with the difficult working mother who writes her check, but that same mother has to accommodate a hidebound boss. "Microinequities apply to everyone," says Young. It's just a question of making people see that universality, which Young says is possible. One of his proudest moments, in fact, came after a training session several years ago. As two high-ranking white male executives walked out of the room, one said to the other, "For the first time this HR stuff was really worthwhile."

So how does Young get two powerful executives to identify their own microdomineering tendencies? One method is by playing a training video—a staged office meeting—that's a festival of microinequities. The boss nudges an employee sitting next to him (clearly his favorite); he doesn't pay attention to some underlings, neglects to identify others by name, and doesn't focus on one's presentation.

Afterward, Young asks the group to describe what happened. The school administrators agree that the boss—a microperp extraordinaire—needs to seriously examine the messages he's sending out, and they correctly identify a number of his power blunders. "If you're in a leadership position," Young says, "you have the power to change the tone of the room, simply by using microadvantages." He gives examples, such as paying attention, maintaining eye contact, not interrupting, and soliciting input from everyone during meetings. (Remember, after all, what happened to those poor, unlistened-to principals.) He says that responding to someone's idea with a question—"How would that work?"—is more likely to keep communication flowing than the boss in the video's knee-capping response of "That's a bad idea." He also notes that a boss could invite someone to sit next to him who wouldn't ordinarily choose that seat. He reminds the group that it's the responsibility of the person in power to be conscious of her facial expressions. If you're furrowing your brow, letting your eyes drift, you're sending a signal, he says. Even silence—as was the case for Mary Rowe's colleague at MIT—can be loaded. "We send more messages to the people we like and agree with," Young explains, "so if you're not getting the message, you're getting a message."

By the end of Young's seminar, managers are shocked to have discovered their inner microperps; recipients of microinequities are relieved to finally put a finger on the imperceptible slights and obstacles they've had to stumble over. One principal, leaving the Princeton meeting, seems slightly awestruck. "This is powerful and frightening," she says. Indeed, Young acknowledges, "This gets to the DNA of culture change. But if we want to be a caring democratic society, what choice do we have?" ◖

> "If you're in a leadership position," Young says, "you have the power to change the tone of the room."

How to Be Wildly Successful

If at first you don't succeed…ask yourself, *Am I an otter? A squirrel? A mouse?* The answer could spell the difference between things going swimmingly and squeaking to a halt. MARTHA BECK helps you find your own winning style.

It was a problem I'd never anticipated: My brainy daughter was having trouble in school. Katie began teaching herself to read at 15 months and tested at a "post–high school" level in almost every subject by fourth grade. Yet her middle-school grades were dropping like a lead balloon, and her morale along with them. I cared more about the morale than the grades. I knew Katie was quickly losing something educational psychologists call her sense of self-efficacy—her belief that she could succeed at specific tasks and life in general. People who lack this trait tend to stop trying because they expect to fail. Then, of course, they do fail, feel even worse, shut down even more, and carry on to catastrophe.

I couldn't understand what put Katie on this slippery slope. True, some people seem genetically inclined to believe in themselves—or not—but experience powerfully influences our sense of self-efficacy. I knew Katie had been confident as a preschooler, but her current trouble at school was destroying her optimism. I tried to help in every way I could. I created homework-checking systems, communicated with teachers like bosom buddies, doled out penalties and rewards. Mostly, though, I just kept cheering Katie on. I was sure that if she would stop hesitating, believe in herself, and just throw herself into the task at hand, she'd get past the problem.

Boy, was I ever wrong.

It took years of confidence-battering struggle—for both Katie and me—before I finally got the information I needed. It came from a no-nonsense bundle of kindly energy named Kathy Kolbe, a specialist on the instinctive patterns that shape human action. Kathy's father pioneered many standardized intelligence tests, but Kathy was born with severe dyslexia, which meant that this obviously bright little girl didn't learn in a typical way. She grew up determined to understand and defend the different ways in which people go about solving problems.

The day Katie and I met her, Kathy was wearing a T-shirt that said DO NOTHING WHEN NOTHING WORKS, a motto that typifies her approach. On her desk were the results from the tests (the Kolbe A and Y Indexes) that my daughter and I had just taken to evaluate our personal "conative styles," or typical action patterns.

"Well," said Kathy, glancing at a bar graph, "I see you both listen better when you're drawing."

Katie and I stared at each other, astonished. Bull's-eye.

"And you've both had a zillion teachers tell you to stop drawing. They said you could do only one thing at a time, but that's not true for you two, is it? You have a hard time focusing if there's nothing to occupy your eyes and hands."

Unexpectedly, I found myself tearing up with gratitude. I'd never realized how frustrated I'd been by the very situation Kathy was describing. Katie sat up a little straighter in her chair.

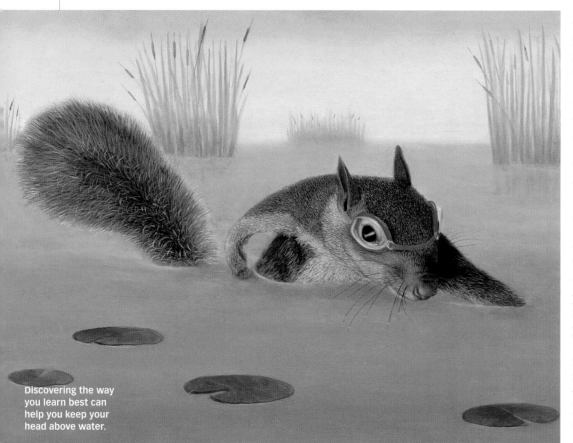

Discovering the way you learn best can help you keep your head above water.

"But," Kathy went on, "Martha, you go about problem-solving in a different way from Katie. There are four basic action modes, and you're what I call a Quick Start. When you want to learn, you just jump in and start messing around."

Another bull's-eye. I cannot count the times I've been defeated, humiliated, or physically injured immediately after saying the words, "Hey, how hard can it be?" But that never seems to stop me from saying them again.

"Now," Kathy went on, "Katie's not a Quick Start. She's a Fact Finder. Before she starts a task, she needs to know all about it. She needs to go through the instructions and analyze them for flaws, then get more information to fill in the gaps."

To my amazement, my daughter nodded vigorously. I've never understood why some people hesitate before diving into unfamiliar tasks or activities. I couldn't imagine wanting more instructions about anything.

"There are two other typical patterns," Kathy explained. "The people I call Implementors—like Thomas Edison, for example—need physical objects to work with. They figure out things by building models or doing concrete tasks. Then there are the Follow Thrus. They set up orderly systems, like the Dewey decimal system or a school curriculum."

"And that, Katie," she said, "is why you're having trouble. The school system was created mainly by people who are natural Follow Thrus. It works best for students with the same profile. Your teachers want you to fit into the system, but you have a hard time seeing how it works. If you question the instructions—which you absolutely need to do—they think you're being sassy."

Katie nodded so hard I feared for her cervical vertebrae. I was stunned. I'd spent years trying to understand my daughter, and a veritable stranger had just nailed the problem in ways I'd never even conceptualized. Katie wanted more instructions? You could have knocked me down with a feather.

BASIC INSTINCT

I've told this story in detail because since meeting Kathy, studying her work, and seeing how dramatically it affects people and their productivity, I've become convinced that many of us feel like failures because we don't recognize (let alone accept) that our instinctive methods of acting are as varied as our eye color. Our modus operandi shapes the way we do everything: make breakfast, drive, learn math. Not recognizing natural differences in our conative styles—assuming instead that we're idiots because we do things unconventionally—can destroy that precious sense of self-efficacy.

Imagine a race between four animals: an otter, a mole, a squirrel, and a mouse. They're headed for a goal several feet away. Which animal will win? Well, it depends. If the goal is underground, my money's on the mole. If it's in a tree? Hello, Mr. Squirrel. Underwater, it's the otter. And if the goal is hidden in tall grass, the mouse will walk away with it. Now, all these animals

can swim, dig, climb, and find things in the grass. It's just that each of them does one of these things better than the others. Putting all four animals in a swimming race, say, would lead to the conclusion that one was better than the others, when the truth is simply that their innate skills are different.

If we're in an environment (such as school, a job, or a family tradition) that asks us to act against our natural style, we feel uncomfortable at best, tormented at worst. Even if we manage to conform, we don't get a high sense of self-efficacy because although we've managed the efficacy part of the equation, we've lost the self. When we fail, we feel like losers; when we succeed, we feel like impostors.

Thanks to Kathy's work (and centuries of psychological work on conation), I've stopped asking others to match my instinctive style. I no longer expect squirrels to swim and otters to climb trees. As a result, I'm better able to support myself, my children, and everyone else I know. Here's a quick primer on how you can do the same:

1. **ACCEPT THAT YOU HAVE AN INBORN, INSTINCTIVE STYLE OF ACTION.** Just learning that there are four distinct patterns of action was a huge aha for me. When Katie and I accepted that we simply had different ways of doing things, our relationship and her confidence began to improve immediately. To identify your own action-mode profile, you can take a formal online test (the Kolbe Index at kolbe.com; there is a charge), or just observe your own approach to getting something done. To give you an example, people with different profiles might respond to a challenge—let's say, learning to crochet—in the following ways:

■ **QUICK START**: If you're a Quick Start who wants to crochet, you'll probably buy some yarn and a hook, get a few tips from an experienced crochetmeister, and jump right into trial and error.

■ **FACT FINDER**: You'll spend hours reading, watching, asking questions, and learning about crocheting before actually beginning to use the tools.

■ **IMPLEMENTOR**: You pay less attention to words than to concrete objects, so you might draw a pattern of a crochet stitch or even create a large model using thick rope, before you go near a needle.

■ **FOLLOW THRU**: You'll likely schedule a lesson with a crochet teacher or buy a book that proceeds through a yarn curriculum, learning new stitches in order of difficulty.

None of these approaches is right or wrong. They can all succeed brilliantly. But someone who's programmed to use one style will feel awkward and discouraged trying to follow another. We can all master each style if we have to, the way a mole can swim or an otter can climb trees, but it's not a best-case scenario.

Many of us have spent a lifetime trying to be what we're not.

So I finally stopped pressuring Katie to act like her Follow Thru teachers or her Quick Start mother. Instead I helped her find detailed information and gave her time to absorb it. She recently devoured a 1,000-page book on Web site design that I would not read if the alternative were death on the rack. It took her a month to finish the book. The next day, she made a Web site. Spooky.

2. **PLAY TO YOUR STRENGTHS.** Once you know your instinctive style, brainstorm ways to make it work for you, not against you. For starters, choose fields of endeavor where you feel comfortable and competent. If you love systematic structure, don't become a freelancer. If you are crazy about physical models, don't force yourself to crunch financial statistics for a living.

To really boost your sense of self-efficacy, think of ways you could modify your usual tasks to suit your personal style. For example, Kathy suggested that Katie might ask for permission to do detailed research reports in place of other school assignments. I nearly threw up at the very thought, but to my astonishment Katie agreed enthusiastically.

Of course, you'll inevitably interact with people whose instinctive patterns are different from yours. Otter, Mole, Squirrel, and Mouse may all show up in the same family, workplace, or book club. Occasionally, it's fine to conform, using styles of action that don't come naturally—but do it consciously and for a limited time, or your sense of self-efficacy will suffer. And finally...

3. **TEAM UP WITH UNLIKE OTHERS.** As long as Otter, Mole, Squirrel, and Mouse are forced to race in the same terrain, at least three of them will be out of their element, looking and feeling like failures. But think what they could do if they pooled their skills. They could access resources from the water, earth, trees, and fields, combining them in ways none of the animals could achieve alone. They could rule the world! (Or at least the backyard.)

This is the very best way to leverage an understanding of conative style—to create useful, complementary strategies instead of disheartening, competitive ones. Many of us have spent a lifetime trying to be what we're not, feeling lousy about ourselves when we fail and sometimes even when we succeed. We hide our differences when, by accepting and celebrating them, we could collaborate to make every effort more exciting, productive, enjoyable, and powerful. Personally, I think we should start right now. I mean, hey, how hard can it be? ⬤

Getting Unstuck

Could that ho-hum job lead to something rich and rewarding down the road— or is it time to get out and follow your bliss? But how do you know what your bliss is? SUZY WELCH—coauthor, with her husband Jack, of *Winning*—gives you the five questions that'll point you in the right direction.

Not long ago, I saw an old friend who recently realized she was—at last—totally happy at work, much to her surprise. "I have finally figured out what I want to be when I grow up," she told me. Ten years earlier, she had moved from Boston to the Midwest because of her husband's job. She didn't exactly kick and scream, but her jaw was surely clenched and she was trying to hold back tears. She had left behind everything and everyone familiar to her, including a rewarding if not perfect part-time position as a hospice worker. Her two sons, then ages 8 and 10, were similarly glum about the move. But move they had to, and move they did.

At first, as the family settled in, my friend stayed home, convinced that her dream of a fulfilling career was stalled, possibly over. But slowly, due to a mixture of financial necessity and boredom, she began to inch back into the workplace. A hospice offer fell through, so she worked as a medical center administrator for a few years and then as a community college admissions officer. She liked aspects of both jobs, but neither felt like a calling. Eventually, with a sigh of resignation, she took a job as a religion teacher at a parochial high school. *I was a philosophy major in college, so this will do for now,* she told herself.

Then a funny thing happened. My friend noticed that the career she'd backed into and settled for filled her with joy. She found teaching teenagers exhilarating—and sometimes downright hilarious. As we spoke, she was moved to tears recounting how she helped the son of a poor Iraqi family, a recent immigrant to the United States, get into a well-known university. She described reading each student's graduation essay, titled "How I Want to Live My Life."

"You should hear these kids," she said with pride. "They've got goals as big as the sky. They all seem to know what they want to be when they grow up. I've only just discovered that myself!"

She is 51 years old.

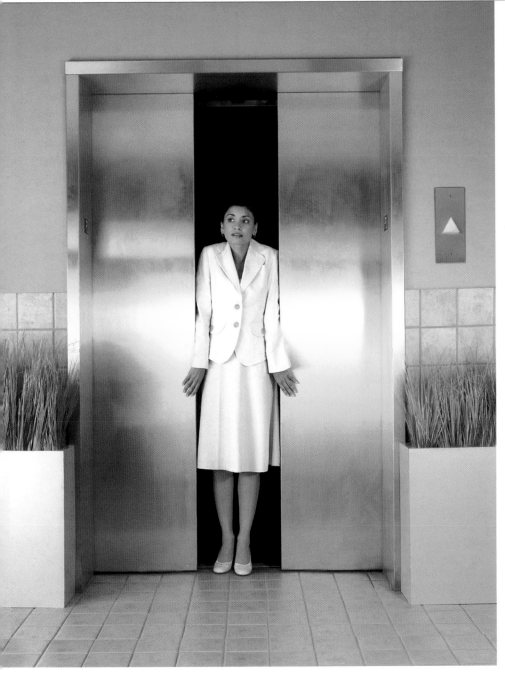

In other words, there are no shortcuts to discovering the perfect job. There is just a journey.

Now, can you hurry that process along and make it less bumpy? Can you actually speed up finding the answer to the "What should I be when I grow up" question?

I think you can, but you need to embrace a practice that requires discipline, candor, and a bit of courage. Simply put: You need to relentlessly ask yourself five questions.

These questions won't tell you if you should become a veterinarian, work in high tech, write a novel, manage a restaurant, or open your own advertising agency. The questions will, however, guide you once your journey has begun, their answers suggesting whether you should stay in a job and give it your all or get up the gumption to move on to something else. Eventually, the questions, which you can ask about either the job you currently hold or a position you are considering, will steer you toward the career that, like my friend's in the Midwest, turns work into joy.

So here they are:

THE 5 QUESTIONS

1. Does this job allow me to work with "my people"—individuals who share my sensibilities about life—or do I have to put on a persona to get through the day?

2. Does this job challenge, stretch, change, and otherwise make me smarter—or does it leave my brain in neutral?

3. Does this job, because of the company's "brand" or my level of responsibility, open the door to future jobs?

4. Does this job represent a considerable compromise for the sake of my family, and if so, do I sincerely accept that deal with all of its consequences?

5. Does this job—the stuff I actually do day-to-day—touch my heart and feed my soul in meaningful ways?

These five questions came to me not as I was searching for my own perfect job (although I think I have finally found it after 20 years!) but as my husband, Jack, and I conducted research for our book, *Winning*. For three years, we traveled around the world talking with people in every line of work about their biggest challenges. In all, we spoke to nearly 250,000 people in hundreds of

And that is exactly how it usually goes. You can figure out what you want to be when you grow up. You just have to be very grown up to do it.

Sure, there are women among us who decide they want to be federal judges at age 12 and get appointed by age 32. But they are more annoying than average. Most women discover their "exactly right" job through a messy, iterative process that involves years of experimentation and reinvention. They grab opportunities when they zip by; they make wrong turns and run twice as fast to correct them; they juggle the husbands and kids who show up along the way; and, very often, they sacrifice a piece of their own dreams on their families' behalf. Most women search, adjust, and search some more for the right career...until one day, it finally appears out of the fog of life's experiences.

wide-ranging Q&A sessions. When we set out on our travels, we expected most of these conversations to be about the usual business topics, like customer satisfaction and foreign competition. These subjects certainly did come up, along with plenty of questions on strategy and leadership. Much to our surprise, however, the people we interviewed wanted passionately to know whether or not they were in the right job in the first place. They yearned for a way to understand who and what they were meant to be in life.

The question of who and what to be is profound, huge in its impact, and by no means limited to the young. Yes, plenty of recent college grads and MBAs we encountered wanted to know how to find the perfect job. But we also heard the "when I grow up" question from executives with jobs that looked, from the outside, to be ideal in every way. We heard it from people who had been running their own companies for decades.

And we heard it—especially—from women in their 30s and 40s who had been working feverishly for years, both at the office and at home, only to find themselves not exactly where they had hoped to be when they set out, all those years ago, to conquer the world.

Their stories were often told with poignant acceptance, but sometimes with deep sadness and confusion. How could they have run so hard and so fast for so long and ended up nowhere near where they wanted to go?

This phenomenon was so common that Jack and I gave it a name: the Everyone's Happy But Me Syndrome.

Women in this situation had arranged their days to be "good enough" at work and "there enough" at home but found they were living in a kind of purgatory, waiting for a time when their own dreams and needs could be met. They didn't dare ask any of the five questions on the previous page—the answers would have revealed a big, aching emptiness in the center of their lives.

Some of the women we met during our travels broke out of the Everyone's Happy But Me Syndrome and found fulfilling careers after a major personal crisis. There was a neurosurgeon in Virginia who admitted to herself, at age 40, that she had gone into medicine only to please her parents. That was the easy part. To realize her authentic life dream—she had always wanted to be a portrait photographer—she had to ask her husband to change his job to make up for the substantial loss of income. He made the sacrifice willingly, the woman told us, "but to be honest, I know he misses his old company and his friends there, and that has left a little hole in our relationship." Gone, too, are the vacations the family used to love. Yet, she said, "everyone in the family is happy that I am finally happy. They wouldn't go back, and neither would I."

In Detroit we met a woman who'd spent 14 years at a prestigious international accounting firm but at age 45 found she just couldn't bring herself to go to the office another day. "For one week, I stayed in bed and cried," she said. "I realized I was working to pay the mortgage on a beautiful house. The job bored me,

"You can figure out what you want to be when you grow up. You just have to be very grown up to do it."

and my life was passing by. That Friday I sent my resignation by e-mail." She sold her house, ended a long-term relationship with a coworker who opposed her decision, and took a job teaching in an inner-city elementary school. "The first year was hell," she told us. "Teaching was not the fantasy I had imagined. The kids were hard on me; I was raw and inexperienced. I missed my boyfriend a lot. I even missed my house. A day didn't go by when I didn't wonder if I'd lost my mind." She stuck it out and today runs a charter school for immigrant children in another city. "My work finally feels important," she said. "It took a while, but I have no regrets."

These women turned their lives upside down to be what they wanted to be; their journeys weren't just bumpy, they were tumultuous and painful for themselves and their families.

That kind of pain, we came to see during our research, was avoided by a small number of women who, along the long road of their careers, never stopped asking themselves the five questions. And once they uncovered the answers, they had the courage to adjust accordingly, moving to another job or field. Some changes were small, others large—but they all moved the women toward the job they were meant to have. And that is how the journey goes.

Let's look at the questions in a bit more detail.

DOES THIS JOB ALLOW ME TO BE WITH "MY PEOPLE"? I will never forget a happy firecracker of a woman we met in Florida who told us, "When I graduated from college, all I knew was I wanted a job—any job—where I could wear high heels and carry a briefcase! For a country girl like me, that meant you'd made something of yourself." She threw herself into nabbing a position as a junior analyst with a buttoned-down New York consulting firm. The "marriage" lasted exactly two years. "It was torture," she recalled. "No one laughed at what I laughed at. No one thought it was okay to argue now and then if you needed to get some issues on the table. No one even enjoyed the same kind of music or TV shows I did. I'm not saying it was a bad place; it just wasn't my kind of place."

This woman zigged and zagged through three more careers before she ultimately found success and fulfillment in the world of (believe it or not) aquarium administration. She wears a T-shirt, shorts, and flip-flops to work and hasn't owned a briefcase for 20 years. Most important, she says, "I love the folks I work with. We agree about what matters—I mean, we just see the world in the same way."

The facts are: No job or profession will ultimately be right if it requires you to work with people who don't share your sensibilities. If you are a brainy introvert, you should work with brainy introverts. If you are a boisterous extrovert, find a profession where that's embraced as the norm. You spend most of your life with your colleagues. You have to like them—and feel and act real around them—if you are going to be what you want when you grow up.

DOES THIS JOB MAKE ME SMARTER? Some people gravitate toward certain professions simply because they are good at them. Women who excel in English in college become editors. Women who love children become teachers. Women who can crunch numbers with the best of them go to Wall Street. This feels very natural, and, to be blunt about it, companies love the deal, too. After all, they want nothing more than to hire a candidate who comes fully equipped for the job.

Now, doing what you're good at is not a bad thing, except that it can eventually lead you down a garden path to...utter boredom.

In our research, we found that the women who most successfully navigated themselves toward the right job in the right profession kept looking for work that required them to learn, stretch, and grow. In fact, the women who loved their jobs the most were those who told us that their work always seemed just a little bit challenging all the time.

DOES THIS JOB OPEN THE DOOR TO FUTURE JOBS? Until you have found your perfect job in your perfect profession, you can't stop thinking about next steps. This question requires you to coolly assess whether your current job—or one you are considering—is a launching pad for the next, better one.

How can you keep your options open? The best way is to work for a company with a strong national "brand"—hundreds and hundreds of companies are in this category—or for an organization with a great reputation locally. One woman we met in Southern California parlayed her low-level job at a well-known regional bank into a managerial job in her state's treasury department. "I was trusted walking in the door for the interview," she said. "The bank gave me a kind of halo."

Job halos are like little angels; they help a lot when a journey is long.

DOES THIS JOB REPRESENT A CONSIDERABLE COMPROMISE FOR MY FAMILY'S SAKE? This question is tough; it forces you to confront just how long it might be before you find the career you've been waiting for.

Almost ten years ago, I took a job—as an editor at the *Harvard Business Review (HBR)*—in large part because it wouldn't require me to travel.

It was quite a change. For years I had been a management consultant, and I loved it. The work was fascinating and the people at my firm were kindred spirits, but I was often away three days a week on business, and even when I wasn't traveling, I worked long hours.

I had three children and was pregnant with my fourth when the *HBR* job came up. My family needed me home, especially since my husband at the time, the family's main wage earner, also traveled extensively.

I made the trade-off. I'm not saying I didn't like my job—I enjoyed many aspects of the work. But *HBR* was a nonprofit monthly magazine, and I never stopped missing the fast-paced excitement of the competitive business marketplace.

Still, I would make that choice again. Sometimes you have to take or keep a job because the people who love you need you to. Eventually, though, circumstances change. Your kids grow up. Your husband gets more flexibility in his job. Your older sister steps in to care for your mother. When the moment arrives and you can stop compromising your own dream, seize it.

FINALLY: DOES THE JOB—THE STUFF I DO EVERY DAY—TOUCH MY HEART AND FEED MY SOUL? This is, in the end, the most important thing you need to ask yourself. Very simply, you will never be what you were meant to be if you aren't having fun.

The perfect job is perfect because it makes you happy inside. Something about it—the thrill of making a big sale or making something work just right for your customers, the camaraderie of hitting a deadline with your colleagues, the reward of coaching new employees—turns your crank. Your work matters to you, and, on a visceral level, it just delights your soul.

The answer to this question is a feeling—a feeling of excitement and sense of meaning. When that's what's going on inside, you know you've finally reached your destination.

It's almost never where you expected it to be.

Remember my friend in the Midwest? As a girl, she dreamed, albeit briefly, of being a surgeon like her father. She also imagined writing poetry and becoming a social worker. She had no idea the best job for her was helping teenagers reach their dreams—until she was doing it.

I met a woman recently who, as the head of development for a state college with 10,000 students, raises millions of dollars a year to fund buildings and scholarships. She has her tough days, but when I asked if there was something else she would rather be doing, she gasped. "This is the perfect job," she said. "I literally couldn't do anything else. I'd miss it too much!"

Fund-raising—and loving it—is just about the last thing she imagined she'd be doing when she began her career 25 years ago. She was the only daughter in a traditional Irish family; her parents mortgaged their home to send her four brothers to college. After secretarial school, she landed a job as a bank teller. She might have stayed at the bank forever, she says, if she hadn't needed to get out of town when her husband began physically abusing her. A bitter divorce left her broke, and so she quickly became a licensed nurse practitioner. "All I knew was that I could get a job as a licensed practical nurse," she recalls.

Four years later, needing more income, she went back to school at night to become a registered nurse. It was there that she took a class in communications and loved it. When she graduated, she found an entry-level position in public relations. That job led to several more jobs and promotions in the PR field, which led to a job as a legislative aide to a congressman, which prepared her perfectly for her current job.

"Looking back now," she told me, "I think, *How sad that all those early years as a bank teller and a nurse were wasted.* But then I realize they really weren't. I couldn't have gotten here if I hadn't been there. I learned something about myself and about work every step of the way."

And that's the key, ultimately—learning. To find your perfect job, you have to relentlessly gather the lessons of the journey.

Just keep asking questions. Does this job allow me to be myself? Does it make me smarter? Does it open doors? Does it represent a compromise I accept? Does it touch my inner being?

If you listen closely enough, with time, patience, and the courage to act, the answers will lead you to the very place you were always meant to be—when you finally grow up. ◐

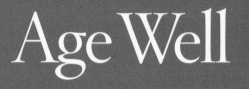

Age Well

Age Brilliantly, Beautifully, Happily

BY VALERIE MONROE

Has it happened to you yet? Because it will. You wake up one morning, rested and calm and deliciously comfortable, and then, as you open your eyes, raising your arms for one last, deep, luxurious stretch, you notice—*what? what's that? what?*—the skin on the insides of your elbows looks frighteningly...loose.

Blinking hard, you'll look again: Damn, loose! *Waaait a minute,* you'll want to say, as if Mother Nature, sly girl, has pulled a fast one on you. But the hand on your alarm clock will tick inexorably from 8:04 to 8:05, and when you arise from your bed, it will be in a different body from the one you went to sleep in.

It sounds a little like a horror movie, doesn't it? That's because in some ways, it is. The sagging skin, the thinning hair and bones, the decrepitude—what one friend calls the ick factor—it's hard to believe that's ever going to happen to robust, fructiferous you. Until it does. Then: *Booga! Booga!* You're old.

Or at least getting there. And there's no going back; not ever. Maybe that's the scariest part, abandoning the hope that you can stop the aging process, reverse it, avoid it. But that abandonment is exactly where the happy ending lies. In her book *When Things Fall Apart,* Buddhist nun Pema Chödrön quotes one of her teacher's remarks about life: It's like getting into a boat that's just about to sail out to sea and sink. There are no life rafts, no floats; no one gets out alive. Rather than try to ward off the inevitable, why not accept it and enjoy the trip?

Easier said than done, you say? Maybe, but it's more possible now than ever. Both physical and social science studies show that aging is not simply a process of decay but also one of growth. For example, though it was once believed the brain was incapable of generating new cells throughout life, researchers have recently found that, at least in some areas, regeneration does occur; and that staying mentally active can cause the brain to sprout new connections between nerve cells. George Vaillant, MD, professor of psychiatry at Harvard Medical School and director of the Harvard Study of Adult Development, reports in his book *Aging Well* that studies using brain imaging techniques of healthy octogenarians and nonagenarians suggest that normal brain shrinkage is less than originally thought, and that much of cell loss is a kind of selective "pruning." In researching wisdom at the Max Planck Institute for Human Development in Berlin, Paul Baltes, PhD, codirector of the institute, found that people can gain wisdom as they age if they think about the how and why of events

(understanding them in context rather than thinking of them as good or bad) and remain open to new experiences. And studies of cognitive functioning among older people have found differences in fluid intelligence (the ability to quickly use new information) and crystallized intelligence (the ability to use information accumulated from past experience). Fluid intelligence declines with age, but crystallized intelligence increases into your 60s; Vaillant believes it can often be as sharp at 80 as at 30. (That's why it might be easier as you get older to finish a crossword puzzle than to figure out how to use a new cell phone.) Then, of course, there's always the misperception that the older you get, the frailer and sicker you get, but think about that: The older you get, obviously the healthier you've been.

A cornerstone of aging brilliantly is "generativity," the term psychologist Erik Erikson used to describe a solution to the adult crisis in middle age. It means, basically, continuing to be productive and creative, and passing along what you've learned in a way that supports the generation following you. Though having children is perhaps the most fundamental way to ensure generativity, it's also available through meaningful work. Work keeps you socially connected, and a study from the Harvard School of Public Health indicates that staying connected may be as powerful a link to healthy aging as exercise.

> The best news of all is that how we age is largely in our control, less a product of our genes than of how we take care of ourselves.

The best news of all is that how we age is largely in our control, less a product of our genes than of how we take care of ourselves. Vaillant names seven predictors of healthy aging: being a non-smoker or stopping young, not abusing alcohol (defined as a dependence on alcohol), a stable marriage, more than 12 years of education, healthy weight, regular exercise, and mature defenses (practical coping strategies). Also critical are a network of intimate friends, healing relationships, knowing how to play, and subjective good health (meaning that you may have an illness or a potentially debilitating condition, but you don't actually feel sick). The six things that—surprisingly—do *not* predict healthy aging are ancestral longevity, parental characteristics, childhood temperament, sociability, cholesterol levels, and stress. It might also surprise you to know that the old are less depressed than the general population, Vaillant reports, and the majority don't suffer from incapacitating illness till the one that gets them for good.

That boat can give you a devastatingly beautiful trip on exquisite and enchanting seas. Age brilliantly? Yes! Let the band play on, with vigor and alacrity and joy, till the whole thing goes under with a shudder and a sigh, slipping valiantly into the deep. ⬛

The Rise and Fall of My Bosom

They've gone from newish (and basically nonexistent) to oldish and worth their weight in gold. A brief history of CATHERINE NEWMAN'S breasts.

1968

Brand-new, they are as pearly pink as buttons on a satin blouse. They sing the song of girl flesh in such a clear voice, you can hardly imagine that one day they'll be the mammary equivalent of Katharine Hepburn calling the loons on Golden Pond.

1975

I smile from the Polaroid snapshot, missing four front teeth and a shirt. My brown bell-bottoms are era-specific, but my brown torso is the icon of carefree childhood. It is punctuated by a sideways colon: The bosom's duties will come, these two polka dots promise, but later.

1979

"Vat?" my Russian grandmother asks—rhetorically—when I arrive for dinner every week. "No boozems yet?" She runs her hand across my chest: It is a book written in Braille, and all the pages are blank. Her own bosom juts out in front of her like a pot roast on a platter. It always reminds me of meat. When I first hear the expression "rack," I think of her and mentally add "of lamb."

Even a perfect pair can't escape the laws of deflation.

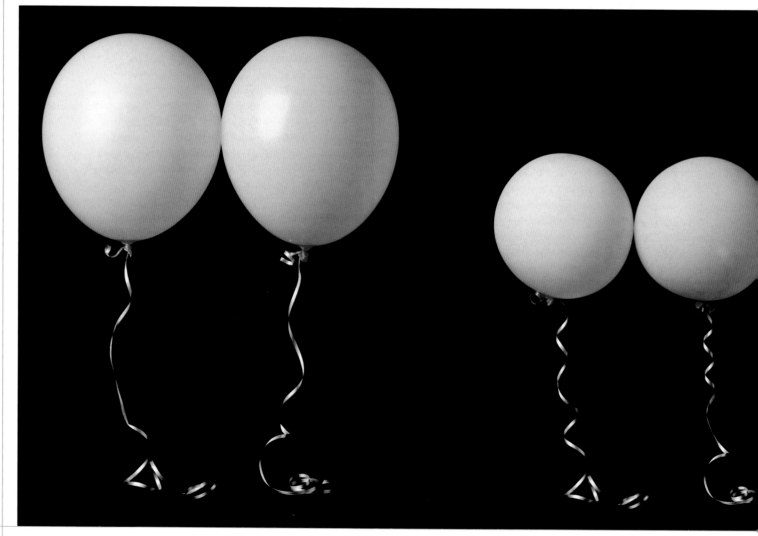

1981

My discreet, optimistic mother takes me to Macy's to buy a satin Gunne Sax blouse and also a brassiere. Can you train something that doesn't exist? This is a philosophical conundrum nobody poses aloud. The bra's cups sit as empty and begging on my chest as alms bowls.

1984

They finally arrive, more impatiently awaited than a mail-order whoopee cushion, and suffer immediate indignities. The sleep-away camp boyfriend—sweet and, later, gay—presses a curious finger to one the way you might check a roast turkey for done-ness. Others grope after them as though they're eggs hidden in a lawn on Easter. The bra's poor clasp! Isn't there an episode of the old TV cartoon *Magilla Gorilla* where he tries to pick the lock of a bank vault with his thick, primate fingers? It's like that.

1986

True young love, and my breasts are stars, my body shining like a constellation I've never even noticed before. It is a revelation of twinkling, currents running from top to bottom as if some hedonistic electrician has rewired me for pleasure.

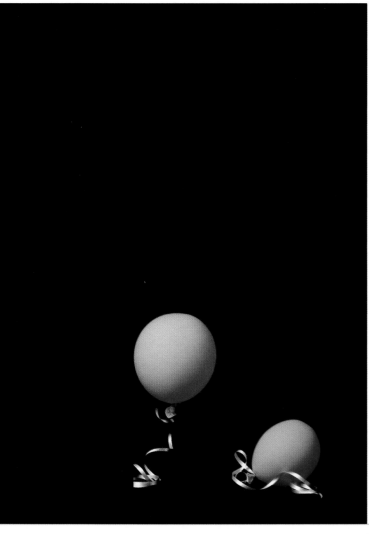

1992

So many disguises: the flattening of athletic support, the bosom like a loaf of Wonder Bread at the bottom of the grocery bag; the peekaboo-I-see-you of black mesh; the bra-framed shine of cleavage over a pool table, a textbook, a houseplant, a frozen margarita, a purring cat, a man. The breasts are upright, if occasionally trampy, citizens of many worlds.

1998

B cup, C cup, D cup. The pregnant bosom swells and threatens to escape, like an overinflated Mighty Mouse helium balloon straining at its tethers in a windy Thanksgiving parade.

1999

You know those early Renaissance paintings where the nursling Jesus perches on Mary's biceps like a miniature old man, suckling from what looks like half a grapefruit sticking out of her neck? Nursing turns out to be nothing like that. Milk sprays from the spigots of my body as urgently as water from a hydrant. My enormous bosom treats the baby like a little pet: It cuddles and feeds him, and he always greets it, panting, as if he thought he'd never see it again. I play voyeur to the milky landscape of their romance: pink moon of cheek, pink mountain of breast, eyelids closing under the dark nightfall of lashes.

2003

Shadows become lumps, and two of my friends are diagnosed, staged, and treated. They suffer unimaginably, and then, through amazing grace, are healthy again. Now their bodies are like living rooms with the big armchairs taken out, only instead of faltering over where to sit, you just notice how beautiful the light is.

2004

My youngest child is newly weaned, and my breasts hang down like banana peels with the bananas all eaten up already. I'm a tube of toothpaste, flat and rolled-up from the bottom, even though just yesterday I was dispensing long, pearly ribbons of paste.

2005

It's like the morning after the party. The balloons have lost their helium and drifted—puckered and loose—down to the floor. In a misguided attempt at festivity, my nipples sprout dark, wiry hairs.

2006

Mine are the brown zipper pulls on an empty leather bag, and now it's my little daughter's silky chest that's graced with the rosy snaps. When I bend over to dry her after our bath, her eyes go wide. "Your nursings are so long," she says, and I laugh. I'm a pair of windsocks hanging in the breezeless afternoon of early middle age, and even though I've loved the wild weather—the swells and the gusts and the changing direction—I don't mind this droopy stillness. Or rather I mind only sometimes. But when he peels me out of a T-shirt, my husband still whispers "Gazongas!" and he's half-teasing, but only half. Because the twinkling is still there—and that's no joke. **O**

RACHEL NAOMI REMEN: "I have to laugh. My life experience is that people with children are often alone in old age. Having children is not a safety hedge. I have friends with three or four kids who live around the country. These friends end up with a couple of phone calls a week, if that. They're often alone in the same way that women who are married might still feel alone. The fact is that everything is impermanent. I think the people who have connected only to their families may be more vulnerable than those who connect more broadly. We need to learn how to be alone. You do that by developing depth within yourself, interests that are yours, a connection to something larger than yourself. You develop your own sense of the meaning of life. Having children is no insurance policy."

"I'm worried about losing my looks and feeling the pressure to have plastic surgery."

DR. MAYA ANGELOU, *77, acclaimed poet and author of* I Know Why the Caged Bird Sings: "The surface, the superficial, the way one looks has become valued too highly in our society. When the skin begins to sag, many women go for Botox. Why on earth would you let somebody stick a needle in your face just to get rid of a wrinkle? Here's the real question: What do we have to do to place more value on age? We have to value ourselves not for what we look like or the things we possess but for the women we are.

"The most important thing I can tell you about aging is this: If you really feel that you want to have an off-the-shoulder blouse and some big beads and thong sandals and a dirndl skirt and a magnolia in your hair, do it. Even if you're wrinkled."

JOAN HAMBURG, *radio host of* The Joan Hamburg Show, *WOR Radio in New York:* "Would I have a facelift? No. I'm sure I'd be the one whose nose would end up on my boobs! I might be the only person in America who feels that way. I just came back from a 60th-birthday party, and I said to my husband, 'My God, I'm going to be the oldest living human being. Look at these women—they're all sucked and pulled and tucked.' But you can tell. In my head, I'm still 20. Yes, my body could use a zipper, but that's okay with me. When I get up in the morning, I look at all my parts and I think, *This is good. This is good.*"

BARBARA EHRENREICH, *64, political essayist, social critic, and author of* Nickel and Dimed: "I've had fears about my body changing, and I've dealt with that

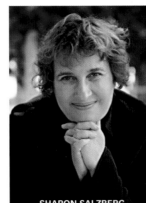

SHARON SALZBERG

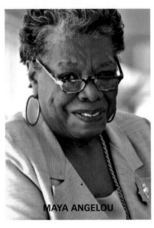

MAYA ANGELOU

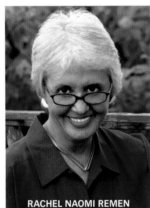

RACHEL NAOMI REMEN

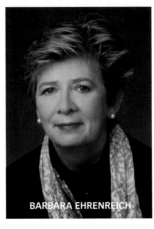

BARBARA EHRENREICH

by becoming kind of a jock. During my early 40s, I developed terrible back problems. I thought, *This is just a completely downward trajectory unless I change my life.* So a friend dragged me to a gym—I had always disdained fitness as a yuppie obsession. But once I began, I thought, *This is great.* I'm actually much stronger and more fit now than I was 20 years ago."

ELIZABETH LESSER, *52, cofounder and senior adviser of the Omega Institute:* "I've realized that aging is the younger cousin of dying. Is my face sagging? Is my body creaking? These questions just bring up the ultimate one: How much time do I have left? We become aware that we're on the downside of the mountain, coasting toward our final days. I was with my mother as she was dying last year, and I became aware that yes, indeed, it's true: Each one of us does have a short time on earth. The wrinkles and the double chin are smoke screens for what we're really afraid of—mortality. I happen to believe that our souls continue after we're gone, and that makes life on earth less fearful. We're here for a reason, and challenges are handed to us so we can grow and become more of who we're meant to be. So I deal with my fear of aging and death by making it my spiritual practice. Not turning away from it, not pretending it doesn't exist, not slapping on a cosmetic Band-Aid. But by taking on a more fearless attitude toward what really is happening to my body and my life."

"I dread the feeling of becoming invisible. What if I never have sex again?"

ABIGAIL THOMAS, *63, fiction and autobiographical writer and author of* Safekeeping: "I wouldn't even go back to as young as I was yesterday. Being this age is completely freeing. To walk out of the house without wondering who's looking back at you makes it possible to focus on what you really want to focus on. It makes it possible to get your work done. For a long time, all I thought about was, Who's looking at me? Who's interested? I didn't even really look at what I felt like looking at on the street. That's what I called sexual power. About ten years ago, exactly what I'd feared came to be: My 'sexual power' changed. For so long, how I looked represented everything to me: who I was as a woman, my power, how I could engage. When it was over, I discovered so many other things. I began to write. I started to see that I wasn't at the world's disposal—I call the shots, and what I'm interested in is what I'm interested in. One day in my 50s, I just woke up and realized I really didn't care about any of the rest of it and hadn't for quite a while. The heat was gone, and what replaced it was an avid desire for life."

MAYA ANGELOU: "At 50 I began to know who I was. It was like waking up to myself."

> "We've got to get in the habit of constantly learning something new."
> — *Joan Hamburg*

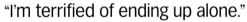

"I'm terrified of ending up alone."

FLORENCE FALK, PhD, *psychotherapist and author of* On My Own: "Historically and prehistorically, women have existed in a context in which, because they bore children, they stayed together while the men were out hunting. So in terms of our collective unconscious, we have a history of being in some kind of connection with other people. We've been nurturers in an earthbound role, so it's difficult for our psyches to contemplate anything else. What's it like not to be tethered with the responsibility of a mate and children? We haven't had a template for that. Of course, it's a human reflex to want to be connected to others. But for women, we expect the connection to make us feel more realized, whole, alive. This is where many women get caught: wanting to be in connection but at the same time resenting it."

"What if I leave my jerk husband but find myself too broke to survive on my own?"

ELIZABETH LESSER: "I've gone through a divorce and the terror of leaving a marriage. I know what it's like to feel stuck in something that is draining your life force, to stay because you're afraid of what's on the other side, especially financially. Helen Keller has become one of my heroes. She was blind, deaf, and mute, and you'd think she'd sit cowering in a corner. Yet this is what she once said: 'Security...does not exist in nature, nor do the children of men as a whole experience it. Avoiding danger is no safer in the long run than outright exposure. Life is either a daring adventure or nothing.' I often think, *If she could live life as a daring*

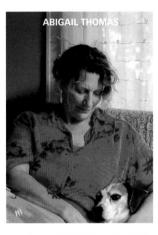

ABIGAIL THOMAS

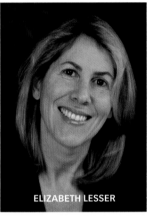

ELIZABETH LESSER

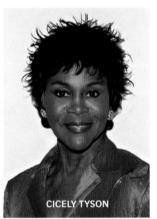

CICELY TYSON

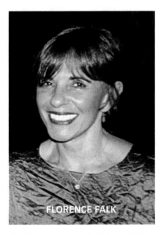

FLORENCE FALK

adventure, then any of us can. I used that when I finally made the decision as a 32-year-old mother to become a single parent and to leave a marriage that had been difficult for 14 years. It was about going for quality of life as opposed to security. It's not just in marriages that this decision is required. It's in everything—your job, where you live, how you relate to people. Much of the time, choosing security isn't a good idea."

JOAN BORYSENKO, PhD, *59, cofounder of the Mind-Body clinical programs at two Harvard Medical School teaching hospitals and author of* Minding the Body, Mending the Mind *and* Inner Peace for Busy People: "I've left a couple of husbands, and here's what I've learned: If you cannot support yourself, you set yourself up to be a prisoner. We can't stay home like June Cleaver and expect a man to take care of us financially. The world doesn't work that way anymore."

JOAN HAMBURG: "Even some of the smartest married women don't know their financial standing. I once talked to a bunch of women at a bank in Staten Island, and I asked, 'Do you know what's in your husband's will? Do you know where his papers are? Do you even know what you're worth?' Not one woman knew. The truth is that we're very complacent when it comes to seizing control of our finances. It's part of that old syndrome: Be the best girl possible, make people happy, and Daddy's going to take care of you. That's over. For women, dealing with money doesn't seem graceful. Many see it as sort of embarrassing to know about money. It's time for us to step right up to the plate and learn. One reason women are so totally unprepared for the financial devastation that can come after a divorce is that they have no clue how to handle their money."

"I'm anxious about the burden of caring for aging relatives."

CICELY TYSON, *actress, most recently in* Diary of a Mad Black Woman: "I've cared for my mother, my father, my sister, my brother. I've lost everyone in my immediate family. And when you're faced with those situations, despite the fact that you feel, *Oh, God, if it ever happens to me, I won't be able to handle it,* you don't know how you'll actually respond until you're in the circumstance. I never anticipated that I'd be the sole surviving member of my family. And I found that when the time came, I did what I had to do. I think all human beings would do the same thing."

Making Friends
with Your Money

The Anxious Woman's Guide to Financial Serenity

ANNE LAMOTT'S been rich and she's been poor, and frankly, she's uncomfortable both ways. A self-confessed money neurotic talks about guilt, envy, fear of being envied, why we allow money or the lack of it to define us, and how to buy a little peace of mind.

Yesterday my son and I were at an airport heading back after our annual visit with his father. I did not have any cash on me to pay for our cab home, so I went to the ATM and tried to withdraw some money. It said my request had been denied, even though I knew I had plenty in my checking account. And it did not occur to me for a second that there was some dumb and benevolent explanation. No, I instantly believed that all my money had been stolen or that my bank had failed or that I was the victim of identity theft, and that my savings and my IRA were gone, too. Kaput. Game over. Fini.

Two weeks before, I had received a letter from the IRS and found myself at the mailbox staring ahead like someone needing the Heimlich maneuver. It did not help that most previous letters from the IRS have been envelopes for my quarterly payments or notices that I had underpaid by $17.34. What an envelope from the IRS means is, Arrest! Liens!

I've done so much healing and restoration in so many areas of my life—around relationships, my body, my sexuality, mothering, daughtering—but this business of financial reality makes all that look easy. Sometimes I feel like I'm trying to put an octopus to bed. As soon as you think you have those other arms tucked in nicely under the sheets, the money arm pops out from under the blankets and flails around.

I am terrified of not having enough, of losing what I have, and of having more than enough—an unfair amount and advantage over most people I know, who do not have enough. I am afraid of all the people I love going broke and needing to come live with me, or of having to bail them all out and thereby losing everything I have and having to go live at the Rescue Mission, which I am not remotely stable enough for.

I am afraid that after the next terrorist attack, I will be worthless because I did not convert my savings into one-ounce gold Krugerrands and store them under a floorboard. I'm afraid when I am doing well financially that everyone secretly hates me, and when I have been struggling that people think I'm a loser. I'm afraid because I used to always say, "If you want to know how God feels about money, look at whom She gives it to"—but now I have some money. It's probably true that everything I enjoy is acquired on the backs of people in sweatshops or with black lung disease. So should I switch to hemp clothing, wood-burning

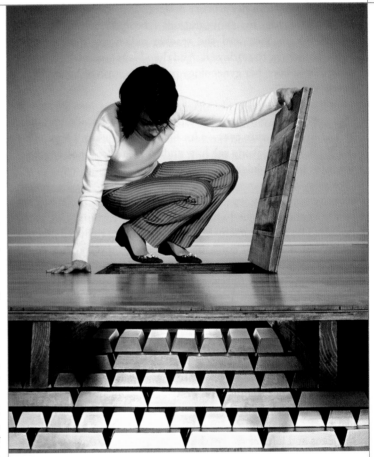

stoves, tempeh chocolates from Berkeley?

I just want to say, I come by this neurosis about money honestly.

My parents had terrible problems economically from birth. My mother was born poor in Liverpool; my father was born to pleasure-denying missionaries in Tokyo. So they were both a little anxious financially.

We lived in a stone castle in Marin County my parents bought for $20,000 in 1960, when I was 6, and there was never quite enough money. During a particularly stressful financial time, when we had to have all the 100-year-old floors torn up, my mother dealt with the tension by charging a Persian rug. When that did not bring her lasting security and self-esteem, she charged two Louis XIV–style chandeliers.

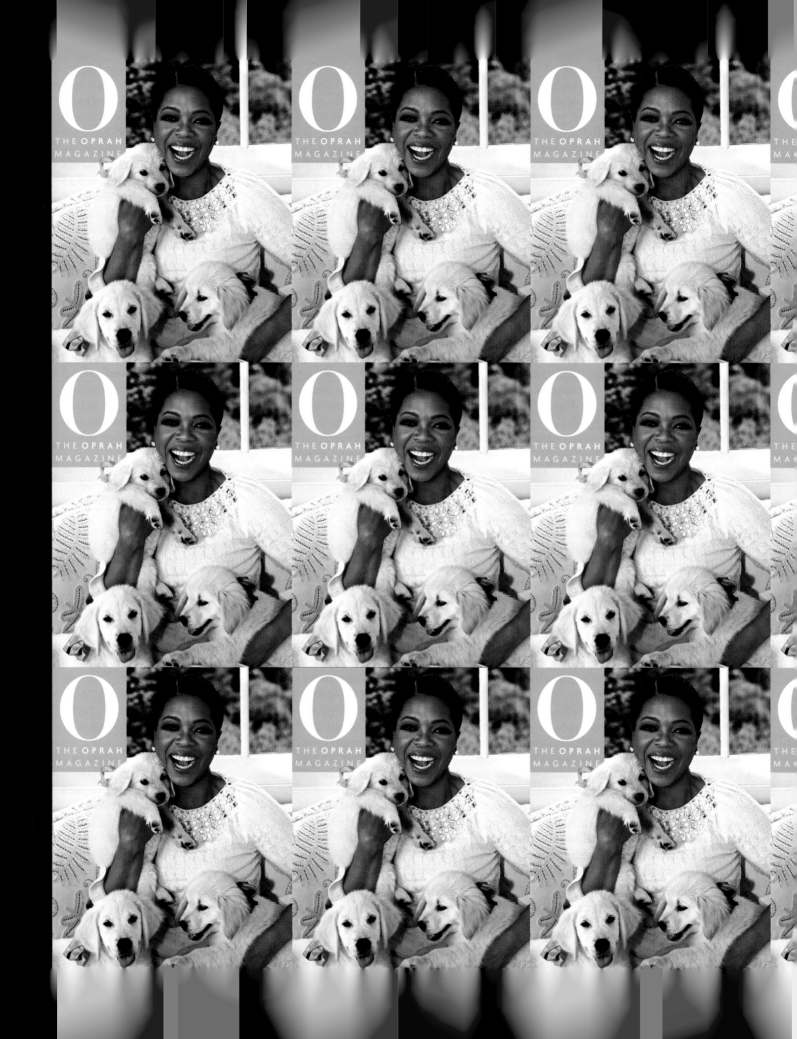

Relationships

The people in your life soothe you, replenish you, remind you why you're here—and sometimes drive you completely around the bend. Here's advice for every parent, sibling, daughter, friend, partner.

Couples

The Love Breakthrough

"I'm right; you're wrong." "You never check in with me first." "You ignore me in public."
News flash: These ordinary little annoyances are potentially ruinous for 80 percent of couples.
Is there any way to stop the downward spiral? Couples therapist BRENT ATKINSON, PhD,
argues yes, but first you'll have to do the one thing that's hardest for you....

Somebody please get me out of here! Grace had to check to be sure that she hadn't actually blurted the words out loud. She'd come to this wedding reception as a favor to her husband, Adam, whose friend from high school was getting married. Adam was sitting at the main table, laughing and having a great time, while Grace was stuck listening to a plump, middle-aged woman chatter about her poodle. Grace thought, *This is the last place on earth I want to be right now.* She looked repeatedly in Adam's direction. Finally catching his eye, she motioned for him to come over. But Adam shook his head and mouthed "I can't!" *Bullshit,* thought Grace. She'd already seen other members of the wedding party leave the table to talk to their families. *This is so typical,* she thought. *He drags me here, then abandons me.*

After what seemed like an eternity, the dancing began. Grace's irritation yielded to a sense of anticipation as Adam smiled and began walking toward her. But he never made it across the room. He was intercepted by three friends who insisted that he go outside with them to smoke cigars. Adam held up one finger, signaling to Grace that he'd be there in a minute. Before she could register a protest, Adam disappeared out the door. Grace sat and stewed, planning what she would say to him when he returned. Ten minutes passed, then 20. After a half hour, she walked out of the reception, got in their car, and went home. Adam eventually returned and searched for Grace. It dawned on him that she had left. He called her cell phone, but she didn't pick up. He shook his head, muttered "What a baby!" and then went back to the party. At 4 o'clock in the morning, Adam slipped into the bedroom, grateful that Grace was sound asleep.

His eyes popped open at 9 A.M. to the sound of the coffee grinder. *Uh-oh,* he thought. *It's time to face the music.* He crept behind his wife and gave her a hug. She endured it silently until he gave up and released her. Playing dumb, Adam asked, "Why did you leave last night? I was looking for you." Grace rolled her eyes and replied, "Yeah, you were looking really hard, weren't you?" Her sarcasm let Adam know he was in the doghouse—a place he was all too familiar with.

Adam was still reeling from the abrupt change he'd seen in Grace since they'd gotten married three years before. Her independence was one of the things he had found most attractive about her, but as soon as they said "I do," she morphed into a demanding, controlling nag who constantly required his attention—or so

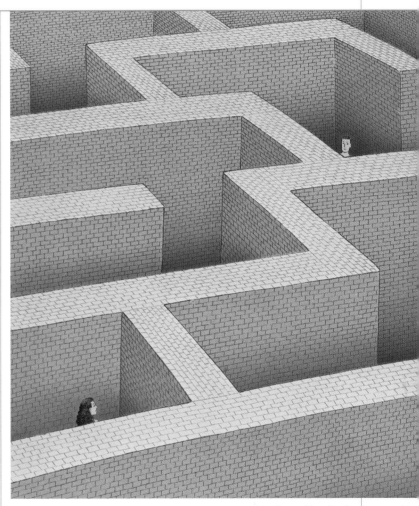

it seemed to him. Adam let out an exasperated sigh and backed away, thinking, *Here we go again.* They didn't speak for the remainder of the day or the following morning. In fact, when they came in for their therapy session three days later, they still hadn't spoken.

Most people believe that certain ways of behaving in relationships are correct and others are incorrect. This is true to some degree. We would probably all agree that physically assaulting one's partner is wrong. But marriage researchers have found that the vast majority of things couples argue about involve areas in which there is no evidence that one partner's standards are better or "healthier" than the other's.

Take selfishness—most of us think it's bad for relationships. The problem is that there are so many potentially legitimate yardsticks for measuring piggishness, and we tend to use our own, not our partner's. Grace believed that Adam's behavior at the reception was selfish—he was thinking only of himself. But Adam believed that Grace was the one who acted badly. He wouldn't dream of restricting her desire to be with her friends.

In my office, I explained to Grace that if she wanted to believe that Adam's actions were wrong, she had every right to. But in doing so, she'd be putting herself in the company of those who are destined to fail in their relationships. The choice was hers. I wouldn't try to stop her. But I could and did tell her that evidence from studies spearheaded by John Gottman at the University of Washington suggests that if Adam and Grace continue with their critical attitudes toward each other, the chances of their marriage surviving over the long haul are less than 20 percent.

I also explained that Adam's responses weren't any more effective than Grace's. He had made it clear that he thought Grace was overreacting and that her expectations were out of line, but Adam needed to know that beliefs like this are highly predictive of divorce. Partners who succeed in their relationships recognize that conflicts are not usually about right or wrong, they're about legitimately different expectations. I told Adam it was important he recognize that Grace's needs at the reception were just as legitimate as his.

I could see them struggling with this information. To Grace, dropping the idea that Adam was wrong would be like letting him off the hook. If he wasn't the bad guy, did she really have a right to be upset?

It's natural to feel agitated when your expectations are ignored, I explained, and she had every right to insist that Adam take her feelings into account. But Adam would be more able to do this if she could give up the idea that he did something wrong and instead explain to him how she felt. Once Grace realized her critical attitude was working against her, she saw the value in not blaming Adam. Instead she confessed that she felt unimportant to him and was afraid he cared more about his friends than her. This was a bold move on Grace's part, leaving her vulnerable. She braced herself for his response. But Adam's eyes softened immediately, and he offered an unsolicited apology, assuring her that he would try to be more sensitive to her feelings.

I wasn't surprised. I've spent 20 years as a marriage counselor, witnessing the profound rewards partners like Grace and Adam reap once they've adjusted their attitudes toward each other. The way our brains are wired, the most effective way to solicit understanding and cooperation is not by attempting to prove oneself right at the other's expense. It's by exposing vulnerability. This is a difficult adjustment for anyone to make when feeling threatened, but in relationships where an emotional bond exists, evidence suggests that our brains are set up to respond to vulnerability with empathy.

A week later, Adam and Grace sat sullenly on my couch. The day before, Grace had decided to surprise Adam by showing up at his office to take him out to lunch. Adam wasn't as pleased as Grace anticipated because he'd already planned a working lunch with a colleague who was helping him with a project. Reluctantly, he broke his plans and went out with Grace, but she was incensed by his attitude.

What happened here? The couple had experienced firsthand the enormous benefits of abandoning critical judgments of each other, yet less than seven days later, they were locked into the same defensive attitudes that had created the impasse at the reception.

Grace and Adam aren't unique. I've spent years patting myself on the back after helping couples experience heartfelt changes during therapy sessions, only to watch them show up the next week as miserable as ever.

Why do people so easily forget the lessons they pick up? Recent neuroscience studies suggest that new insights often don't last because they aren't integrated into the brain states that become active when the insights are most necessary. Finding a new way of thinking when we are calm doesn't necessarily transfer to moments when we're upset. When we feel threatened, our brains automatically kick in to modes designed for self-protection—not relationship bliss. During studies dating back to the 1950s involving electrical stimulation of the brain, researchers were able to see the moods, desires, and concerns of patients change dramatically. For example, upon stimulation of a specific region of the brain, a patient in a study conducted by Robert Heath at Tulane University threatened to kill the physician nearest him at the time. In a similar experiment, the patient couldn't explain why he was so sure he'd been wronged only a few moments earlier. He knew the electrical stimulation had made him feel angry, but when the self-protective mode in his brain was electrically activated, he trusted his perceptions more than logic.

Neuroscientist Joseph LeDoux at the Center for Neural Science at New York University has identified the neural mechanisms

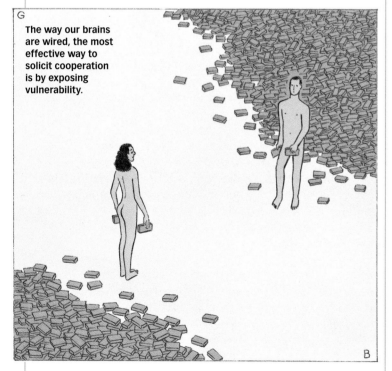

The way our brains are wired, the most effective way to solicit cooperation is by exposing vulnerability.

that help explain how this happens. Relying mostly on findings from studies on animals, LeDoux discovered that emotion has a privileged position of influence in the brain. His studies suggest that our brains are set up so that self-protective emotions can hijack the conscious mind for periods of time, driving us to act in ways that we may later regret. Although Grace left the previous therapy session armed with new knowledge about how to bring out the best in Adam, when he balked at going to lunch with her, Grace was seized by an impulse to criticize him. She couldn't apply the new way of thinking she'd learned the previous week because she was in an operating mode that was programmed for self-protection—not mutual understanding. When she questioned Adam's priorities, his walls went up immediately.

Fortunately, our brains are not only equipped for self-protection; we're also wired for love. Neuroscientist Jaak Panksepp and his colleagues at Bowling Green State University have found neural pathways for four specialized social brain states that produce feelings that draw us closer to those we love: One state produces a feeling of vulnerability and a longing for emotional contact, a second produces feelings of tenderness and urges to care for others, a third produces the urge for spontaneous and playful social contact, and a fourth activates sexual desire. While it's possible to engage in caring actions without the activation of these mood states, such actions often feel fake, lacking the heartfelt quality that gives them meaning. Caring acts are simply that: acts.

> Finding new ways of thinking when you're calm doesn't necessarily transfer to moments when you're upset.

When relationships are going well, the intimacy states are naturally active—and the feelings they produce are contagious. When one person is feeling sad, tender, playful, or lustful, it's easy for the other to feel something similar. For example, Panksepp has found that distress cries of young animals automatically activate the caretaking circuits of nearby adult animals. UCLA researcher Marco Iacoboni believes that this may be because of "mirror neurons" recently discovered in various areas of the brain. Mirror neurons allow us to feel what another person is experiencing. This is why we cry at the movies when we sense the emotions of the characters, even though we don't know them. Mirror neurons help our brains re-create the feelings inside ourselves, allowing us to be powerfully affected by others.

In our first session, when I helped Grace move from her critical stance to a more vulnerable place, I had bet on Adam's mirror neurons, and I wasn't disappointed. When she disclosed that she was feeling unimportant, Adam's brain automatically responded with tenderness.

Counseling can help clients like Grace and Adam develop the ability to shift from critical and defensive postures to more unguarded internal states. Nearly all neuroscience researchers agree on one thing: The mechanism through which the brain acquires new habits is repetition. One of the most enduring concepts in the field of neuroscience is Hebb's law, which states that when brain processes occur together over and over again, the connections between neurons involved are strengthened, so these processes are more likely to occur in conjunction in the future. I knew that if Grace and Adam could think differently *while* they were angered, and if they could do this enough times, the new thought processes would begin spontaneously every time they became annoyed with each other, and they'd stand a chance of eliminating their knee-jerk reactions. Rehearsing new thoughts alone would not do the trick. They'd have to practice new ways of thinking under game conditions—that is, when they were actually furious.

The problem was that when Grace and Adam fought, they seemed completely unable to avoid their usual interactions unless I was there to help them. Near the end of our second session, Adam remarked, "I wish we could take you home with us!" I replied, "Maybe you can." I made Adam and Grace each an audiotape that they promised to listen to every time they found themselves ready to smack the other upside the head. This isn't unusual; the way our brains work means most of us require outside input when we're enraged. Prerecorded audiotapes are a great way to get an unbiased perspective exactly when we need it.

Grace first used her audiotape just three days later. Without consulting her, Adam made arrangements to watch *Monday Night Football* at a friend's house. When he called Grace to tell her, she was miffed but shrugged it off. As the evening wore on, though, she was flooded by thoughts like *He was single so long that he doesn't know how to be in a relationship* and *This man is an emotional moron!*

She decided that maybe it would be a good idea to listen to the tape I'd made for her: "Grace, if you're listening to this, you're probably feeling that Adam has been inattentive or selfish in some way. It probably feels like he's ignoring your wishes. I'm making this tape because I want him to be as concerned about your needs as he is his own, and I won't be satisfied until he is." My words helped Grace relax somewhat, although she still felt angry. "Grace, remember in our last session how I was talking to you about the fact that 96 percent of the time, the likelihood that a person's partner will care about how she or he feels depends on the attitude that she or he has in the beginning moments of the conversation? Your attitude can have a powerful effect on Adam, even if he has a bad attitude to begin with. Right now you probably feel that Adam's actions or thinking is wrong or out of line in some way. If you enter the conversation with this attitude, you can kiss the chances of getting Adam to care about how you feel goodbye."

This statement infuriated Grace, and she turned the tape off. But after a few minutes, she decided to go back to it. "Grace, is it possible that if the roles were reversed, Adam wouldn't be as mad at you?" She had to admit that Adam wouldn't be bothered if she made plans without contacting him.

At 11 o'clock, Adam's car rolled into the garage. Grace took a deep breath and waited for him to come inside. As he walked

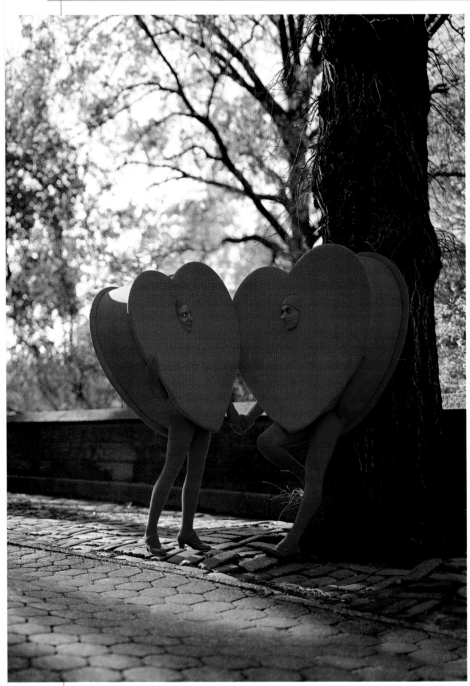

lighthearted to say. "Think of how much you'll save on hair gel!" No. "Hey, it works for Bruce Willis!" Oh, dear God, *no.*

This is the problem for most of us: We have no idea how to regroup after one of these little attacks. Both Goldstein and Miller suggest the best thing to do is to minimize embarrassment and change the subject. "Anyone want a second helping?" works, "How 'bout those Knicks?" is an old standby, or my personal favorite: "Who needs a refill on the wine?"

What's even more difficult than dealing with other people's cutting remarks can be recognizing when you're about to launch one of these covert missiles. If this behavior seems uncomfortably familiar—or if you've felt an uncomfortable pause descend after a spouse-targeted remark—Miller advises practicing a little mindfulness. Before you blurt out that your partner failed the bar (for, hey, the third time in a row), examine your motive. Is it to entertain? To shock? Are you mad about something he said or did earlier? If your partner made a similar remark about you, would you cringe? "Rather than being lost in a kind of automatic behavior," he says, "you've got to step outside yourself so you can catch yourself in the act."

I myself have been guilty of zinging. Once, at a family gathering, I was telling what I thought was a knee-slapping story of how my husband and I met: He had been terribly quiet but doggedly followed me around a party while I ignored him. I imitated his clumsy attempts at conversation, complete with stammering. "So, then, ah, wh-where are you, um, where are you from?" I stuttered, while my family chortled away.

Later he pulled me aside. "You're an outgoing person, so you think that shyness is charming," he said. "It's called 'painfully shy' for a reason."

Goldstein says he has a point. "You were trying to make yourself look good at his expense by showing that you were pursued and the life of the party," she says bluntly. And you know what? She's absolutely right. If we're starkly honest with ourselves, most of those little zings can be boiled down to the most childlike of impulses: "I was showing off" or "I was mad because she gets more attention" or "I know him better than anyone else."

Once I became aware that I was fricasseeing my husband for a few laughs, I stopped. It dawned on me that couples are privy to tender information about each other, and, as Goldstein says, a mate is supposed to protect that knowledge, not employ it as a joke or a bludgeon.

That's the ironic thing about those stealth humiliations. When someone needles her partner, her hope is that others will rally to her side. Remember my friend Janet, the one who said her husband got his jollies from phone sex? She did it expecting we'd all be clucking in sympathy. But when we were heading home that night, it wasn't his bad habit that we were talking about. ◘

Then there's the insensitive miscalculation, in which you breezily underestimate your partner's vulnerabilities. As an example, Goldstein offers her own husband, who told friends that it took her 45 minutes to scrape off her makeup at night. "I'm like, 'Excuse me. People aren't supposed to know I'm working hard at trying to look glamorous,'" she says.

That reminded me of a friend who recently announced that her husband was trying Rogaine, while he blushed to the roots of his rapidly retreating hairline. "Well, it's no big secret that you're going bald," she pointed out. During the hideous silence that followed, my husband examined the pattern on his napkin as if it contained a secret code, while I looked everywhere but at the poor schmo's high forehead and searched my brain for something

What Men Wish You Knew About Them

They laugh! They cry! They need to be alone! They want to be your hero! *O* asked some famously perceptive male writers, "If you could let women in on one secret about men, what would it be?"

THE HEROES INSIDE US

WALTER KIRN

This is the secret. This is the great truth.

We don't particularly value our own existences.

It starts around age 3 and never stops: the process of rehearsing all the ways in which we might gloriously die. We've barely been born when we start mock-perishing. The first time I bit the dust was in an ambush by three or four boys who'd armed themselves with sticks that were either machine guns or swords, I don't remember. Nor do I remember which force of evil I alone was resisting that fateful day when I first fell backward on the grass, clutched my heart, and let out the sigh that tells a man's foes that they may have killed his body but they'll never vanquish his spirit. I was only 5 years old, but the whole performance felt instinctive.

Women are encouraged to give life. Men are encouraged to give it up. The basic scenario, of course, involves standing up to the bad guys on behalf of some innocent person or high ideal. The other basic scenario involves being one of the bad guys—the baddest of all. Either way the ending is the same. We fall, we sigh, there's a pause, we get back up, and then the next day we pretend to die again.

We don't always die in combat. That's just one way. Sometimes we die from exposure or starvation while exploring the arctic or trekking through the jungle. Sometimes our rocket ship crashes en route to Mars or our race car hits a wall during the last lap of the Daytona 500. Sometimes the smoke inside the burning house that we've rushed into to rescue the little girl's kitten is just too thick and toxic to withstand. And sometimes we die from simple overwork while laboring selflessly to support our loved ones or save the ranch from bankruptcy.

What doesn't change is the satisfaction we take—in our fantasies, that is—at going down fighting, with our boots on.

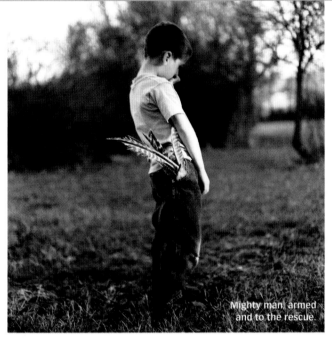

Mighty man, armed and to the rescue.

What also doesn't change is our suspicion that we might not be mourned as deeply as we imagine or honored for as long as we might hope. That stirs a certain resentment in some men.

Since kindergarten we've been demonstrating our willingness to die at practically any moment for virtually any cause, and the women who will outlive us don't appreciate it. Yes, today we're grouching about the phone bill or failing once again to mow the lawn, but tomorrow we may be out defending the homeland or pursuing an armed robber down a dark alley. Women shouldn't forget this. What looks like a husband napping on a sofa is really a hero of tomorrow dreaming of his own selfless demise.

The least a woman can do is let him sleep.

WHY WE CRY AT THE ODDEST TIMES

JONATHAN LETHEM

I'm going to try to put this as simply as I can: What women don't quite get about men—at least the men I'm qualified to speak for—is that we're pretty much constantly on the lookout for an opportunity to cry.

Or should I call it an excuse to cry? But look, that hesitation of mine—do I mean opportunity or excuse?—is probably itself a good example of the sorts of knots we men tie ourselves in as we negotiate this issue. See, we've got these tears rattling around inside us, tears that are the typical by-product of walking around alive and with our senses open on planet earth. Tears of loss, tears of joy, tears of empathy, and also those inexplicable epiphanic tears that signify our sudden apprehension that we're living beings clinging to one another in an endless sea of time and space, a fact that anyone may at any time find unexpectedly beautiful and sad.

But unlike the tears of the females with whom we share this planet, and to whom we cling, our tears largely refuse to emerge at the times when they're called for, traditional moments like weddings and funerals, moments of wonderful or terrible news arriving suddenly by telephone, and so on. And this is what the women must think: *You heartless jerks.* And for some strange reason, this is exactly why the tears have chosen to hide—so that we can get away with being mistaken for heartless jerks. The rickety construct that is the male self-image has a strong preference for being taken for heartless, rather than weepy. Go figure.

But that leaves the problem of those uncried tears, which are always plotting escape bids at unexpected moments when the patrol relaxes, much like the prisoners of war in a World War II movie. For me, my best chances, the best openings for my tears to flow, are certain moments during the watching of baseball games, mostly in the postseason (basketball or football, for whatever reason, doesn't cut it). Also certain songs by Bob Dylan, Willie Nelson, Al Green, and a handful of others. And, most reliable of all, certain movies. A great example being *The Great Escape,* starring Steve McQueen. Personally, that movie always leaves me wrecked, that moment when he tries to jump his motorcycle over the barbed-wire fence dividing Germany from Switzerland....

Also, one other thing: We read women's magazines, hoping to find out what women think of us, anytime we're left safely alone with one.

IT'S NOT ABOUT YOU
WILLIAM HENRY LEWIS

Some years back, I was a goalkeeper for a soccer club competing for a league title. We lost a key match. That evening my wife-to-be stopped by my place. She had in mind to share a beer, tend to my kicked shins, and massage the tension of the game from my shoulders; perhaps the day would give way to our sharing mushroom risotto, wine, and dessert between the sheets.

But I put all that on hold with a mumbled "I just want to be on my own tonight," which in my mind had everything to do with the awareness of my bad mood and nothing to do with not wanting to be with her, looking lovely and inviting in a white cotton sundress that caught the saffron shafts of late-day sun angling into my bedroom. But there she was, showered, scented, sundress beautiful.

She would tell me much later that my wanting to spend the evening alone sparked in her the possibility that I was not so interested in her. For a moment, she saw less of my blues and more of what she feared might be the typical commitment-phobic man's I-need-space maneuver. She is a woman with a big, open heart and thought to ask me what I felt about her.

I could have relieved her worries, but I just wanted quiet. Ever since I was 5, the two-headed soccer demon of euphoria and torment had burned in me so fiercely that any loss was bound to make me unhappy. At 36 my better-playing days were gone, and every new game was a stepping away from what I cherished as my manhood. It was not a good time to sip wine and rub noses. Being in my foul mood, I did not assuage her worries, and she did not leave me to be alone in that moment, to steep in my stoic and sullen solitude, like some pitiful Hemingway protagonist.

What we missed then was the opportunity to understand that I loved her like the sun that lit her dress, and given a later moment, we could talk about how my mood had nothing to do with her.

It wasn't about her.

It was about a man realizing the loss of his youth; it was about me feeling vulnerable, but, being male, not risking the words to reveal it. That interior male moment needed nothing more than a bit of time to see itself, but we engaged instead in a strained discussion about the relationship that was evolving. Some couples begin their ends attending to such ill-timed anxieties.

My wife and I look back on this as a moment of disconnect. From this looking back, we have a stronger sense

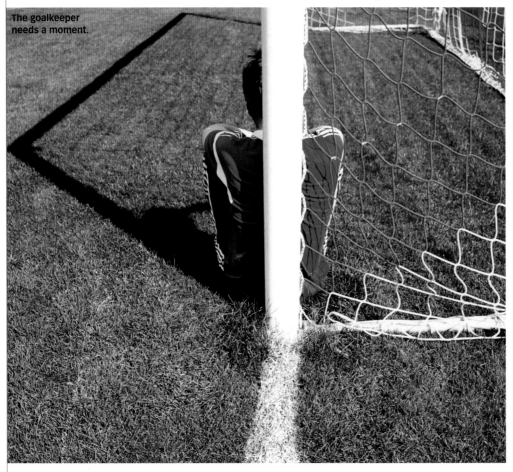

The goalkeeper needs a moment.

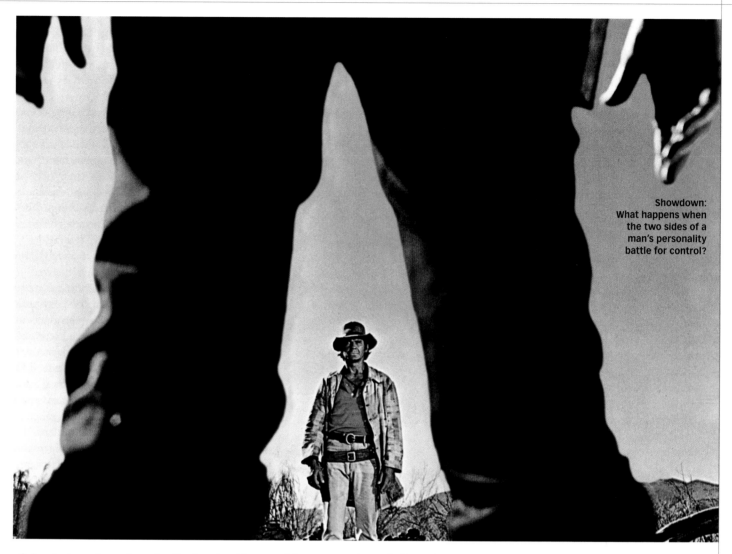

Showdown: What happens when the two sides of a man's personality battle for control?

of the timing of touch and talk that fortifies our life as great friends and lovers. Since then there have been many more games won and lost, many saffron-bright sunsets and risottos and, yes, many wonderful desserts.

WHY MEN GO NUTS

MARK LEYNER

The most fundamental way a woman can misunderstand a man—and the misunderstanding with the most far-reaching consequences— is to think that she can understand him at all, to think that she can even know who that person is lying beside her in bed or sitting across from her at some restaurant.

There's a terribly misleading myth in our culture that men— as psychological entities—are solid, unyielding, and immutable, and that, conversely, women are more fluid and amenable to change. Nothing could be further from the truth. Just look at old yearbook photos. There's Jane—student council president, literary magazine editor, varsity swim team, beaming with ebullient optimism and self-confidence. And now here's a photo of Jane in the business section of today's newspaper. Why, look, she's the CEO of some obscenely successful company. She hasn't changed

at all. She's the same old Jane—beaming with ebullient optimism and self-confidence. Let's peruse the yearbook again. There's Dick, president of the Chess Club, founder of the Origami Society, lettered in lacrosse.... Now look at that newspaper. Isn't that Dick's photo, accompanying the article "Deranged Psycho Goes on Shooting Spree in Upstate Mall"? Dick's changed.

Just this morning in *The New York Times* there was an article about Richard J. Roach, a blustery, hot-tempered Republican district attorney and vaunted antidrug zealot who would brag about the draconian sentences he'd wring from juries down there in Roberts County, Texas. And what became of this real-life Dick? He ended up dosing himself with Levitra and injecting methamphetamine in the presence of his office secretary (who was wearing a wire). Government officials had also been investigating him for pornography and weapons possession.

Roach's explanation? "I just sort of...went nuts."

Men are going nuts all the time. Men are in a perpetual state of repentance, rehabilitation, and recidivism. And I really don't think most women completely understand that.

There are such wildly contradictory impulses and exigencies tearing at American males that they are rent asunder and fragmented from boyhood on.

Marriage

Astonished by Love

Who knew that "in sickness" could do more to deepen a marriage than "in health" ever did? ELLEN TIEN reports on the bizarre, out-of-the-blue illness that rocked her world.

How?" I cried as my husband lifted and carried me into the hospital bathroom, stopping to hoist my dead weight with his knee, my inert body rolling, unpredictable and clumsy as melons in a sack. Arms dangled helplessly from my sides, someone else's arms. For a moment, midhoist, someone else's fingertips grazed the linoleum floor. "How can you bear to see me this way?" I asked as Will cradled and wiped and washed my paralyzed being and hauled me back to the bed. "How can you stand it?"

He laid a cool hand on my forehead, hot from the rage of corticosteroids that were rushing through my bloodstream in an attempt to bring my engorged spinal cord down to functioning dimension. "Ellen," he answered. I closed my eyes in the dark and leaned against the sound of my own name.

"I was paralyzed when I met you," he said, placing each word faceup, like a card, "and you made me whole. You showed me that it was all right to be happy. So if I have to do this every day for the rest of my life, I'll do it gladly, because you made me see that I could."

I was paralyzed when I met you.
When I met you.

But I get ahead of myself. Begin at the middle.

By all accounts, it was a fine marriage. Not, perhaps, a googoo-gaga, chase-me sort of marriage, but a fine one. Over 12 years, the number of long, moist embraces in corners and ravaged, yearning looks at breakfast certainly waned, replaced instead with trips to Whole Foods and updates on work and sharp kicks under the table when Will forgot he wasn't supposed to mention the time the hostess, a fashion editor, had suffered a nervous breakdown and shown up to an important editorial meeting in her pajamas and slippers.

It was fine, though. We were fine. It is possible that we each sensed, in ways both acute and distant, that there might be something more out there, something thrilling and transforming. But the journey between out there and in here is formidable, and it can be difficult to navigate one's way between those two points. So we persevered, maybe without as much yearning and embracing and moistness, but we persevered with perseverance, stolid and forward facing.

How?
How can you stand it?
Begin closer to the beginning.

> By all accounts, it was a fine marriage. Not a googoo-gaga, chase-me sort of marriage, but a fine one.

We were an unlikely couple and the likeliest couple on earth. William Betts Dana was a Connecticut-born Yankee with all the rules that this implies; Ellen Jean Tien was an overachieving daughter of Chinese immigrants, with all the breaking of rules that this entails. Will Dana struggled to communicate; Ellen Tien struggled not to. Will analyzed; Ellen intuited. He let things go; I clasped them close.

When he stumbled over words trying to convey how he felt, I laughed heartlessly at him and told him to stop communicating and intuiting—to get off my turf—and to just let go.

Although we had known of each other in the way that anyone who pays attention to mastheads or bylines feels a kinship to a name on a line, we officially met on a bitter winter night in 1991, at a party in a SoHo loft. He was rumpled and charmingly tongue-tied but managed to squeak out an invitation for me to visit him in Chicago, where he had recently moved. On a whim, out of a feeling of listlessness or destiny or both, I flew there and visited him. I visited him again. Then again.

On one visit, in the bargello of demicoastal flights that would embody our courtship, we were draped on a battered brown sofa when I noticed the time on a digital clock: 11:11. "Quick, make a wish," I prompted.

We wished.

At 11:12, I asked him, "What did you wish?"

"That I could fly," he said, shrugging when a sudden laugh pricked the corners of my mouth. "It's the wish I always used to make when I was a kid. In a pinch, the words popped into my head: I wish I could fly."

This struck me as so pure and so good, I married him.

You showed me that it was all right to be happy.

I married him, not for his looks or his money although he had a tolerable supply of both. Nor did I marry him for his devotion or tenderness since I was neither tender nor devoted and was unable to accept what I couldn't give back. I married him for his brains. Not for his *brain,* which was an altogether too complicated and tortuous arrangement of rooms with bad lighting. No, for his *brains*—his braininess, his kinetic body of knowledge, his vigorous intellect, his undisputable dominion over facts and theories and givens.

"Ask Will," my girlfriends would say when, in a conversation, we reached a place of puzzlement. "He knows everything."

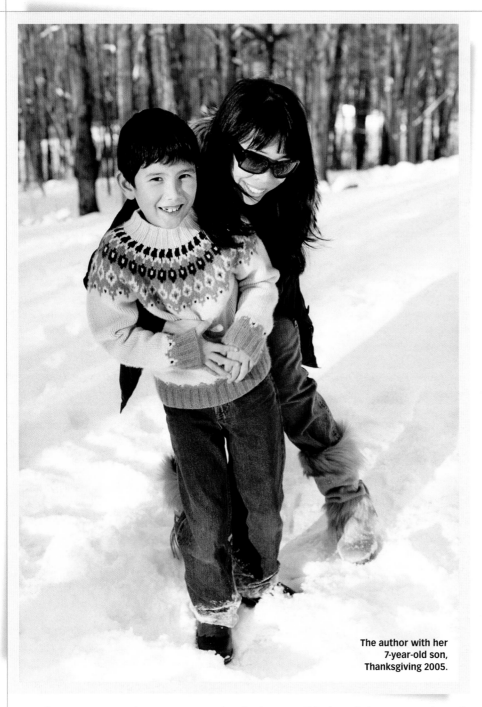

The author with her
7-year-old son,
Thanksgiving 2005.

"You would be the best medical examiner ever."

"They should hire you to run *The New Yorker.*"

Once, after he had declared that I would make an exemplary prime minister, I pointed out that he *always* said that I would be the best such and such and, frankly, it seemed a bit indiscriminate. "Untrue," he protested. "I've never said you would make the best underwater tunnel digger."

That's where he was mistaken. Before we met, I was one of the greatest sandhogs of our time.

But if the Man Who Knew Everything believed that I could do anything, then maybe I would have to believe it, too.

You made me see that I could.

We bought an apartment on 22nd Street.

We adopted a dog who looked like a fox.

We had a son.

We used to joke that the arc of our life would move from "Did the dog poop?" to "Did the baby poop?" to "Did *you* poop?" and then—finished. Done. A complete life together, charted in three easy-to-answer questions.

Except that somewhere between the baby pooping and me pooping—June 17, 2002, to be precise—I got cancer.

Now I grant you, when you're already 1,146 words in, cancer can be rather a bomb to drop on a story, especially when it serves only as more exposition and is really somewhat beside the point. Allow me to detonate: I was diagnosed with a breast cancer; it was small and intense and manageable.

Of course, when I say *manageable,* I mean by me. At the ping of diagnosis, Will's busy brains etiolated into vapor. It wasn't that he couldn't cope—it was that he wouldn't. My girlfriends went with me to doctor consulta-

If we were not soul mates, we were kindred spirits. We shared the religion of language, a belief in words and the strength of their composition. He was an editor and I was a writer and we became each other's eyes. He read every piece I wrote. His were the eyes I turned to first; his were the brains I relied upon.

You made me whole.

More than that, he had a greater faith in me than anyone had ever mustered—greater even than my parents, deeper even than my son. He maintained an unflagging confidence in my abilities, real or imagined: Whenever a discussion arose that involved any type of high-functioning career, he invariably gestured toward me and enthused.

"You would make the greatest Supreme Court judge."

tions; my best friend, Jacquie, accompanied me to my surgery. My surgeon, Dr. Nowak, assumed that I was a single mother. I am pretty sure that my oncologist, Dr. Tepler, thought I was a lesbian. The former had referred me to the latter, and I pictured the two physicians, running into one another at breast cancer conferences, exchanging small talk.

"By the way, I've started treating that patient of yours, Ellen Tien."

"Oh, right—the single lesbian mother?"

When my radiation treatments began—8 A.M. appointments at Weill Cornell's Stich Radiation Center—Will officially took his bolt of denial to the tailor and had it made into a three-piece suit.

"Look at you, all dressed and ready to go," he would say gaily on a Monday morning (he is a morning person in the worst way). "Where are you headed?"

Radiation, I would say.

Tuesday: "Where are you off to on such a nice morning?"

Radiation, I would answer darkly.

Wednesday: "What are you—?"

Radiation!

It was the same for six weeks.

If I have to do this every day for the rest of my life.

But if there is a gist to this part of the story—and I am a terrific fan of the gist—it is that in a marriage, what seems like a brute transgression on the outside can transliterate to merely a workaday blemish on the inside. The gander's indolence or neglect might appall the flock but may barely register with the goose.

We had an ordinary marriage; cancer made it extra ordinary.

The blizzard passes; the ground is still white, only more so.

If I couldn't quite commit to forgiving Will for his absenteeism, I could, in a specialized way, get it—or at least I would have to say I did unless I was willing to play the fool who stayed with the fool who played her for a fool. Getting it was the toothpick that could save the card house, the international symbol for truce. How many times had I oppugned Will for a perceived disregard, a forgotten quart of milk, a veiled insult from a member of his family, only to be neutralized: Okay. Okay. I get it.

So the business of living went on as usual, although now slightly hobbled by the realization that life was no longer a simple matter of three poop questions. But since the evolution of a relationship is less about forgiveness and scatology and more about the accumulation of real estate, we forged onward and bought a weekend house in the jungles of Connecticut. For the next year, we excitedly huddled together in the glow of a collective project, connected by the inherent promise found in paint chips and carpet swatches and fixtures.

It was Memorial Day weekend 2004, our first weekend in the new house, and we were in an Ace Hardware store when the magma burst loose and Pompeii was buried.

I was paralyzed when I met you.

I was paralyzed.

A crushing pain blossomed cruelly in my chest and back—I staggered back between the spools of chain-link and the bags of peat moss, and knew instantly that something was wrong. We made a dash for the car and drove to a hospital in nearby Torrington. I remember Will tersely counting down the miles.

Only seven more miles to go.

Only six more miles to go.

I doubled over in my seat, negotiating for air. I started to lose feeling in my fingers and toes. At one point, I turned and looked in the backseat and saw my son—his chubby 6-year-old hands clenched in fear, tears silently streaming down his face—mumbling to himself, "Don't make a sound. Don't get in the way. Don't make a sound. Don't get in the way."

I think that was the worst part of all.

Only four more miles to go.

We arrived at the hospital in Torrington, the morphine was plugged in, the bottom dropped out of reality, and I stopped being able to chronicle the events in any organized fashion. At some juncture, the chief neurologist walked in the room and declared herself "completely unqualified to diagnose the problem," which was reassuring. There was talk of airlifting me back to New York but, concerned that the paralysis would spread to my lungs and they would not be able to intubate me midair, an ambulance was deemed preferable. Will's cousin Kate picked up our son so Will could ride with me.

By the time we were racing past Westchester, I was paralyzed from the shoulders down.

When we pulled into the ambulance entrance of Weill Cornell Medical Center on 70th Street, I remember Will musing, "Wow— we made really good time."

The doctors—these being rather more qualified than the ones in Torrington—swiftly arrived at a diagnosis: acute transverse myelitis, a rare idiopathic condition in which a body's immune system attacks the myelin sheath around its own spinal cord. It was unrelated to the cancer, a second fluke, a brilliant stroke of unluck.

I was assigned the top myelitis specialist in the city, Dr. Apatoff, a wiry man in a bow tie with a hyperintelligent face and the bedside manner of a schnauzer.

There were high-dose IV steroids and MRIs and spinal taps and more steroids.

The IV tree grew thicker and thicker with bags. There were drugs to calm the drugs that inflamed and other drugs to calm the calming drugs and then new drugs to counteract the overcalmingness of the drugs before them. The narcotics dogs chased their tails up and down my veins until my mind was burned into the blue-white burst of a flashbulb, all heat and muffled explosion and floating spots.

I remember weakly joking to Will, "What next? Thrush?"

The next day, I got thrush.

A few days after that, steroid-induced edema blew me up like a human blister. In 72 hours, I gained 40 pounds of water weight; as the fluid rushed into my face, my eyelid and the right side of my nose—weakened by a host of secondary infections—collapsed in a heap somewhere above my mouth.

How can you bear to see me like this?

I was no longer presentable or sane, yet a throng of visitors persisted in making my room a ruthless party, the strange manic gaiety of which pushed me deeper into confusion.

Food and flowers formed a slag heap along the windows.

I was afraid to sleep alone in the room.

My stomach, bruised from daily multiple injections, turned the deep, mottled maroon of a tortoise cowry.

My friend Elizabeth baked an enormous pink buttercream cake.

I snapped at Will in front of his mother, and the next day

> Will had a greater faith in me than anyone had ever mustered.

when she called—a nurse propped the phone on a pillow next to my ear—the whole room could hear her anxiously wailing, "You must be nicer to Willie! You *must* be nicer to Willie!"

Sheesh, someone in the room said. Pick your priorities.

Everyone laughed.

My son went to a carnival, and I worried that he might horse around during a ride and lean too far one way and his body would be crushed between the metal cars.

Jacquie brought me a Porthault bathrobe, and I wept because I bled on it.

I asked Will repeatedly if the dog missed me.

Pick your priorities.

I wish I could fly.

Time stacked atop time. I was moved out of the ICU, first into the neurological ward and then upstairs to a grimly cheerful physical rehab unit called Baker 17 that had a shiny Pergo wood laminate floor, peevish nurses, and orderlies who flatly refused to change sheets.

Two weeks later, Will and I came home with a wheelchair and walker.

Three months later, I could walk on my own but had no sensation down the left side of my body.

Nine months later, Will drove me to the office of Dr. Daniel Baker, a plastic surgeon, who painstakingly began to give me back my self, reconstructing my face in a series of surgeries, each four months apart. After the first surgery, in which my collapsed face was fattened with cartilage grafts, my nose foreshortened and upturned, I looked like a pig. After the second surgery, I looked like exactly half a pig. This was all according to plan.

Next month I will schedule a third surgery, after which I will, with luck, resemble not a barnyard animal at all.

At the one-year mark, the function in my hands had improved, but I had no use of my thumbs or my right index finger.

I still can't tie a shoe or write legibly or play the piano.

End at the beginning.

"How?" I asked Will as he bathed and dressed and fed me for weeks upon weeks, matter-of-factly and without complaint, as if this had always been the arrangement.

I was paralyzed when I met you.

"How can you bear to see me this way?" I asked him as he laid ice packs across the stitches around my nose; cleaned the brittle, bloody lacquer pooled behind my ears, which had been pillaged for cartilage; tried—oh, how he tried in his clumsy, ignorant, manlike way!—to help me brush my hair or fasten jewelry or even put on makeup in a grotesquely comic attempt to simulate a regular human facade.

You made me whole.

For the better part of a year, I declined all but the most obligatory social events. Subjecting my distorted, crumpled features and bloated girth to public gaze was too awful to be borne: the startled expressions, the quick aversion of eyes, the way that people I had known for years no longer recognized me.

He never averted his eyes.

You showed me that it was all right to be happy.

"How can you stand it?" I asked him, when he came home from work at night, only to have to tackle an additional mountain of accrued tasks. There was mail to open, books to put away, printers to fill, food to warm, buttons to unbutton, presents to wrap. I once relied on his eyes, his brains. Now I needed his hands, too.

If I have to do this every day for the rest of my life.

He started bringing me scissors—sewing shears, meat scissors, paper cutters, clippers with specially designed handles, spring-loaded cutters—until I found a pair that I could operate. He bought me fat magic markers that I could grasp in my fist and a buttonhook. Every morning he unscrewed bottles of water, de-foiled cups of yogurt, opened cartons of milk, and then closed them up and put them back in the refrigerator so I could have access to them later. All this he did without fanfare or comment. All this he did so I wouldn't always have to feel stranded.

You made me see that I could.

Begin at the end.

This is not a story about how crisis can rejuvenate love or whisk us to new heights or strengthen and improve a relationship. Sometimes it does and sometimes it doesn't, but more often than not it eventually just blends in like paint, stroked smoother and longer and wider, until it disappears into the plain—remembered but not perceived. The landscape reverts to sameness. In a society that exalts the special and the different, do we dare to posit that sameness may be our salvation?

There is a fortitude in something that has always stood.

Marriage is sameness. It is a contraption, at times creakier than others, with a discrete set of ropes and pulleys that two partners pass back and forth between each other until they can no longer. It is a fabric with a fixed set of threads weaving in and out of the patterns, showing up here, then showing up there, again. The fibers weave a sameness, the very sameness that impels some people to divorce, others to mate for life.

I will never make a complete recovery. This is a hard sentence to say, an even harder sentence to write. But this is not a story about me. This is the story of a marriage, a marriage that granted, in every state of change, sameness. A marriage that, when people asked, "How are things?" allowed me to answer, "The same."

By all accounts, it was a fine marriage. It saw two big bumps, but it has seen even more paved road. And so Will and I continue to pass the same ropes back and forth, to follow the same finite set of threads as they disappear and return.

It is a fine marriage. We are fine. It is possible that we once sensed, in ways both acute and distant, that there might be something more out there, something thrilling and transforming, but now we know that we were wrong. ◖

> In a society that exalts the special and the different, do we dare to posit that sameness may be our salvation?

The Kindness of Strangers (the Rudeness of Spouses)

At work your spouse is the soul of consideration. At night it's all you can do to get him to be civil. And, sometimes, you're the bad guy. Therapist TERRENCE REAL on how to make home a nicer place to come home to.

A couple I'll call Ted and Anne were attending a workshop I was giving on relationship skills. They were there because they quarreled constantly, they said—just that week they had argued bitterly over driving the kids to school. As best I could piece it together, the fight went something like this:

Anne: "Honey, you're going to need to take both kids to school tomorrow. I scheduled a doctor's appointment—"

Ted: "You know I can't do that. I made a plan to run with Jim, and I've canceled twice already. This is called 'How many ways can we stop Ted from exercising?' "

Anne: "You know, Ted—"

Ted [*irritated*]: "Thirty minutes is what I ask for. Thirty minutes out of 24 hours. That's all I want."

Anne [*shouting*]: "And all I want is a real partner for a change. Someone who cares about something besides himself!"

After hearing them out, I asked Ted, "Was there any other time this week when you were equally annoyed with someone but chose to handle things differently?" After some prodding, he came up with a mistake his assistant had made at work. He'd been packing up his papers for an important presentation when Julie admitted she'd forgotten to tell him that the meeting was canceled.

Julie is terrific, Ted told me, but ever since her mother's hospitalization, she'd been letting things slip. Her apology didn't change the fact that this latest lapse cost him hours of valuable time. Still, Ted knew better than to lash out. Looking at Julie's stricken face, he said, his anger drained and he asked her whether she needed time off. When she responded that it was better for her to be at the office, he was touched, and she was reassured.

Placing the two incidents side by side, an obvious question emerged: Why did Ted show more consideration to his assistant than to his wife? For her part, Anne was known as a straight shooter with her friends and at work, but with Ted she allowed resentment to build until she blew up in a rage. As shocking as it might sound, Ted and Anne reserved their worst behavior for each other.

Helping couples for more than 20 years has brought me face-to-face with a sobering truth: Most of us don't treat our spouses with nearly the same level of respect and diplomacy that we extend to colleagues, friends, and even strangers. We give lip service to the idea that marriage takes effort, but in our day-to-day lives we think, *I don't want to work this hard.*

"Look," Ted said to me, "when I'm in the office, I have to manage my staff. But I don't want to think of my marriage as a job."

Ted was pleading the case for what I call the Popeye syndrome: "I yam what I yam!" His fantasy was to come home, loosen his belt, pop open a beer, flip on the TV, belch...and be loved. Men might have gotten away with this a generation ago, but now it's quite likely that as we pull up in our driveways after a hard day at work, our wives pull in behind us. If we want our marriages to be happy, we don't get to come home and just "relax"—which to most of the men I work with means "be left alone."

Anne had her own version of Popeye—I want what I want, but I don't want to ask for it. She told me that her anger at Ted came from an abiding feeling that "he just isn't there" with her and the kids. "Ted is the kind of guy," she said, "who will come home, step over a pile of stinky diapers to give me a kiss, and not even think to pick them up. I have to manage the house, the kids, our social calendar." She summed it up with a phrase I hear over and over again from women: "I feel like I don't have a partner." I asked Anne to spell out what more partnering might look like ("I shouldn't have to tell him what to do!"), and then I asked if she could think of any ways to help him rise to the occasion.

"But that's just the point!" she said. "Why do I need to take responsibility for Ted's behavior? I spent years in therapy learning how not to do that. Are you kidding?"

"Well—" I said.

"I yam what I yam": Popeye syndrome is a couple's nightmare.

"I am not going back to that codependent stuff. Why should I make his problem my concern?"

"Because you love him?"

"Right," she snorted.

"Okay, then. Because you live with him. You have to deal with him."

She shook her head.

"I don't know, Anne," I said. "I didn't pick him. You did."

Anne's refusal to give her husband direction came from an understandable and healthy impulse to stop taking care of him. But there's a difference between babying someone and helping him out. Anne's new stance was rooted in the same old underlying assumption as the most traditional fairy-tale vision of happily-ever-after—a good husband shouldn't have to be told what I want. "I'm sorry," I said. "But Cinderella is dead and Prince Charming most likely just got out of rehab. If you're going to get your needs met, you're going to have to state them effectively."

I believe the quality we bring to relationships with friends and coworkers but leave on the front steps at home is thoughtfulness. I don't mean remembering birthdays. I mean reining in your annoyance when you know someone's going through a tough time, or giving the other person the benefit of the doubt, or saying, "Let's figure out a solution together." Spontaneity is great for positive emotions, but handling life's challenges takes care and skill. And contrary to the idea that we shouldn't have to be so calculating with our mates, we need to be even more conscious, more on our toes, because no one pushes our hot buttons better or more often.

In the workshop, Anne laid the blame for her bad behavior squarely at the feet of her partner. She admitted to yelling, calling Ted selfish and uncaring, and even throwing things—but only, she said, because he was so difficult. Hers wasn't the only destructive response to conflict that I've seen in my practice. Another woman might have blamed herself; someone else would have withdrawn from Ted or tried hard to "fix" him. As we all do, Anne brought her characteristic reaction to difficulty into the marriage with her. She could have married Mahatma Gandhi, and sooner or later the plates would have flown.

Anne's default setting, what I call first consciousness, is rage. But with a little coaching, she could develop an inner voice that would help her choose a more constructive response. She could take a moment— the time it takes to draw a breath—to practice using second consciousness, a learned, adult way to react.

"Guys are enormously skilled at dealing with a woman having a fit," I said. "They duck under the wave, let the storm pass,

then go on doing whatever they want. What guys are not used to is moderate firmness that doesn't back off." I asked Anne to practice speaking to Ted in a way that conveys she genuinely wants a partner (rather than simply venting): "Ted, I feel lonely and overwhelmed. When I say I need you to take the kids, you don't have to make a big fuss about it, okay?" With encouragement, she listed four specific changes she wanted Ted to make: Take over the burden of checking in with the kids' teachers; call his mother every week rather than relying on her to do it; plan a family outing once or twice a month; treat her now and then to a night out or flowers. To her surprise, Ted agreed to all four. Then Anne asked the million-dollar question, "What can I do to help you deliver?"

Ted took an aggrieved tone. "You can tell me what I'm doing right," he said peevishly. "Don't just scold me."

Anne, provoked, began to wind up, but a look from me stopped her. She took a deep breath, let go of her first consciousness, and…smiled. "Deal," she said, holding out her hand.

"Go on," I told Ted. "Shake on it, partner."

In a follow-up letter about two months later, Anne wrote: "I'll come home and see Ted sacked out on the couch and become enraged. Every particle of me wants to rip into him, but a voice in my head says, 'Stop!' I breathe and make myself settle down. Then I wake up the lazy bum and tell him, respectfully, that his participation in our family is not discretionary." Now Anne gets heard: "Instead of the issue turning back to 'How Anne spoke to poor Ted,' my husband actually gets off his butt and pitches in. And on those few occasions when he tries to pull that victim stuff—'Anne, you're so hard on me…blah, blah'—I don't buy into it anymore. I'm not being hard, and I know it."

Anne got into a habit that I encourage my clients to develop. Before opening your mouth, ask yourself two questions:

1. What do I really want? It may seem appealing to prove him wrong, pay him back, leave in a huff, or cave in to keep the peace, but what you probably really crave is healthy intimacy.

2. Is what I'm about to say or do right now going to get me closer to what I want? If you honestly feel your next word or action has a shot at success, go ahead and try it. But if it isn't going to be constructive, then don't do it. It's that simple. When Ted told Anne she could be more supportive and less scolding, it wasn't hard to imagine any number of juicy responses she might have shot back, like "I'll reward you when there's something to reward" or "Can't you be a man and not base your actions on my approval?" Such zingers would have been fair, given the way Ted was behaving.

But what Anne wanted most was a thoughtful partner, so instead of picking a fight, she dared to take yes for an answer, accepting his suggestion even though it wasn't delivered as graciously as she had wished.

You might say that cultivating second consciousness means learning to act in your own best interest. Or you might simply call it learning to love like a grown-up. ◐

Looking Out for #2

Her first marriage foundered. What made her think the second would be an improvement? LISE FUNDERBURG on what she's learned and what she's doing differently this time.

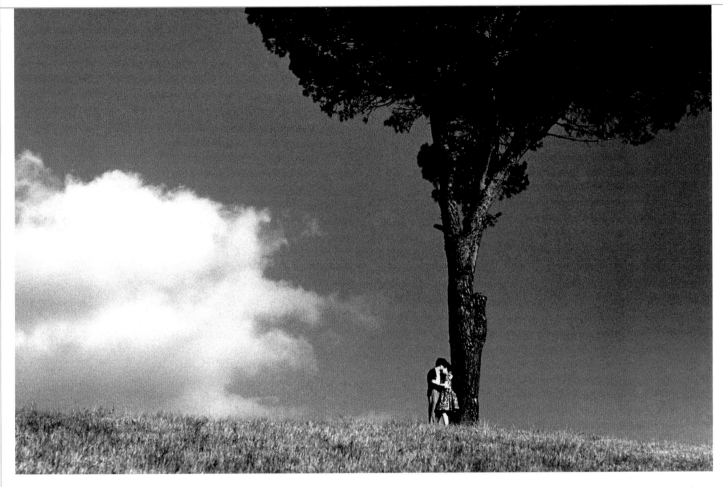

It wasn't until I decided to marry again that I realized how completely uncertain and illogical marriage is. The second time around, you can't hide behind romantic innocence. You already know how easy it is to take another person for granted. You know how hard it is to live with someone else: to build intimacy over years, to grow without stealing all the available sunlight and food, or to simply like that other person day in and day out despite chore wars, seat-up/seat-down debates, and other domestic disputes, such as appropriate use of mayonnaise in sandwich-making (never versus always). The second time around, you already know how easy it is to fail.

Forget corroborating statistics that show up in print (divorce for almost 50 percent of first marriages and 40 percent of second); anyone can see that failure lurks on the other side of the next financial downturn or conflict in life directions or mountain of careless, bruising words. All around, marriages are crumbling, families are splintering, people are retreating into corners, making do, putting up, shutting off.

And yet even before I met John, even as I combed through the ashes of the first marriage, looking for what to discard and what to salvage, I realized the idea of marriage didn't repel me. The problem had been in thinking that it marked the arrival at a destination instead of signaling a point of departure. It wasn't marriage that had failed my first husband and me: By expecting it to maintain itself based on one sunny April afternoon of exchanged vows, we had failed it. For eight years, we left those promises untended, impending ruin masked by compatibility and goodwill.

In its aftermath, people, friends, and acquaintances seemed to anticipate bitterness—they expected bile and brokenness when breaking the news of other people's nuptials. They got neither. I had a greater respect for the institution. I was humbled by the enterprise I had come to see as demanding courage and hope and a relentless investment of self. I was in awe.

When John and I both recognized the irreversible pull between us—the astounding affinity, the willingness to understand, the tenderness, the fun—we started to consider a future. We fit as a couple; we fit in the larger context of each other's lives. He actually liked my eccentric family, the forces of nature that they can be. And I was crazy about his 17-year-old son, who lived with him and who stepped off the path of adolescent individuation rites long enough to allow me glimpses of his kind heart and sharp mind, as well as a chance to find my way around that phenomenon I'd never understood—the teenage boy.

John and I shared a striking number of interests (urban living, pork) and traits (bossiness, get-up-and-go). What we didn't share we admired, and what we didn't admire we accepted. My brilliant therapist had been telling me all along that a mature love is one in which the beloved can have flaws but still be considered a perfect match. *Oh,* I thought, *I get it now.*

After two years of tumbling and inching toward each other, John and I married. It was a summer wedding, in my (now our) backyard, with 150 witnesses and 40 slabs of barbecued ribs, a mess of side dishes where a first marriage's gift table might have been, and a feeling of pleasure that was quiet and sure. In front of a village of loved ones (and platters of pork), we pledged our troth, and I felt with equal conviction that I (a) was doing the right thing and (b) had no idea what I was getting into.

The paradox of those realizations prompted what John calls a BFO: a blinding flash of the obvious. Suddenly, I understood that marriage is, as it has often been said, a leap of faith. I had just made the leap; now came the faith. In that moment, I saw that my best hope for defying statistics and building a strong union was to consider marriage an expression of faith, a spiritual act that requires devotion and practice and the same naked honesty that people seek between themselves and their god(s).

I am not religious in the conventional sense, certainly not what some of my relatives would call churched. I grew up in a religious minority's minority, a birthright Unitarian, and in my adulthood I have—if it's possible for Unitarians to do so—lapsed. But I attend weddings and funerals and civil commitments, baby dedications and bat mitzvahs and any number of holidays and ceremonies. My Methodist, African Methodist, and Colored Methodist relatives have not left the church, and so I have had the opportunity over the years to witness the faith of others, a stirring and beautiful thing.

Among the friends and relations whose spirituality I admire, I've noted that their practice is not restricted to a particular day of the week but applied to the twists and turns of everyday life. Likewise, my commitment to this marriage is not something I dust off at anniversaries or in the wake of troubles. It is a close

and constant touchstone. I am conscious of this promise I've made to John to cast my lot with his, to be a guardian of his unguarded heart as I offer up my own.

Consciousness introduces a higher plane on which to relate, retreat, take solace, and find answers, to rise above the petty fray. Unfortunately, it's not a complete guarantee against quotidian tangles. It would still kill no one to put the toilet seat back down, to know where the vacuum is stored and act upon said knowledge. Or to remember that he has more than once explained to me in assiduous detail the virtues of the Norton 850 Commando, which was one of the fastest production motorcycles you could buy in 1973, when European motorcycles still dominated the market for performance and before Japan's Honda 750 four cylinder hit and immediately took over, pushing Norton out of business within a few years, followed shortly thereafter by the death of Triumph.

Faith demands belief in what you can't see. I know, for example, that I must have my own version of the Norton Commando story even if I can't see it. And believing that allows me to be more patient. When John goes on about some great passion of his that I rank up there with paint drying and software downloading, I remind myself that this is an opportunity I'm being given to challenge my own limits, that it is a gift to share in someone else's enthusiasm and imagination, and that this is what happens when you live with someone day after day after day. If all else fails, I use the time to reflect on our spring trip to France, how perfect the weather was, how wonderful it was to rummage through country flea markets together, and how we kept our sense of humor when all the charming hotels and *gîtes* were booked during the week of the Ascension and we ended up in a charmless motor inn overlooking a big-box mall.

Faith is a way to step outside yourself, to remember that this anecdote, too, shall pass; that being a team is more important than which exit he takes off the highway; that you don't need to balance the checkbook the same way in order to prove that you're evenly yoked and well suited; and that annoyance and blame are often the result of misplaced anxieties, which, if clearly identified, could most likely be addressed and resolved without leaving open or festering wounds. We are all, as the psychotherapist Deborah Luepnitz writes, porcupines. We seek the warmth of others but soon tangle ourselves in one another's prickly quills.

Faith, among the faithful I know, is not about perfection. It's about knowing, as Quakers would put it, that there is an inextinguishable light inside everyone that is holy. It's about valuing the holy in the face of the flawed, about leaving room to grow, to fall down, then get back up again, all with equal dignity. And so, I find after more than a year of practicing, is a good marriage. ⬤

> In front of a village of loved ones, we pledged our troth, and I felt with equal conviction that I (a) was doing the right thing and (b) had no idea what I was getting into.

You Got Nailed!

Going through pockets, checking collars for lipstick, hiring a seedy gumshoe to tail the louse—*so* retro! Today's suspicious wife has an arsenal of spyware that can slip her right into her husband's computer, read his incriminating e-mails, and track his clandestine Web visits. But is cybersnooping smart? Ethical? Is it even legal? LIZ BRODY meets some women who've caught their husbands with their virtual pants down.

I love you...very, very much...I want you so much." Brenda took in the words on the screen. She was alone at her husband's computer in their home office, using a new program that let her see chat room messages he'd sent earlier. The writing didn't sound like him, and the smiley face icons punctuating the sentences were not his style. She looked closer at the monitor.

And then she saw the "Sue"—"I love you, Sue, very very much." He also called her "baby," an endearment he had never used for his wife in 32 years of marriage. Names can never harm you, the saying goes, but that "baby" hit Brenda like shrapnel.

I'm on the phone with her two weeks later, having met online in a group called Internet Chat Infidelity. "Honey, I got plenty of time," she says, taking a deep drag on her cigarette. After a sudden uneasy feeling, at 54, two kids, two grandkids, and three dogs, Brenda (who, for reasons that will become obvious, can't reveal her last name) loaded her husband's computer with all the latest electronic spyware she could afford. And with it, she's been watching every key he strikes, every message he writes. Sounds like a Sting song, and a sting operation it is.

She tells me that she first got interested in her husband's PC seven years ago. At that time, she was managing a convenience store. "My life was great. I thought I had a happy marriage; my daughter was expecting her first child," she says. "Well, one day he was clicking away on his computer, and I felt, *Something's just not right*." She barely knew where to find the "on" button, but while he was at work, she scrounged around his desk, discovered passwords on Post-its, and got into his e-mail. He was corresponding with five different women, using a special program called ICQ Voice Message to send his spoken affections, one of which Brenda managed to record. She plays me a snippet:

"Baby...I want to tell you about my voice"—his tone comes over the receiver low and intimate, the kind of smooth persuasion known to unhook a bra, and he confesses that he's taped the message numerous times to get it right—"I love you more than anything in the world. Please don't do anything to ever change that."

Just listening to this betrayal floors me with a sickening rush I imagine Brenda felt when she first heard it, the sensation of glancing down from a great height, knowing with a swift vividness that you could fall a very long way. "This," she says, "is what brought me down to ground level. I went over the edge." Raging,

she confronted him, pounded her fists into him—"I was gasping for air; I was so angry I could hardly breathe," she says—and he finally admitted to playing around online. There was nothing more, he swore. He would stop. And for the next seven years, he did, or he seemed to, until just a few weeks ago, when Brenda had that second intuition.

Now he's back to his old games, and she's worried that his activities may be carrying over into the flesh. But she isn't counting on Post-its to find out. Through friends who happen to be detectives, she got wise to the new spy equipment, and her arsenal now includes a keylogger, a tiny device that plugs in where the keyboard hooks up to the computer and captures whatever he types; Internet surveillance software designed to record both sides of the dialogue; and a data recovery program for resurrecting deleted files. Just for good measure, she planted a GPS tracking unit the size of a pack of chewing gum inside his truck so she could monitor where he goes and how long he stops.

The evidence of his cyberlife is painful, like the e-mail he wrote to one woman telling her he'd applied for a different position at work—"He never said a word about it to me"—which cut deeper than all the "nasty little pictures of men and women doing things" she found him swapping with e-mates. Brenda is not sure how long she can continue to live with this, but 32 years of marriage are hard to throw away. In a sense, she's waiting to catch him crossing a line that leaves no question. Meanwhile doubt spreads like rot through everything she does. And as much as she hates all this prowling around, feeling that the truth is within her grasp, she says, "is putting my mind at ease."

Too many of us know the anguish of suspecting infidelity—the sink of the gut that says yes, it's happening, while the mind and the man placate, "Don't be so neurotic; nothing's going on." Monogamy, unfortunately, seems to malfunction with alarming frequency. And when it does, honesty is not exactly on the tip of a philanderer's tongue, which leaves the other party either to sedate herself on denial or to start searching for evidence. But the days of rooting through suit pockets for receipts and checking collars for stray lipstick stains are over.

I first heard that the infidelity business had gone high-tech over dinner with my cousin, James Mintz, not long after his private investigative firm, the James Mintz Group, with its industrially hip Manhattan digs, was written up in *The New Yorker*. (He's got six offices and, over the years, has had clients like the city of New York, Morgan Stanley, and the Beatles.) I was thinking about a friend who'd recently walked in on her fiancé pants-down with the dog sitter, a story I found particularly disturbing because my husband is working 3,000 miles away and it's hard not to wonder what kind of overtime he's up to.

Jim's poker face never quite hides the mischief in his eyes, which somehow makes him an easy guy to confide in, much to the chagrin of the many shady characters who've ended up confessing their worst misdeeds to him.

"So," I ask, peering over the Greek menu. "What does one do if she suspects her husband of being unfaithful and wants to have him followed? What's the protocol?"

"It's expensive," he says, trying to decide if he wants the squid.

"Say the person could pay." I throw him a meaningful look.

"We don't do domestic cases," he says, with a look back that means the "person" better not be me. He's got operatives, obviously—he mentions a guy by the name of Buddy Bubaloo, something like that. "But," my cousin puts down his menu and says, in his best slide-it-under-the-table sotto voce, "tailing is old-fashioned. These days it's all about the computer."

He points out that people having affairs now inevitably e-mail or make arrangements on the Internet. And, he says, in the hands of someone like his computer forensics guy, an adulterer's hard drive can become a lurid libretto of guilt—full of detailed messages, text documents, Web sites visited, directions MapQuested, all retrievable long after they've been deleted. An electronic memory, after all, never forgets. "People are shocked at what you can bring back," he says.

Other experts in the secrets-finding trade agree. "Virtually everyone who cheats will do it electronically," says Sharon Nelson, Esq., whose firm, Sensei Enterprises, in Fairfax, Virginia, handles computer forensics for about 100 divorce cases a year. "What we read scorches our eyebrows much of the time.... I mean, it's not poetry, prose, flowers. Most of it is extraordinarily explicit and damning." And professionals aren't the only ones dragging hard drives for clues; in the past five years or so, a whole do-it-yourself spyware industry has also flourished, allowing doubting spouses to become at-home detectives.

On the weekends, you can usually catch Beverly (she, too, thought it wisest to keep things on a first-name basis) at a rodeo, watching her boyfriend ride bulls. The 44-year-old has no cowgirl ambitions herself, but she's never been afraid to take a beast by the horns. Four years ago, when she was living in the South, raising two children, her husband of more than 11 years, James, started visiting his mother with dutiful regularity. "They didn't speak for months, and all of a sudden he's going to see his mom three weekends in a row?" Beverly asks incredulously. She also stumbled on a suspicious e-mail—one of those

> "I go downstairs to the computer. The wood floors are creaking; my cat is meowing. I'm whispering, 'No, no, Manny; be quiet.'"

"If I call two times and hang up, you'll know it's me" sort of messages. She confronted James about whether he was seeing another woman, and he confessed that he was, she says. "I was devastated because all my family and friends had been asking, 'Do you think there's somebody else?' And I kept going, 'No, I really don't think so.'"

They decided to split up. If Beverly had been in a stupor about her husband's infidelity, she was jolted awake when he decided to fight for custody of their daughter and son, 8 and 10 at the time (she wanted to take them back to her home state; James felt strongly that everyone should stay put). Fighting back, she hit the Internet. "I did a search looking for spyware so I could see what he was doing," she says. Spector was the program she chose—a powerful surveillance tool that records e-mails, chats, instant messages, keystrokes, and Web sites visited, and takes continuous screen shots so you can view exactly what the person has seen (there's even a version you can covertly install on someone else's computer simply by e-mailing it, although the company states that you are violating its license agreement if you don't own that machine). While James was at work one day, Beverly slipped her new software disc into his desktop and hit download.

Most nights James unwound with games on the computer that was in their son's room, two feet from the boy's bed, according to Beverly. When she went to see what Spector had netted, she discovered that James and his Yahoo! Dominoes partner were playing something a little dicier than dotted blocks. The partner was, in fact, his girlfriend. "I was able to read a lot of the stuff they were saying to each other," Beverly recalls. "She would ask personal things about me. Very personal things. One time she asked about my bra size, and he's like, 'Well, gee, I don't even know.' He says, 'Hold on, I'll find out.' He goes and checks in my drawer. She also wanted to know how much I weighed, how tall I was. That bothered me, probably a whole lot more than when he admitted to me that he was seeing somebody."

She found it tough, too, when he wrote to the girlfriend that this wasn't the first time he'd cheated on Beverly—"and it had happened before I thought anything started getting bad," she says, her voice tight. But the real dirt—the evidence she could use in court to fight his custody suit, Beverly thought, was James's forays onto the Internet. As he clicked and clattered away, surrounded by their son's toy cars and Pokémon figures, he was visiting Web sites Beverly describes as "extremely inappropriate." And from the exchanges he was having with the girlfriend, it was clear to her that "there were things going on with his hands besides just typing—you'll have to read between the lines—and he would have had his back to my son's bed, so he would have had no way of knowing if the child woke up and could see the computer screen."

James didn't have any idea he was being monitored until his deposition. His attorney still can't believe it: "After her lawyer

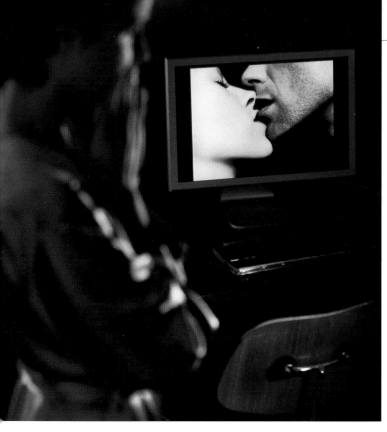

asked all the basic questions, 'Where do you work, how's your health?' blah, blah, blah, he goes, 'Are you interested in writing' "— he pauses to draw out the next word—" 'pornography?' My client goes, 'What?' And the lawyer pulls out a stack of papers the size of a phone book, which were conversations between him and his girlfriend, and puts them on the table and says, 'Would you look at these?' It was the shock of the century."

James, who had never heard of spyware, says he felt as if he'd been "punched in the stomach." If the raunchy printouts might have cast doubt on his future as a father figure, however, the court said: Not so fast. Spector's intelligence gathering had run up against the Florida wiretapping law, which states that intercepting a communication while it's in transit is a crime. The judge threw out Beverly's evidence because it had been collected illegally and in August 2003 awarded James custody. She appealed.

At the next hearing, the lawyers and their experts duked it out over what came down to a technological hanging chad: James's side charged that Spector intercepted his messages. Beverly's lawyer argued no, the spyware retrieved the information after it had been received and stored in the computer. In trying to rule, the court had to acknowledge that the time period in question was "evanescent." "Nobody really knew how this thing worked," James's attorney says.

Judges, however, tend to bristle at anything smacking of eavesdropping, and Beverly had clearly snooped. In February 2005, she lost her appeal and any chance of custody. James says there were other reasons he got the kids, including the fact that she left the state before the case was over to take advantage of a job opportunity. "To be honest, had that testimony been admitted, would it have been embarrassing and damaging? Yes. Would I still have won? Yes. She let whatever activity was taking place on that computer go on," he says, denying her implications about his hands being off the keyboard. "If she was so concerned about the children's safety, she would have nipped it in the bud. She didn't."

Beverly is now teaching pre-K and discussing marriage with her rodeo man. She gets the kids for the summer and every other weekend. "Things just didn't go my way," she says.

I'll say they didn't—the court denies her evidence over a hair so fine it's "evanescent"? Suddenly, my cousin's parting words are ringing in my ears: "Before you do anything," he'd said, "talk to a lawyer—there are issues about whose computer it is and what you can do to it."

After talking to a number of lawyers, I learned that Beverly was actually lucky: Though losing custody may seem harsh, the fact is, she could have landed in jail. When I asked New York divorce attorney Ken Warner whether using a program like Spector is basically illegal, he said, "Not basically. It's illegal. It's illegal to intentionally tap into or hack into the computer account of another person that is closed and where the hacking is unauthorized or not permitted." He stopped to cite New York penal law (Section 156.10, to be exact), relevantly titled Computer Trespass. "And it's a class E felony, which is punishable by up to four years in prison." With electronic evidence increasingly making its way into divorce court, the American Bar Association saw fit earlier this year to devote an entire issue of its journal *Family Advocate* to articles like "Spy v. Spy: Snooping by Husbands, Wives, and Lovers." Even if spousal sleuthing doesn't break wiretapping laws, simply invading someone's privacy (say, by sneaking past a password) can subject you to damages. Yet every state is different, and many cases are cutting new ground.

When Mary Lenahan had her husband's computer professionally searched six years ago, it was her attorney's idea. This was after Mary found a letter to his girlfriend in the sunroom, and she knew her 19-year marriage was beyond repair. Like Beverly, she'd been soldiering through for the kids, three boys in their teens. But when her husband made it clear he wanted a divorce and full custody, any remaining civility erupted. "I'll never forget standing in our bedroom, and he just looked at me and said, 'I will destroy you,' " recalls Mary, now 50 and a nurse liaison for a large hospital in Summit, New Jersey. "Those four words are what got me through the whole thing. I was not going to let that happen."

When her lawyer, Phyllis Klein O'Brien, suggested they see if there was any evidence on the computer that might discredit his parenting skills—the letter to his girlfriend indicated it was a good possibility—Mary agreed. "So we surreptitiously had a private investigator copy the entire hard drive," says Klein O'Brien, a partner at Donahue, Hagan, Klein, Newsome & O'Donnell. She was taking a risk. In most cases, a lawyer won't go near the other party's PC without a court order, but this was 2000, and there was no precedent in New Jersey. "I didn't know if the judge would understand the technology well enough. I was afraid he would say no."

The hard drive contained e-mails to the girlfriend, according to court records, as well as "images" he'd viewed on Netscape that Mary can only say made her "upset" (she and Klein O'Brien are barred from discussing further details). "You look at the person you married and had children with, and you feel like you don't even know him anymore." Klein O'Brien, meanwhile, was dealing with her own upset. The opposing counsel had slapped her with a motion accusing her of violating the state wiretapping statute—again, intercepting and copying messages—which she knew could put her behind bars. She'd spent hours poring over that statute—practically scrubbing it clean, she read it so many times—before suggesting Mary hire the PI and was convinced that, in this particular case, they'd done nothing illegal. "I can still picture myself at my desk, freaking, and calling in my associate, saying, 'Read this with me. Read this statute with me again,'" says Klein O'Brien. "'Aren't I right? Aren't I right?'"

She ultimately convinced the judge that she was. The key was that Mary's husband had inadvertently set up his AOL account to save e-mails to the hard drive (normally AOL saves everything to its own server), which meant that there was no interception or illegal access in retrieving them. Furthermore, because the computer was one the whole family used and the e-mails were not password protected, there was no privacy invasion. The couple ended up settling and agreeing to joint custody, with a larger chunk of time going to Mary. Klein O'Brien could finally breathe. "I didn't know any of this before," she says. "I was scared to death."

A half-hour drive out of Jacksonville, Florida, is a spanking new development of houses, some not yet sold, with driveways laid out neat as pleats along a circular drive—the kind of place that offers good golf and barbecue. I've come to meet the Mintz Group's computer forensics expert, curious to see what a real pro can do with a hard drive. John McElhatton and his wife, Tina, a newly retired teacher, bought here a year ago to have somewhere to vacation. His base in Virginia, just outside Washington, D.C., is where he does all his digital dissections, but he's got enough equipment here to show me a few things.

After 26 years in the FBI, McElhatton, dressed in easy-fit jeans and leather moccasins, has definitely got the art of the background-blend down. He helped start the FBI's computer forensics unit with another agent in the early nineties. In the beginning, it was just the two of them; now the department numbers almost 300. "Initially, we were doing financial crimes, a lot of healthcare fraud," he says, admitting they were working by the seat of their pants, developing their own techniques as they went along. Things heated up when Aldrich Ames, a CIA counterintelligence officer, went down as a Russian spy, thanks in large part to what McElhatton's team pulled from the entrails of his computer. ("It's classified," he says, when I pump him for details.) His technological chops helped solve other cases—murders, kidnappings—but in the mid-nineties, he says, something else started washing up in the flotsam of retrieved bits and bytes: child porn. Pedophilia was nothing new, obviously, but computer forensics opened a larger keyhole, through which many in the field say they've seen too much. "Imagine going in every day and working that stuff. You have kids...," he trails off, perhaps thinking of his three. "I wouldn't say that was the reason I retired, but it was one of them for sure."

As a free agent, he started his own business in 1997 and for the past four years has been working with my cousin. McElhatton invites me into his airy den. All that time spent on the dark side of human nature may account for the bright Butter Up yellow of the walls. I can see he's got more than the average home PC: His computer is custom-made, with five hard drives and a couple of keyboards, although they slide and stow in a pretty ordinary way. A portable PC built into a hard black carrying case is much more 007—he can sneak off in the middle of the night, hook it up jumper-cable style to a suspect's computer, then "suck the data right out to a drive that's on this one."

McElhatton, booting up his system now, is talking about making a "mirror image," which is an exact replica of a hard drive (if it were yours, you'd have no idea you weren't on your own computer—think: clone). Computer forensics experts typically do their investigations on such a copy, running sophisticated utilities that open-sesame through passwords and revive data from the dead and deleted. Like Raquel Welch in that old movie *Fantastic Voyage,* where she gets microsized and travels inside a human body, McElhatton enters each re-created computer and follows a stranger's logic along arteries of circuitry, searching for clusters of bad behavior.

"So what are we looking at here?" I ask. On his screen, I see a MapQuest for directions to a street called River Road (he clicks the mouse), then a flight reservation (click), rental car. He explains that we're on the computer of a real estate agent who was soliciting potential sellers for himself, not the company he worked for, going to see people he wasn't supposed to be meeting with. McElhatton clicks over to Google and pulls up a long history of search terms the man had entered: "Escorts." "Virgin Islands." "Cyndi." "Trish." "Jessica." (I had to promise to change the names.)

"Right. So—yeah," he says, "it's very interesting what people are searching for." He remembers an FBI case where a woman OD'd on pills and left a suicide note. When they investigated her husband's computer to see if he'd typed the note himself (he'd recently taken out an enormous insurance policy on her), they didn't find one, but they did ferret out searches he'd done for undetectable poisons. He confessed to killing her.

McElhatton moves on to deleted files. Easy game. They don't actually get erased, he explains, just overwritten when the computer runs out of space. But with PCs now powered by 60, 80, even 100 gigabytes, this often doesn't happen. "A ten-gigabyte hard drive—which is nothing today—holds the equivalent of about 15,000 paperback books," says McElhatton.

E-mail may or may not be salvageable, I learn. Suffice it to say, whatever you write on corporate e-mail goes down in history. AOL, on the other hand, "is problematic for the forensic examiner," says McElhatton, because it automatically saves everything to its own server (unless, like Mary's husband, you choose to save it onto your computer); Yahoo! and Hotmail are easier to dredge up. But all e-mails have a chance of landing in something called residual space.

"Residual space is some of the most fertile ground for computer forensics because people don't know about it, have no access to it, and have no control over it," says McElhatton. Say you type a letter (and I'm brutally simplifying here): Often that doesn't fill the space allotted for the file you've created. The computer, efficient as it is, goes, "Oh joy, here's a dresser drawer that has a little extra room," and stuffs in random data that's hanging around—deleted e-mails, photos, scanned documents, and, who knows, maybe a smoking gun.

McElhatton says it's even possible to recover information that's been deliberately eliminated. One time the Mintz Group was called in by a firm that suspected an employee of stealing proprietary data—they thought he might be planning to start his own business. The man, however, got wind that they were onto him and quickly had his company laptop completely reformatted. "This guy thought he was pretty smart," says McElhatton, "but we got the equivalent of maybe 20 printed pages' worth of documents and e-mails he'd written."

Later when I ask my cousin about the case, he says, "I remember it. The e-mails, unfortunately, weren't damning as much as suggestive. But the employee had a nickname for the guy he was corresponding with. He called him Q-ball." When Jim went to interview the suspect, he brought along the stack of printouts. Peeling the first page off the top, he held it up and said, "I know all about you and Q-ball."

My cousin laughs. "The guy looks at this pile of paper and thinks we've got everything he'd done on his computer. He rolls over."

Before I leave Florida, McElhatton tells me about one other nifty way to trace electronic fingerprints: metadata, technically data about data, like the time and date a document is modified, the program that creates a file. It sounds so mundane, but, he says, metadata is what finally cracked the case of the sadist BTK ("bind, torture, kill"), who played cat and mouse with the Wichita police for 30 years while he murdered at least ten victims. "Check it out," McElhatton says.

On February 16, 2005, in a cramped Kansas cubicle, Detective Randy Stone was nervously staring at his laptop—that's how he remembers it when I call him to follow up on this BTK thing. The message on the screen simply read "This is a test." It was BTK's 11th communiqué and had arrived on a floppy disk, along with a victim's necklace and some printed material. Stone, who's with the forensic computer crime unit of the Wichita police, was skeptical he'd find any clues on the disk. Nevertheless, when he started his meticulous probing of metadata, "Christ Lutheran Church" came up (the message had been created on a version of Office registered to the church) and—Stone couldn't believe his luck—"Dennis," the name used to log on to the computer where the document was last saved. Stone Googled the Christ Lutheran Church in Wichita, clicked a link on its Web site, and right at the top of the next page he saw it: Dennis Rader. He was president of the congregation.

"I'm sitting there looking at his name on the monitor with a crowd of people behind me. I turn around and poof, everybody's gone, just running in different directions," Stone recalls. Nine

days later, on February 25, 2005, BTK was arrested.

That was a great moment for computer forensics, but Stone fears the rapid advance of technology is conjuring up crimes so new, the legal system is at a loss when it comes to prosecuting them. "Husband and wife get a divorce," he starts, describing a real domestic case. "He moves to Wyoming, goes online, and puts an ad on an adult sex site. In this ad, he claims to be the ex-wife. Says, Here's who I am, here's my phone number, here's where I live, where I work, what I drive, here's my picture, and my fantasy is to be stalked and raped.

"A local guy in Wichita answers, thinking he's corresponding with a woman. The ex-husband says, 'Yeah, this is my biggest fantasy, ha-ha. If you do it, I will pretend to resist because it just enhances the excitement.' He says, 'On Wednesdays I leave the sliding glass door unlocked for my son.' So the dude shows up, goes in through the sliding glass door, rummages around in her drawer and steals some underwear, lays a rose on her bed, and leaves." After he sent her a dozen roses at work the next day, the woman talked the local flower shop into divulging his name and phone number, arranged a meeting, and brought the police. But what is his crime? Stone asks. "In his mind, he does not have the criminal intent to commit a rape—he's just continuing a mutually consensual fantasy. So how do you charge him? And what do you charge the ex-husband in Wyoming with? You could actually engineer a situation where something happens to your ex and you are not liable even though you set all the wheels in motion for harm to occur. We've had several cases like that."

I ask Stone if he's come across a lot of cheating spouses in his extensive gigabyte travels. He tells me about a woman who, in his opinion, found something worse.

March 10, 2004, was Lent. John Coleman had fallen asleep upstairs in his suburban home outside Wichita when his wife came in from church and first heard about the pictures. Married for ten months, Pam and John had met on a blind date about four years before they wed—he, a police officer, she, an accountant at the local air force base, both the type of people who see things in black-and-white, right or wrong, according to Pam, now 43. This was the second time around for each, and between them, they were raising five kids. "He was a huge family man," she says.

Pam was in the kitchen when her teenage stepson told her there were pictures on his dad's computer she should see, and he'd save them on a floppy disk for her to look at later. She had noticed a change in John since they'd all moved into that house together. Before, he thought nothing of whipping up dinner or mowing the lawn. But lately he'd lost interest in helping out. "I'd come home, and he'd be on the computer down in the basement where the family room was," says Pam. "I could tell he'd just run up the stairs when he heard me in the garage." She'd ask about dinner. "He'd say, 'Well, I didn't know what you wanted me to fix.' The point is, I'm not picky. It was like he was engrossed in something else."

When Pam got a free moment, she opened the floppy and saw

> Checking the car—
> "straws with lipstick,
> underwear"—
> became part of her
> nocturnal rounds.

the child. "It was like running into a brick wall," she says. A girl. Naked and sexually posed.

Pam's own two children, now also John's stepchildren, ages 8 and 12, were girls.

She started going through some of the other disks in the filing cabinet next to his desk and found they all contained similar photos of little girls. Wondering if downloading such pictures was even legal, she called a friend who worked for an attorney. It was Friday and the friend said she might not be able to find out that day. Over the weekend, John seemed like his old self, talking about doing projects around the house because spring was coming, says Pam. "Now, this," she thought, "is the person I fell in love with and married." She didn't mention the disks.

Back at work on Monday, she got a call around noon. It was her friend's boss on the line saying the DA had already been notified. "He tells me, 'You're right, it is illegal. And John knows it's illegal. Things are going to start happening.' And I no more than hung up the phone than it rang." This time it was an officer from the Wichita Police Department's Exploited and Missing Child Unit (EMCU), who wanted her to come down to the station to make a statement. On the basis of her interview, without seeing the pictures, two detectives drove off to arrest John at the nearby Park City Police Department, where he worked, while three others went to the house to seize his computer and floppy disks. After Pam met them back home, during all the commotion the phone rang. "One of the detectives said, 'It's probably him. Don't answer it.' And it was," says Pam. "His message was something to the effect of, 'Didn't know if you'd answer the phone or not.' Pause. 'I'll talk to you later. I love you.'" She broke down in tears.

John's computer ended up in the hands of Randy Stone. Part of his job was to confirm that Pam hadn't planted the porn, always a concern in a case like this, particularly since John was a cop. Through the metadata, Stone could show that the pictures were loaded on Tuesdays and Wednesdays, when John had his days off and Pam was at work.

The detectives had to talk to Pam's daughters as well. When the eldest told them that one night she'd woken up and John had his hand under her shirt—she turned over and he went away—Pam went into a tailspin. "Because now I'm questioning myself. What did I do to my kids, what did I get them into? How come I didn't know?" By that time, she'd already begun filing for divorce.

"I saw a horrific side of my husband that I never knew existed," she wrote in a statement she prepared for the court. "I never expected John, as a person, but especially as an officer of the law, to unashamedly violate the laws he was employed to enforce."

On December 3, 2004, John Coleman was sentenced to 32 months in jail for sexual exploitation of a child (the charge related to fondling his stepdaughter was ultimately dropped). "There were about 1,000 photos—explicit sex acts involving children and men wearing leather masks," says Assistant District Attorney Marc Bennett. "The stack was about four or five inches

> "He just looked
> at me and said,
> 'I will destroy you.'
> I was not going to
> let that happen."

high. The judge was appalled." Pam, who hasn't talked to John since the day of his arrest, remembers his final comments. "He said, 'I'm sorry to all my friends and family and the communities that have been involved in this. I was wrong. And I lost a lot, too. Lost my job, my career.' Almost the very last thing he said was, 'I lost my best friend, my wife.'"

Pam has used her anger to move on, although she's working against an undertow—her love for him, her loyalty. "Why," she asks, as if she's speaking to him, "didn't you say something so you could get help?" Then to me, "But I'm mad."

Suzanne Baughan, the wife of another cop, is also mad. For most of her decadelong marriage, the 32-year-old was white-knuckling the suburban dream so hard she neglected to pay attention to the rumors that her husband, Wade, had a mistress. Or to the threats she says he started making over the past couple of years, telling her "he would break my face or kill me if I didn't do what he wanted." Aside from his being very controlling, she says "the worst thing was forced sex." A lot was at stake. The Baughans had a nice house—a traditional colonial in Haymarket, Virginia, outside Washington, D.C.—the yard, the dog, and a side business in residential real estate, which allowed Suzanne to stay at home with their 6-year-old son, Mason, whom she hoped would soon have a sibling. "I never wanted to be labeled as divorced. I guess I'm very prudish and old-fashioned," she says, "and I was in love with him." But in the earliest days of 2006, as people everywhere dragged their Christmas trees to the curbs, something shifted.

Suzanne could not ignore the January cell phone bill. One number was all over it, including a call after midnight on New Year's Eve, just around the time Wade said he was going to get something out of the car (neither Wade nor his lawyer returned O's calls). He'd quit his job as a police officer in November and was now working part-time as a Prince William County sheriff's deputy so he could spend more time pursuing real estate deals. When one of Suzanne's girlfriends suggested phonebust.com (you give them the number, even if it's unpublished, and for a fee, they tell you whose it is), she discovered that the one decorating her phone bill belonged to a female police officer Wade used to work with, the woman the rumors had been about.

By this time, it was February. He was barely home anymore, she says, often coming in late, hopping on the computer, and then hitting the sack. One night after they'd gone to sleep, Suzanne very carefully slipped out of bed. She'd just come home from the hospital after having back surgery. "I'm barely able to walk, and I have to go downstairs," she says, remembering how she rued her dislike of carpet that had left the steps bare. "The wood floors are creaking; my cat is meowing. I'm whispering, 'No, no, Manny; be quiet.'" The office was directly below the bedroom. When she finally managed to sneak in, she saw not only that the computer was going but that Wade was still logged on. "He was so convinced I was an airhead, he believed he could get away with anything," she says. A former teacher with a master's in special education, Suzanne deftly went to "history" and clicked on one of the Web sites he'd just been visiting, and the tidy future she'd planned for herself imploded.

"It was a picture of him and his mistress. He's sitting on a couch—I don't know what couch. And he has his shirt off. And she's on top of him, just in underwear, straddling him. And he's about to kiss her bosom." The Web site hooks people up for group sex. According to the member profile that went with the photo, they are a fun couple—straight (him), bicurious (her), and married to each other—looking for other women preferably above 5'8" (Suzanne is 5'6½").

"My heart sank," she says. "No words can explain how I felt. I mean, it was hard enough knowing that he was unfaithful and betrayed me. But this is really risky behavior. He was putting my life on the line here. And he obviously didn't care."

She hit print. *Print. Print. Print.* Over the next month, she made several more furtive missions, often at night because that's when he'd just been on the computer and she could surf in his wake without passwords. As the pages slid out of the printer, she'd shove them under a rug until she could hide them in a box of baby clothes. Meanwhile, she tried to fend off his sexual advances—if putting up with them was hard before, now it was dangerous. One of the first things she did was get an AIDS test, and then she used her back surgery as an excuse. The few times he did insist they have sex, she says, "I told him I would do something to him, versus him touching me. And that worked."

After a couple of weeks, she stepped up her investigation into a full commando surveillance operation. He never let her have access to his Range Rover, she says, but she picked it up from the shop one day before he could get there and got the key copied; at the same time, she installed a hidden GPS device (she'd hired a PI to tail him, but her husband's driving style—"he's a police officer and pretty much goes 80 in a 25-mile-an-hour zone"—made him impossible to follow without blowing one's cover). Checking inside the car—"straws with lipstick, extra clothes, extra underwear," Suzanne sighs—became part of her nocturnal rounds.

The cell phone was another data mine. When Wade asked her to mail back his old one because he'd been sent an updated model, she said sure. "But I kept it." The problem was it had no battery, and when she went to the mobile company, they wouldn't give her a new one; they would ship it only to her husband's address because he'd bought the phone. Twice she had to shoo the UPS man away when Wade was home; on the third delivery try, however, she got the battery and popped it in. There were all sorts of numbers that she believes were his sex buddies—"names he'd put 'F***' by." Suzanne also found his calendar on the phone, going two years back. "Each time he would have sex with his mistress," she says, "it was marked down."

As unhinged as she was by discovering the kinky, sordid details of his organized deceit, Suzanne's undercover work turned up something else: evidence suggesting that Wade was forging documents for a big commercial real estate deal he was hoping to close.

By the time she went to the police—the same department he'd worked for—they were already investigating the matter. On March 9, 2006, detectives swarmed the Baughans' house, taking his computer, among other things. "I told Wade we were officially separated and he'd just lost the best thing that had ever happened to him. And I told him I knew about the affair," says Suzanne, "which he denied."

A year later, Gene Wade Baughan was sentenced to four months imprisonment plus four years probation for four felony counts of forgery. And Suzanne, to her surprise, is looking forward to being divorced. After years of worrying about what he's up to or what he might do to her, she says, "there's just been a big peace."

The verdict is in: You can run (around), that's for sure, but you cannot hide. Yet I'm still struggling with a question or two. I'm struck by these women, with their intrepid ingenuity, their high-techery and derring-do—and at the same time, it's a little unsettling to be reminded that just about every naughty impulse has become a searchable, readable, printable part of the record. It's another example of how public our lives have grown as we keep losing personal details to the whoosh of the information highway, leaving us baldly exposed.

Legal issues—clearly considerable—aside, I wonder if, given a good reason, I would load up the spyware. Where do you draw the line between your right to know what he's up to and his right to privacy? I make a quick call to Randy Cohen, whose ethics column I read every week in *The New York Times Magazine.* I can feel his neck hairs bristle over the phone—no fan of intimate espionage here. "But," he reasons, "if there is real evidence I've been catting around and you've tried more than once to say, 'Look, we really have to talk about this,' and I've refused to be honest with you, then I think you're permitted to take more extreme measures."

Just one more call. "So what are you asking me?" *O*'s life coach columnist, Martha Beck, tries to clarify at the other end of the line. I've rung her up for—she's right, for what? Maybe reassurance? I replay Cohen's scenario. Beck has known a few neurotics in her time. Couldn't all this computer peeping exacerbate an overly suspicious nature, even become addictive, I pose? "If you're obsessed with spying on your spouse, that's not love," she says. "That's you trying to control another person so that you won't get your feelings hurt, ever ever ever. And it creates exactly what you fear." Generally, however, Beck gives a hearty thumbs-up to following your hunch: "When someone lies, the body reacts violently, and the other person picks it up," she says. "So if he's lying to you and he keeps insisting nothing's wrong—and it is—you inevitably end up thinking, *I'm crazy.* And that feeling is even worse than knowing that someone is cheating on you." Reality, harsh as it is, offers relief.

In the end, truth simply trumps. And Suzanne Baughan is thanking the technology goddesses for leading her to it. "To be looking at this stuff and think this man is my husband," she says, "is unbelievable. There must be a lot of women out there who know something's going on but are too scared to do anything about it. I was one of them.

"I could still be in the dark." ◨

Sex

Let's Talk About Sex

Sex isn't just about earth-shattering orgasms. It's about the awesome,
sense-awakening, sometimes meandering trip women take to get there.
Hilda Hutcherson, MD, tells LISA KOGAN how to get comfy in the passenger seat.

I'm Sauvignon Blanc-ing with my friend Laurie when she announces that after almost seven perfectly respectable weeks of movies, dinners, and walks in the park with "adorable, divorced, one-kid-lives-in-Brooklyn, struggling architect guy," the two have finally gone to bed together. "And did the earth move?" I ask.

"Lisa," my slightly rattled friend replies, "the duvet cover didn't even move."

I do the only thing a person in my position can do: signal the waitress for a dessert menu as my beautiful, size 8 friend admits that he wanted the lights on so he could see her and she wanted the lights off so he couldn't.

Sex—when it's meaningful—can be a sublime expression of love. When it's not, well, it can be even better. And do you know why that is? Neither do I, but that's exactly my point: Sexual pleasure is an elusive little critter. Just when you think you've got it all figured out, something happens—you realize you're in your no-human-being-must-ever-see-these-panties panties, he accidentally elbows you in a way that may require a kidney transplant, the dog appears to be staring, the other people on the subway appear to be staring—well, you get the idea....

Hilda Hutcherson, MD, codirector of the New York Center for Women's Sexual Health at Columbia University Medical Center, is a firm believer in pleasure. In fact, she's written the

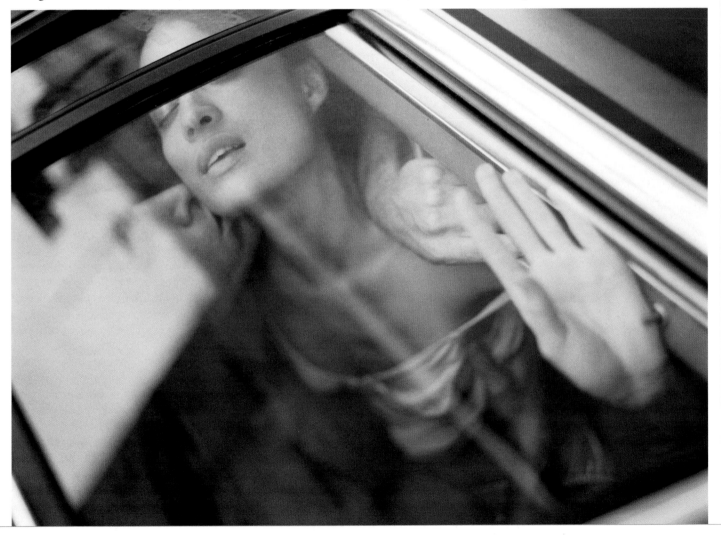

book on it—*Pleasure: A Woman's Guide to Getting the Sex You Want, Need, and Deserve*. We sit down at the little blond wood table in her slightly academic, slightly comfy, very lived-in office and cut straight to the chase.

"I'm mad at women," I tell her.

"Something we said?"

"Sort of. I'm just so sick of nearly everyone I know—myself included—walking around feeling crummy about our bodies to the point that it's actually hard to accept pleasure."

"I know what you mean. If you don't feel at ease with your body—this package that carries your mind and your soul around every day—then how can you really enjoy anything, especially sex? You're as close as you can be to another human being and instead of feeling his lips, and his fingers, and his heartbeat, you're thinking, *Oh my God, he's near that spot of cellulite by my thigh* or *He's going to realize that my boobs are drooping, that they're not the same size....*"

I make a mental note to buy a new bra immediately, and she continues. "It's pretty amazing. I've had patients say, 'I'm only 37, but I can't have oral sex because I've got gray hair down there and he'll think I'm old.' The things we obsess over."

"So do you prescribe Clairol for those patients?"

"I say, 'Honey, if he's down there doin' that, the last thing on his mind is a little gray hair. He's looking to give you pleasure, and it's up to you to let go and be in the moment.' Another thing I get all the time is, 'I can't have oral sex because I don't think I smell right, or it won't taste good.' I always say, 'Please, tell me how it's supposed to smell. I don't care what those commercials say, it's not supposed to smell like a spring rain or an English garden...unless, of course, you're trying to attract bees.' Lisa, do you know what a vagina should smell like?"

"The thing is, Hilda, my parents are still living...."

"It should smell like a vagina! It has a natural scent, and that scent is there for a reason; it's an aphrodisiac. It's part of the mating ritual. As far as taste goes, how many women have actually taken the time to taste themselves?"

"Ummm, I'm gonna say...eleven?"

"I encourage women to taste their own secretions, rather than constantly worrying about them. Self-knowledge makes you more accepting of your body."

"But," I say, both in complete agreement and in desperate need of a subject change, "all the knowledge in the world still doesn't guarantee a girl an orgasm."

"You know," she says filling our coffee cups, "orgasms are intensely pleasurable, but you can't go chasing them. You can't work on them, you can't will them. You can't say, 'Okay, if I try really, really hard, I'm going to have an orgasm'—it doesn't work that way."

"How exactly does it work?"

"You have to really concentrate on what all five of your senses are experiencing." Hilda sees my skepticism and elaborates: "When

> "The thing is, if you tell your partner what you want, most of the time you'll get it."

I was in college at Stanford, I liked going to Los Angeles to party. I used to hop in my car and race to get to that party." She smiles. "Then one day, I decided to take the scenic route. It was longer, it was slower, but, my God, it was incredible! I remember pulling over, listening to the ocean, looking at the seagulls, smelling the air. I actually forgot all about L.A. I mean, this was the kind of place that makes you believe in a higher power." She seems momentarily lost in the memory. "Anyway, if I had missed the party altogether, the trip would not have been a failure because I took in so much beauty and I had so much fun."

"Okay," I say, getting back to matters at hand. "In order to achieve orgasm, it might be a good idea to...take the Pacific Coast Highway." We clink our mugs together and laugh.

"All I'm saying," she continues, "is that pleasure comes in many forms. Your partner may be kissing your earlobes and stroking the back of your knees, but if you're thinking, *He's gotta make me climax* or *This isn't great sex,* then you're missing out on some extraordinary sensations because your head just isn't in the game. I've got a whole other group of patients who actually do have orgasms but are upset because they're not having *Sex and the City* orgasms."

"What's a *Sex and the City* orgasm? Is that where this sort of lightning bolt comes roaring through you at a Manolo Blahnik sale? Because I once saw these fabulous suede boots in navy, and for a minute there..."

Hilda interrupts: "*Sex and the City* was a double-edged sword, and I think we're still feeling its effect. That show obliterated many taboos and got women really talking, but it also made us question ourselves: *How come I've never had that female ejaculation thing that Samantha had?* or *Why aren't I able to achieve multiple orgasms the way those women seem to?*

"I always ask, 'Did the sex leave you feeling good about yourself? Did it leave you feeling connected to your partner?' If the answer is yes, then I say quit looking for multiple anything, celebrate the pleasure you *are* having, and go to sleep in his arms."

"Hilda, how did you get so comfortable with all of this?"

"Oh, I was a real prude." She sees I'm not buying it. "I really was! The first man I slept with was my first husband. Like a lot of us growing up, I watched my mother wait on my dad hand and foot. If he cleared his throat, she would be rushing to get him a cold lemonade. So in my mind, it was all about making sure your man was satisfied, because," she says with a sigh, "that's what you have to do for your husband."

"What changed you?"

"A couple of things. One day I filled out one of those 'how well do you know your spouse?' surveys in some magazine. And I was feeling very proud of myself. I went to Harvard. I went to Stanford. I mean, I'm a smart girl. I know his favorite foods, favorite color, the last book he read, what kind of underwear he likes...." Her voice trails off. "Then it hit me: I had no clue what book *I* had last read, *my* favorite food, *my* favorite color—it was all a blank. I had no idea what kind of underwear felt good against my skin—I just bought whatever was on sale. Isn't that something?" she asks, still a bit mystified. "I knew everything about how to make *him* happy, but I didn't know anything about myself."

"Then I guess you're not really allowed to be mad at him for not knowing anything about you."

"Exactly. Why should he? I simply didn't feel entitled to pleasure. That realization was a life-altering revelation."

"Was it also the end of that marriage?"

"Yes, once I woke up, there was no going back to sleep. The next moment came," she says brightening, "when I started my ob-gyn practice. Women would say to me, 'I've heard about this thing called a clitoris, but I don't know how to find it.' Or they'd ask for advice about anal sex, or they'd want to know if there's a vibrator I like. Believe me, I could go on and on."

"I believe you," I say quickly.

"These women forced me to face my own demons. I had to look at all the negative messages that were fed to me over the years. I realized the only way I could help people deal with their issues was if I dealt with my own. So I educated myself into feeling good about my body, good about sex, and free to talk about

everything under the sun. I tell my patients, 'If I can go to a sex shop and buy a vibrator, then so can you.' "

"You learned to ask for what you want in bed."

"That's right. And there are all kinds of ways to ask for what you want. Sometimes it's as simple as saying, 'Darling, let's try something new.' Sometimes it's going out and buying a book of erotica. Sometimes it means putting his hand right where you want it to be and showing him the pressure and tempo that feels good to you." She refills our cups and goes on. "The thing is, if you tell your partner what you want, most of the time you'll get it."

"And if you don't?"

"If someone isn't open to giving you pleasure, then I'd say you're probably with the wrong person." We sit and sip for a minute. Out the window I can see the sky streaked with gray and the students looking a little eager, a little anxious—as though they were born with too much homework. Hilda is the first to speak: "There are an awful lot of reasons in the world to feel bad right now," she says finally. "But how amazing is it that we each have this remarkable built-in capacity for pure joy? Women have to realize that sexual pleasure is our birthright." ◘

Something Wilder

You might expect your sex life to wither in your 40s and 50s. But no. If you're up for a little adventure, this is exactly when things can—and should—blossom. Psychoanalyst Gail Saltz gives NINA BURLEIGH the whys and hows.

An editor at a national magazine once called me into his office to discuss a story about aging female movie stars. With a picture of his much younger wife and toddler on the shelf behind him, this 50-something man said he hoped each star would talk to us about a very specific moment: "I want to know what it felt like when she realized she'd reached an age where no man was ever going to want to kiss her again."

Although I never wrote the story, I've never forgotten that middle-aged man's casual assumption that women inevitably become undesirable. It offended me—and as I passed my 40th birthday, I feared it might have some truth to it.

Then I met New York psychoanalyst Gail Saltz, who begs to differ. At 44, she exudes a sexy, healthy energy in a trim suit, tastefully low-cut blouse, and light makeup. If women become less sexually active as they age, she says, it's more likely because they've lost their desire, not their desirability. "That's the most common issue I see in 40- and 50-year-olds," says Saltz, a clinical associate professor of psychiatry at New York–Presbyterian Hospital, author, and contributor to NBC's *Today* show. "Statistically, it affects one out of three women."

She cites a "conspiracy of forces" that diminish libido: anxiety, depression, exhaustion, and relationship conflicts. Middle-aged women face some disturbing challenges: "They have elderly parents and worries about their own health and life changes. We are talking about loss, which is exceptionally stressful." Less often lust is zapped by hormonal changes. When a woman comes to Saltz with no sex drive, she sends her first to a gynecologist. Low testosterone can be a culprit, but Saltz contends it's rare. Likewise, dropping estrogen thins the vaginal wall, "but of the vast number of women with diminished desire, there's only a small percentage of cases where it's due to hormones alone."

Saltz advises women to tend to what she calls the biggest female sex organ, the brain, by indulging in more fantasies and allowing themselves to explore new, possibly unorthodox erotic avenues. "What you liked when you were 20 may not be what you like in your 40s. I see women who say, 'I liked to do it standing up on the table, and now it's so much effort; I prefer it on my side, or something more relaxed, and I'm having a hard time saying what I want.' I've also seen the opposite, women who were inhibited in young adulthood are now thinking, *I would try doggy style*

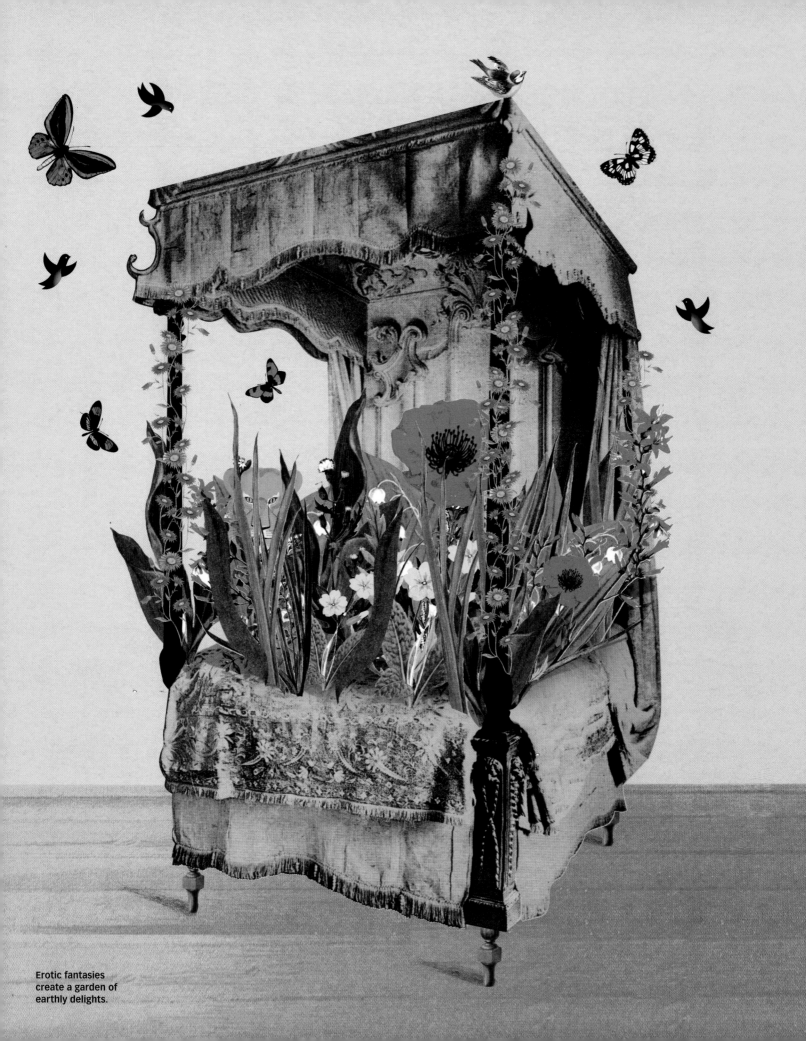

Erotic fantasies
create a garden of
earthly delights.

or anal sex, but they're too embarrassed to ask. And it is really important to ask." The good news, she says, is that as men age, they're usually more willing to listen. "So you probably have a more receptive partner."

When it comes to sexual requests, Saltz, who has been married for 17 years and has three kids, thinks "direct is always best." If you can't bear an explicit conversation, she suggests writing a note, drawing a cartoon, or leaving out a toy or prop you'd like to use.

Bear in mind that his desires and abilities may be changing, too. "He might wish he could hold you up against the wall, but he can't anymore," she says. "Maybe he used to enjoy having you on top, but now he needs a different position for his erection to hold. If a woman doesn't know that some loss of erectile strength is normal, it can start a whole cycle of not wanting to be in bed because it's humiliating."

Fantasy, she says, is crucial to maintaining a healthy sex life over time. She contends that a lot of women lie there contemplating what they should make for dinner because they're afraid to imagine domination or animals or the guy down the street. "But it's fine to fantasize—if it works in the service of your sex life with your partner, great. There's a big difference between thinking about the soccer coach and getting a motel room with him."

If you're like me, with so many distractions at work and home that the mere idea of sneaky sex with a soccer coach is laughably exhausting, Saltz recommends picking up Nancy Friday's voluminous collection of fantasies, *My Secret Garden*. Women should also masturbate more, she says. "It's hugely important, because your body is changing, your tastes are changing, and you need to figure out what stimulation works for you." And she's in favor of vibrators, saying, "Only 20 percent of women reach orgasm through intercourse alone."

Mechanical problems that sometimes come with age are, surprisingly, easier to resolve than emotional ones. Surgery or medication can help incontinence, uterine prolapse, and other medical issues that make sex difficult or embarrassing. The most common complaint in menopausal women is vaginal dryness. Saltz recommends having a lubricant on hand and not being shy about applying it. "Women are really nervous now about taking estrogen. That means they are struggling with dryness and atrophy, and let me say, if it's dry and it hurts, you are not going to feel like having sex," she says.

Frankly, you have to use it or lose it: "The vagina is a muscle," she says. "I urge women without a partner to insert something. Otherwise, the vagina shrinks and might never get back its original elasticity. Women need to know this. They need to take care of their bodies."

What about those who worry that gray hair, saggy breasts, and flabby arms mean the end of fun between the sheets? Hollywood still isn't giving us any aging female sex icons, although 60-year-old Charlotte Rampling is giving it a good go in France.

> "It's fine to fantasize. There's a big difference between thinking about the soccer coach and getting a motel room with him."

Yet Saltz believes we can choose to maintain our sexuality. "What matters is what's going on between you and your partner and how you feel about your body," she says. She's not opposed to plastic surgery: It helps some of her patients enormously, especially those who have a lifelong "trouble spot" fixed. "But if the issue is really about needing to keep a 20-something body, it can't be done," she says. "If you try, you'll be in conflict with yourself, and then you won't fully enjoy sex."

Some of Saltz's patients have the misfortune of being with men like that editor who found older women unattractive. "In that case, you need couples therapy. The idea is to come together and talk about what's important to both of you, and in that process your partner will either decide that he values you as a person and can find sexiness in you or remain so mired in perky breasts that the marriage may not be salvageable. I have worked with women who've been dumped by men having a midlife crisis—they must have that sports car and an affair. What's terrible is that most of these women blame themselves."

Fundamental differences between men and women can exacerbate sexual problems in middle age. Men tend to use sex to shed stress and increase intimacy, but when women are strung out, they're not in the mood—plus, anxiety in a woman prevents orgasm, Saltz says. Women also have a different definition of closeness than men, often craving what Saltz calls "talky-talky bonding." Basic plumbing disparities present another hindrance: Men can reach orgasm in four minutes; the average woman needs at least 20, and older women on certain drugs such as antidepressants, antihypertensives, or ulcer medications might require up to 45.

Saltz is adamant that women not give up. When people come to her office complaining about general unhappiness in life, she almost invariably discovers that they're not enjoying sex anymore. "They'll say, 'I'm okay with that.' And I'll say, 'Lack of good sex is part of the reason you're depressed.'"

I ask whether she isn't putting yet another layer of pressure on aging baby boomers by insisting they continue to romp in the sack. She roundly disagrees. "If someone told you to do exercises with your mind to avoid dementia, you'd do them, right? If you put in the effort with sex, life will be better in many respects, including how you feel about yourself and your relationship, and how you deal with the world. The bottom line is it's not all gloom. Yes, there are changes. But many women do find their way. They have figured themselves out and have seen that sustaining an evolving sexual relationship is extremely gratifying. It makes you closer and closer to your partner," she says. "Women who like sex and have worked to make it good for themselves tend to be very confident people." �‍

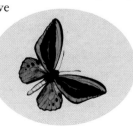

Confessions of an Ex–Sex Kitten

In her teens and 20s, she saw sex as a simple game of conquest—and whoever had the most boys at the end won. Today she'd rather stay home than wake up with a stranger. What changed? LISA DIERBECK traces her evolution from vamp to veteran.

I don't believe in casual sex. It's not that I'm opposed to it exactly, it's just that—in my own experience—no such thing exists. If it's not emotional, I'm not interested. For me, sex without feeling is an empty ritual, a cold, mechanical exchange that leaves me lonely and depressed. Given the choice between that and solitude, I prefer to be alone.

Even the phrase "casual sex" has a hollow ring that bothers me. It's a contradiction in terms. Where's the casual part? I've thrown casual dinner parties, serving Chinese takeout on paper plates. I've worn casual clothes to plush offices on Fridays. But applied to relationships, *casual* is a code word for apathy. If someone says, "This is only physical," my translation is: "I don't care about you." Forget casual. The more accurate word is *heartless*.

Sex strikes me as too intense a venture to be taken lightly. Thrilling and uncertain, it involves baring your soul, not just tearing off your clothes. Because sexuality is a powerful, anarchic force over which we have little control, it's soothing to pretend it's no big deal. I used to be blasé about it. I treated sex like a swimming pool. Instead of hesitating, I always plunged right in. Now, as a reformed tramp at 40, I look back at my wild ways and wonder what planet I was on. I have more respect for sex, its hazards and surprises. Watch out for that sweet dark-eyed hunk at the watercooler; he may turn out to be a mean, manipulative jerk. And if you're hell-bent on a casual liaison, you might miss that shy, bespectacled geek at your local library who could set your heart aflame and worship you. Either way, a sexual experience is unpredictable. Offering a rare chance to feel transcendence—an ecstatic state that transports people outside themselves—the sexual embrace has a strong spiritual side. Whatever happens, having sex with someone changes you.

I didn't always think this. For a long time, I saw sex without strings as the key to independence. I was raised in 1970s New York, a rollicking, amoral, sex-crazed place. The decade introduced freedoms undreamed of by my grandmother Lillian, who'd been taught to close her eyes chastely during intercourse and

> If you're hell-bent on a casual liaison, you might miss that shy, bespectacled geek at your local library who could set your heart aflame and worship you.

contemplate her rose garden. Claiming the right to an appetite was a critical step forward for women. But in our eagerness to take the guilt out of sex and let it be natural and healthy, we might have gotten a little carried away. During my childhood, the rules were suspended while the Sexual Revolution swept through town. Our teenage sisters lurked in hotel lobbies, stalking rock stars. Our moms and dads frolicked at key parties. Our high school teachers took their students to bed, and no one got sued or fired. My friends and I roamed the streets of Manhattan incautiously, a reckless pack of underage girls dressed to kill in platform shoes and hot pants. My single burning ambition was to be a sex kitten. As ambitions go, it was pretty easy to accomplish.

It took me many years to figure out that I wasn't who I was pretending to be. Outwardly, I'd become a bold, brazen adventuress who made a habit of propositioning men she hardly knew. I'd hand my phone number to a guy at a party, arrange to meet him on his doorstep, spend an hour or two in his apartment, and slip away. Every time I did this, I felt a curious combination of victory and devastation. I was afraid of something that I couldn't pinpoint, and I wasn't nearly as frisky and footloose as I acted. I was a confused young woman who had trouble trusting men. Easy sex was a tactic to keep men at arm's length by treating them as conquests. If this sounds like something a guy might do, it was. Alarmed by the power imbalance between men and women, I thought sleeping around would even up the score. I wore my sexuality like a protective suit of armor. My swaggering bravado was a put-on. I led a rather sad, disconnected life—until I mustered up the courage to let my guard down. I can't help wondering now if maybe there are some women out there, like me, putting on this same kind of act, suppressing their passion and vulnerability. I believe women today are under pressure to reinvent themselves, to conform to a bed-hopping, no-strings ethos that's in vogue.

Now that the love affair has been replaced by the booty call, it's fashionable to treat sex as something without weight or meaning. Our aggressively modern culture has chipped away at

RELATIONSHIPS

our collective faith in romance. Decades ago, *The Joy of Sex* made history with its illustrated, step-by-step recipes for lovemaking. It was a useful, practical source of information, except for one colossal error. Unlike cooking, sex isn't a hobby. People aren't playthings. They're richly intricate creatures full of good and evil impulses, psychological conflicts and contradictions. Sometimes we insist upon a "casual relationship" to deny the uncomfortable truth: Sex is complicated.

As a society, we've tried to simplify things by separating physical pleasure from emotional attachment. At the same time, we've started to confuse sexiness with physical perfection. While we're running off to our plastic surgeons for Botox injections and breast implants, we've forgotten that what's really sexy can't be bottled. It's an inner spark that's as distinctive as your personality. Being hot is a state of mind, and it's subjective. It takes two to generate heat. Desire demands emotion.

In fact, the alchemy of attraction is so personal and inexplicable, no one fully understands it. Poets, playwrights, and novelists have spent centuries trying to grasp it. A how-to guide can teach you how to have a bigger, better orgasm. A vial of Viagra can "enhance performance" so you can have sex around the clock. But there's no secret formula for what floats your boat, or who. Ever since I stopped leaving my heart on the bedside table, I've thought of sex as mystical. Romantics like me may be an endangered species, but instead of trying to blend in at the swingers' party, let's stand up and be counted. ◐

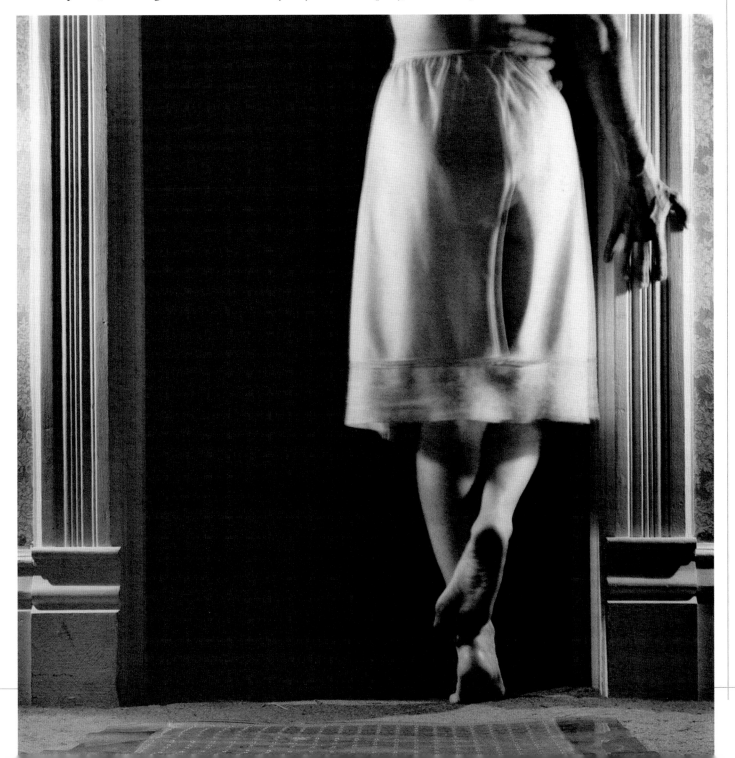

Everything I Need to Know About Manners, I Learned in Bed

Forget Emily Post. **TOM CHIARELLA** makes politeness sexy.

My mother insisted I use my manners. The rules were uncomplicated and clear. Always say please and thank you. Wait your turn. Don't chew with your mouth open. Don't lick your fingers. Elbows off the table. Don't play with your food. No singing during a meal. These things mattered, she assured me. She seemed smart, and she carried a wooden spoon. I got stern looks and cracks on the knuckles. Over time she made me a believer.

Still, I was never an enthusiast. I liked slouching and enjoyed slurping. I could see nothing wrong with reaching across the table for the rolls. Even as I learned them, manners seemed distant, abstract, unconnected to my life. I had the dim sense that I might need them should I visit the White House for a state dinner, or sit down with a sultan, or shake hands with a movie director. But who was I kidding? I was 8 years old. I lived in Rochester, New York. What did I really matter in the grand scheme?

I didn't see why manners couldn't be like a tuxedo or a limousine, something you rolled out on special occasions. I made secret teenage plans to live my way—belching, scratching, and putting shoes on the table by day, locating a more demure self at night, on dates, at weddings, in future sit-downs with royalty. Through all this my mother was pragmatic, encouraging me to think of manners as the best line of social defense. She even sent me to charm school. She felt that I had to do more than wear my manners like a costume if they were going to protect me. I didn't understand what she was so afraid of.

Not until after I had left home, anyway. I didn't understand until late one night, as a 20-year-old college student, when I sat on a single bed in a claptrap college apartment, waiting for a 23-year-old art student to come out of the bathroom before sex. At that moment, I knew this much: I was going to get some. But I didn't know the niceties, the procedures, the expectations for what was to come. It wasn't the mechanics of sex that worried me; it was the question of whether I should get in the bed or wait with my hands folded. I was struggling with how to behave in this room, this space, in this moment, with this person. In a setting stripped of discernible guidelines, I didn't know a damned thing. Not where to sit, or where to put my hands, or lay my clothes, even whether or not to avert my eyes when the art student finally did get out of the bathroom. No one had prepared me. I flat out didn't know the rules.

In the years since then, it has occurred to me that this night marked the beginning of my appreciation of good manners. I'm not saying I learned all my manners in the

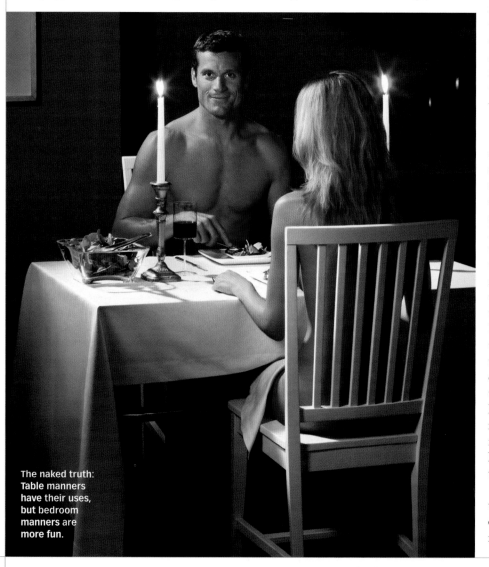

The naked truth: Table manners have their uses, but bedroom manners are more fun.

bedroom. I knew how to hold open a door before that. My point is that I gained a richer understanding of the subtle importance of manners thanks to sex—the most common and, paradoxically, the rarest of human transactions.

There's nothing especially precious about the manners you use in the bedroom. They're not about giving yourself more fully or turning on your heartlight. Rather, they're the block-and-tackle truths of two people dealing with their most private stuff in a semipublic fashion. The manners you learned at the dinner table do come into play (even in sex there is reaching, passing, serving, and knowing when to ask permission). But the manners of the bedroom are less absolute.

The proper fork, the correct technique for cutting your prime rib, the elbows on the table thing: Those are capital-M Manners. Knowing when to defer to the wishes of another, granting kindnesses simply because you can, making a person understand how much you value their presence in your little bed on a Wednesday night in a distant suburb: These are lowercase manners, pure and simple, more subtle and eminently more fun to take on.

The first thing to know about the manners of desire is that it's okay to drop them, at least periodically. The pure energy of sex should subvert them, at least initially. There's a pleasure in giving up social niceties, after a date, after a courtship, after years of circling each other in the office. In a clinch, with both people ripping at buttons and zippers, you give up all the proprieties. All the prescribed distancing—physical and psychological: gone. The carefully chosen words: also gone. And, let's face it, it's a pretty great form of chaos. When you're belly to belly, with each person moving things toward some next step, some new pleasure, some favorite part of the body, manners are slippery. They get squeezed out, the tighter you get, and fall on the floor.

But they wait there on the floor, or at the end of the bed, for the first moment of physical distance, the first tiny nudge of separation, so they can slip back into the equation. Within seconds of climax. I think there is probably an easily discernible set of Manners for people who are lying naked, six inches from each other, freshly uncoupled. You don't talk about work; you don't answer the phone. No reading. No glancing at the clock or brushing your hair. No eating—unless you feed the other person first, and no getting up to get a drink unless you offer the other person one, too. You give a compliment—you find a superlative, you make it known that you are thankful, or affirmed, or whatever it is you feel a person should be after sex. You tell them they are great. Or they are sweet. Fun. Strong. Sexy. Smart about things. That they smell good. Or have wonderful skin. You find something you mean, then you utter it. You give the compliment to the other person because there's a lot of risk in sex, and it's your duty to acknowledge that.

But there is no rule for lights on or lights off; there is only the hand reaching for the switch, to turn it one way or the other. And

I don't know if you avert your eyes when the other person rises; it is a matter of reading the signals that are sent. Speaking as a man now, I would say I like looking at a woman afterward, just after, but I know women who never want to be looked at in those moments. If it were up to me, the rule would be the eyes must linger. But it is not up to me, and that's probably the biggest rule of all. Here is the heart of the matter: It is not up to one person; it's up to both. And that's why manners are more than a defense; they are a kind of language, one spoken through the communication of desire. You cede to the desire of the other. There is no rule for being under the covers or not, or whether or not you wear your underwear to bed. It may differ every time.

If you are making rules, or relying on them blindly, in these first moments of lovemaking, then the fact is you are being rude. The purpose of Manners is, in some way, to codify behavior. In the bedroom, that just plain gets oppressive. You have to modify your manners in accordance with the connection you make. You can't write down manners like these. If that were possible, they would have given you a list in high school and been done with it. You have to teach yourself, then learn some more.

Does the person cover themselves as they rise? Do they rush to the bathroom? Then there it is, the rule. Respect it. Avert your eyes, turn off the light, give the other person what they need. In sex, wishes are rules. And manners are the kindnesses we give without sarcasm, judgment, or expectation.

With the art student, I checked things. I got up and folded my clothes. Respread the blanket so the bed looked neater. But she would notice that, I figured; she would take it to mean that I was calling her a slob. So I remussed it right away. Clothes on? Clothes off? Under the covers? Wait in the chair? I put on my shirt, then took it off again.

I have witnessed versions of this very scene played out in movies for nearly 30 years since then. The guy checks his breath, rearranges the pillows, maybe looks around the room in places he ought not. And I always roll my eyes, because it rarely happens that way, with that much time. But the art student really did take forever. The more time that passed, the less certain I was of anything. Surely there had to be a rule that you didn't disappear into the bathroom. Then I remembered what my charm school teacher had always said: When confronted with something that confuses you at the dinner table—an extra serving fork, a plate of aspic between courses, the random cheese plate—move slowly and with assurance. "It looks more elegant if you seem to know what you are doing," she said, "even if you don't."

So I looked around, found a candle, sniffed it, then lit it. I turned off the light, got in bed, and the art student came to me. Naked. Delightful. She smiled when she pulled back the covers. "I was waiting for you to find that candle," she said, as she settled in next to me, "and turn out those lights. Thank you."

I told her she was most welcome. ◗

In sex, wishes are rules. And manners are the kindnesses we give without judgment or expectation.

Tantric Sex

You've wondered about it. You've read about it. Hours and hours of kissing.
Soul-melding eye contact. Transcendental sex.... Hey, I'll have what they're having!
But what's involved? And what does a weekend workshop in the Poconos have
to do with the real thing? AIMEE LEE BALL comes back with a firsthand report.

An urban legend with the ring of authenticity cites a survey in which tantric sex tops the list of subjects that most interest 14- to 25-year-olds—the prototype MTV generation. Me too, although I'm hardly MTV's target audience. Who wouldn't be curious about a practice that is alleged to foster staring into a beloved's eyes for hours and hours, kissing for hours and hours, making love for hours and hours?

It's not as if we don't already commit enough time and energy to sex in our society—we live in a sexually saturated culture; both Madison Avenue and Hollywood are truly obsessed with the subject—but much of what we read, observe, and experience in our bedrooms seems to be about performance, about attracting a partner and being "good in bed" and reaching some multiorgasmic goalpost. There is now on my desk a small library of books about tantric sex, and while the explicit detailing of intimate behavior might make our grandmothers blush (and might at first be confused with garden-variety porn), the practice of tantra (based on ancient Hindu and Buddhist scriptures) is supposed to facilitate a more meaningful intimacy, an actual spiritual connection between partners. Mark Epstein, MD, a New York City psychiatrist and the author of *Open to Desire: Embracing a Lust for Life—Insights from Buddhism and Psychotherapy,* reframes this concept as the dropping of a veil between "self" and "other." Tantra is not just some postmodern *Kama Sutra* or postgraduate search for the G-spot, according to its aficionados. It is intended to develop the "awakened mind" of meditation in a sexual context. It is, although this sounds incredibly highfalutin, about finding aspects of the divinity in one's beloved.

I don't hang out in X-rated shops, but I doubt there's much pornography that talks about men and women transforming erotic energy into a refined state of consciousness. I don't get HBO either, so I learned only recently that *Sex and the City* (inevitably) seized upon the idea of tantra, veering perilously close to *Hustler* territory. The four main characters (hardly prudes) were embarrassed but crippled by the "inability to look away from a car crash" as they attended a tantric seminar and were instructed how to perform genital massage on a man "as if you are using an orange juicer." Mastery of the technique would make a man faithful, said the coach, "because once they go tantric, they don't go back."

There was nothing even remotely spiritual about this sordid display, but it's not hard to understand the impetus behind the desire for a legitimate tantric experience—the yearning for a passionate bond. The idea that tantra can dissolve the boundaries between two people, that through the body you can meet the essence of another person, is so attractive. The "real" tantra seems to be about connection, generosity, being in the present, and transcending sex as a competitive sport. But go searching for the spiritual dimension of sex, and you'll encounter a lot of gooey rhetoric. "It's the art of disappearing inside each other," says Margot Anand, of San Rafael, California, who uses the term SkyDancing for her tantric workshops. "Lovers are like two instruments before a concert: They have to learn how to be in tune; otherwise it will not be melodic. When a man and a woman practice tantra, they have the tools to go beyond ego, beyond gender, even beyond having a body, like navigating into space."

What exactly are the men and women doing? "Dancing, moving, breathing, visualizing, contracting and releasing the internal muscles, relaxing the pelvis, understanding sexual anatomy, confronting their shadows, learning how to scream, learning how to breathe from the sexual organs all the way to the heart, breathing in a circular fashion with each other, understanding successful communication. These are great secrets that transform couples' lives." Isn't all that muscle work just like Kegeling, taught by most gynecologists to maintain internal muscular strength? And isn't "communication" the key to all good coupleness, not only tantric?

"Sometimes I think I shouldn't call what I teach tantra; I should call it the Margot Anand method," she says, and she gets annoyed when I ask her to describe any more unusual or specific techniques—as if writing is too imperfect a medium for conveying the concept—but finally mentions a game called Yin-Yang, in which partners act as king and queen for the day, taking turns trying to grant the other any wish within reason. "What you get to practice is daring to ask, being supported in the asking, and letting go of your own will to control things," Anand explains.

This newly popularized version of tantra is the Western "repackaging" of an honorable, even scholarly Eastern body of knowledge, according to Michael Witzel, PhD, professor of Sanskrit at Harvard University and managing editor of the *International Journal of Tantric Studies.* "As with yoga, what we get in the West is mostly gymnastics, just body exercises," he says with ill-concealed contempt. And yet there are seemingly sane people who claim to have gotten something valuable from such lessons. When 48-year-old Californian Tracy first went to a tantric workshop, her boyfriend observed that it was exactly what the rest of the country expected of anyone living in Northern California. "We're straight and normal people," says Tracy, a development director of a nonprofit organization. "We were in a fairly new relationship, a second-time-around relationship, and taking the course together sounded like a good way to establish the intimacy I was looking for. But it felt scary and really pushed me to some of my edges." Tracy and her boyfriend learned techniques such as "streaming energy" (one partner bends at the waist, head and arms hanging loosely, and begins to shake slightly, drawing energy up from feet to head as the other partner strokes her back) and "lion's play" (the partners put palms together, growl at each other, and pseudo-wrestle). "One goal of tantra is to spread sexual energy throughout the body," says Tracy. "I get to the point where I feel completely orgasmic, and it feels like it's coming from the genitals all the way up to my head. It's the opposite of rushing to orgasm."

After four years as workshop faithfuls, the couple often decides to have tantric dates, which start with "heart salutations": sitting across from each other, hands brought into prayer position, then leaning toward each other and breathing. "It's a sweet and simple way to mark that we're entering sacred space," says Tracy, who creates a tantric "temple" in their home, cleared of clutter, candles lit, sarongs hung on windows. "We don't ever have alcohol, because it's all about being present, but we might have feathers or chimes. We're attending to each of the senses." One of her favorite exercises is called the breath of love, which she ends with the classic tantric position called yab-yum, the man sitting cross-legged with the woman straddling his waist, her legs wrapped around him. "It doesn't actually involve sex at all," says Tracy, "but it feels more intimate than sex, which is saying something. First you imagine that you're breathing from your sex organs up to your heart; then you imagine a bowl of energy between the two of you that you're both filling up; then you share the energy, looking into each other's eyes and breathing into each other's mouths. At the end, the kissing is electric. There's no penetration, no genital stimulation, but I am so much more turned on than when having regular sex. You get so high, it's amazing."

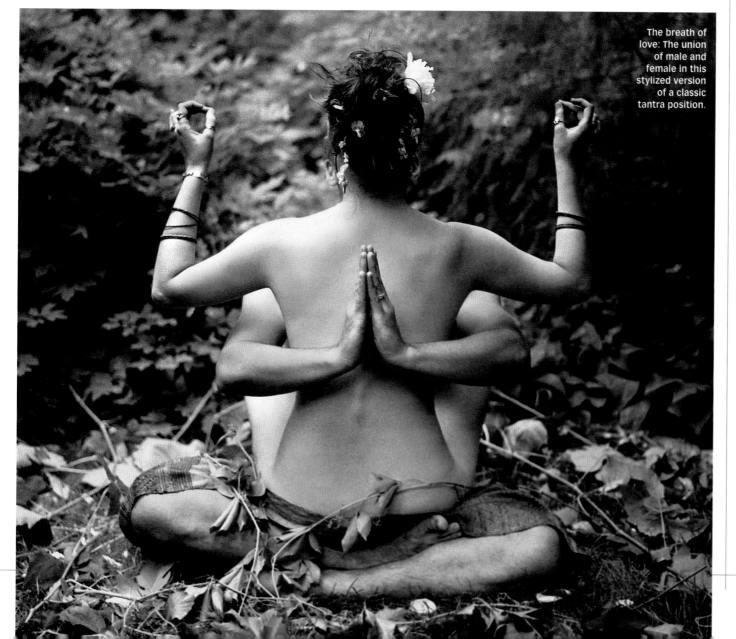

The breath of love: The union of male and female in this stylized version of a classic tantra position.

One basic tantric tenet is that men can withhold ejaculation and prolong erection and that seminal fluid contains drops of vital energy, the spending of which ages the body and dulls the senses. This premise accounts for the boom in Westernized tantra, according to Jonathan Margolis, author of *O: The Intimate History of the Orgasm.* In a chapter called "A Little Coitus Never Hoitus" (a witticism poached from Dorothy Parker), Margolis posits that hours and hours of lovemaking is more about male ego than female pleasure. The idea of a sexual marathon is fodder for a man's braggadocio—"an under-the-duvet power politics play," he writes, and "the long-lost cousin of Viagra," which is "thinly disguised as sensitivity to women." But from an informal scan of tantric sex Web sites, Margolis reports that the withheld orgasm is not as intense—"more like a quiet, 'held-in' sneeze than a full-blooded *ker-chow.*"

Unsurprisingly, the subject has found a welcome reception on the Internet. The Web site tantra.com reports that it gets about 13,000 visitors a day. Visitors to the site are promised "deeper intimacy" with a $14.99-per-month membership and are directed to purchases of books and videotapes, sex "furniture," and rabbit-fur massage mitts. (A popular item is Kama Sutra Honey Dust, a "velvety-soft powder" that comes with its own handmade feather duster.) Much of the so-called expertise bandied about on the Web and in books is hardly distinguishable from ads for escort services. (One site, geared toward men, suggests that visitors "scroll through the complete list of available goddesses." Goddess Grace, for instance, on call from 9 A.M. to 9 P.M. in Southern California, is pictured with hands in the *namaste* prayer position over bare breasts.) Some of it seems eccentrically esoteric or just plain silly ("Tantra is the wild summer thunderstorm…," "Tantra is the mother tiger…"). The World Tantra Association talks about weaving a "magic carpet" with "yarn" from the seven chakras, or energy centers, in the body.

I react badly to such grandiose language. It all just means: You'll feel better. The same could be said for Tylenol. I question such an intense sales pitch. Years ago there was an advertising campaign for something I've now forgotten whose simple and direct tagline was "Try it, you'll like it," and I thought: *That must be a pretty good product.* So this must be a pretty bad one, if it's so consistently overstated. "There's a lot of pseudo stuff," says Mark Epstein, "people trying to create workshop-y types of things. It's a growth industry. Why is it happening in the culture right now? People need help with their sexuality. It's gone so far away from anything spiritual."

Wondering how serious, instructive, and ultimately spiritual the myriad tantra workshops and seminars around the country are, I decide to conduct my own research and head for the Pocono Mountains of eastern Pennsylvania for a weekend of "love without limits." The workshop is led by a woman I'll call Dr. Madge, a psychologist and "leading-edge healer" dedicated to "reintegrating sexuality into spirituality" and "expanding the boundaries of the family." The setting was promised to be a "beautiful mountain retreat center" where we would be "working with breath, energy, conscious touch, and movement to create a glorious space of love, which invites heart opening, sensuality, and spiritual communion." I was e-mailed a list of suggested useful items, including a flashlight, drums or other musical instrument, massage oil, sensual fruit or sweets, and a flowing costume ("a beautiful scarf or two is very versatile"). Despite language that seemed intentionally non-sleazy (and the fact that anything involving sweets is okay by me), I wondered about that massage oil. But before I remitted $475, a phone call to Dr. Madge's California office assured me that the workshop was appropriate for both couples and singles.

The accommodations at the lodge, built for Christian retreats in the 1940s, could generously be called monastic—a clean towel and set of sheets waiting on each bed, with meals served cafeteria-style. The group assembled on floor cushions in front of a makeshift altar with candles and photos of an Indian yogi "no longer in the body." There were four couples, three single men, and three single women—matched sets, I noticed—ranging in age from their 30s to 60s, and we began with Dr. Madge–led breathing exercises. An older woman, who had been exhaling most audibly, announced right away that she'd recently ended 15 years of celibacy and now froze when her partner, a divorced former pastor, touched her anus. Hello, Toto, I don't think we're in Kansas anymore. Another couple had just met the previous day, after a cross-country e-mail correspondence and one night spent at a Best Western: The woman declared herself to be a "pagan" practicing "polyamory," which, Dr. Madge clarified, meant "responsible nonmonogamy." A chunky 30-something guy admitted that he had trouble satisfying women; a Nordic-looking American businessman now living in Europe had recently begun a ménage à trois with his wife of 20 years and another woman—he cheerfully offered to teach us "a great three-way kiss" they had perfected. Two of the singles, a plain Jane who ran an animal hospital and a handsome man who worked in politics, seemed to be tantra junkies—frequent fliers at this kind of workshop.

The maxim about the "wallflower at the orgy" fit me perfectly. I reached for the keys to my rented car several times—this level of intimate talk among strangers wasn't what I'd anticipated, but it was, after all, just talk, so I carried on with journalistic detachment. And as we formed two circles, men and women facing each other, the exercises were innocuous. Everyone was asked to share a story about some wounding life experience—for instance, being taught as a child that sex was dirty. We were instructed to inhale one-third of a breath and then try to lay an egg, feeling the force of pelvic pressure. We were asked to stick our tongue between our teeth and try to complain (all attempts devolved into laughter). We were told to look at the other person without seeing the physical body. And we kept rotating the circles, changing partners, so that even the couples that had arrived paired up were now interacting with strangers. I can't say that I learned anything—because there was no relationship with these others, no basis of information on which to layer more classified disclosures, and I was too self-conscious to have any epiphanies myself—but it was all moderately interesting.

The next day, we moved beyond interesting. Tantra, Dr. Madge explained, means a willingness to embrace whatever shows up, and she announced that we would be breaking down our "genital armory," worshipping each other as gods and goddesses through massage, so everyone should think about partnering up. I in turn announced that they'd have to buy me dinner and a movie first. I wasn't taught that sex is dirty, but I did learn that it's private, and I had no intention of participating in a gropefest on an ancient Sears, Roebuck carpet with a dozen strangers. "Just do the energy work, the breathing," Dr. Madge urged. "You'll get tremendous benefit. The three best tantric partners are fear, chaos, and confusion, because it's only in a state of 'I don't know' that you can learn. You can decide on your own zone of comfort, and if you don't want to see what's going on, keep your eyes closed." She then removed her only article of clothing, a pareu, exposing pendulous breasts and blondish pubic hair, and everyone in the room followed except me and the ménage fellow, who apparently took pity on me and rather sweetly offered to be my (fully clothed) partner. Dr. Madge picked up a microphone and directed the group through seven levels of breathing and rubbing, while signaling time to move on by ringing chimes. I stopped my partner just north of the heart chakra and kept my back to the room. Okay, I peeked. All around us, naked couples were grunting through various kinds of foreplay (the singles with someone they'd just met) while Dr. Madge led them, as if calling a square dance, occasionally inquiring in her electronically amplified voice, "Does anyone need lube?"

After this session, everyone went into dinner: tuna casserole and butterscotch pudding with (I'm not making this up) Reddi-wip.

Now truly ready to bolt, I was persuaded to stay for the evening's festivities, which sounded like a return to civility: the women dancing for the men, the men dancing for the women, with canned music since nobody had brought drums. But I knew my limitations when everyone started getting creative with those sensual fruits, artfully arranging grapes and cherries on the eyelids and in the belly buttons of prone partners before moving on to other places. With a reputation now bordering on Amish, I surprised no one when I beat a path out of Dodge, taking an extremely long shower at the earliest possible opportunity.

I'm rarely shockable, and I'm willing to concede that some of the exercises might be fun to implement in private with a beloved significant other, but the idea of being assigned to select a stranger with whom to be erotic grosses me out. The experience impresses me as the ignominy of a singles bar taken to its penultimate creepiness. At the very least, it seems anachronistic, like something out of the sixties, when sexually bored suburbanites threw their car keys into a bowl at the beginning of a party and went home with whoever belonged to the keys they retrieved. And co-opted tantra does seem of a piece with the current zeitgeist, along with cable porn and 14-year-olds "hooking up" in the Clintonian belief that oral sex is not sex. My reading of the group I encountered is that the couples were basically exhibitionists getting off on public displays of mutual masturbation, and the singles were looking for some noncommittal sexual contact in the guise of enlightenment.

Merely engaging in sex, or attempting more intimacy as my Poconos friends did, doesn't deserve the name tantra, according to Jeffrey Hopkins, PhD, professor of Tibetan Buddhist studies at the University of Virginia and author or translator of 31 books on the subject. "Traditional tantric teachings are aimed at overcoming lust and desire, as opposed to an excuse for having sex," says Hopkins. "Sex is used only as a technique to have a powerfully blissful encounter with another person, to utilize a more deeply concentrated mind that in turn will overcome lust and afflictive desire. The aim is to use lust to overcome lust. It is counterintuitive." In her book about adolescent love, *The Ripening Seed,* the French novelist Colette referred to sensory objects and experiences as "these pleasures so lightly called physical" because they affect us on more than just a tactile, tangible level. I wonder whether such a concept would have much meaning to that 14-to-25-year-old audience so fascinated by tantric sex, although it would seem that the potentially transformative nature of physical intimacy is the secret of real tantra. "White tantra" seems to be code for a more chaste educational experience in the workshop world. But it's a minefield out there, even if your motivation is pure and you choose a literary route to enlightenment.

"There are many good, dull books about tantra and many that are bad but interesting," wrote Wendy Doniger recently in the *London Times Literary Supplement.* "This is true of many areas of knowledge, but tantra is particularly susceptible both to juicy sensationalism and to an overcompensating academic desiccation." Doniger goes on to say that the book she was reviewing, *Kiss of the Yogini,* by David Gordon White, berates Americans who "cobbled together the pathetic hybrid of New Age 'tantric sex,'" who "blend together Indian erotics, erotic art, techniques of massage, Ayurveda, and yoga into a single invented tradition." This amalgam, White contends, "is to medieval tantra what finger painting is to fine art."

So, what if you wanted to find the real thing? There seems to be a prosaic truth about tantra hidden by the hype: Just like religion, it's been commercialized, and just like ads or toothpaste or automobiles, it's been overly sexualized, but there's a great deal more to it than the physical. "Contrary to popular view, tantric practice is not primarily about sexual practices with a partner," warns Robert Sachs, a clinical social worker who wrote *The Passionate Buddha: Wisdom on Intimacy and Enduring Love.* "As prerequisites to tantric lovemaking, mutuality and an affectionate, loving bond between the partners are essential. From the Buddhist point of view, working with subtle energies in the body must be rooted in a morality that demonstrates a caring and regard for all beings, especially our partner." Caring and regard on the floor of a Pocono lodge? I don't think so....

Sachs advises: "Beware of any seminar or crash course promising to make you a tantric lover in one weekend," which reminds me of Thoreau's advisory: "Beware of all enterprises that require new clothes." I'd amend that to: "Beware of all enterprises that require no clothes." ◙

How Men Really Feel About Breast Implants

Seriously. After the initial ogle, what's going through the average man's mind? Is anything going through his mind? Is he awed, intimidated, repelled…or simply grateful for these larger-than-life, attention-grabbing blouse busters? TOM CHIARELLA gets it all off his chest.

ake is a beautifully complicated word. It starts softly, in almost a whisper, then quickly gathers strength on the way to its harsh, nasty terminus. It's employed with equal authority by schoolchildren and accountants, jewelers and philosophers. And it's rife with contradiction. In sports a fake is a move, a tool, a device. In art it is corruption. A fake either works so perfectly that the fact of the counterfeit goes unnoticed, or it is so poorly executed that it fools no one and does not work at all. Noun. Verb. Adjective. The word has range.

I always laugh when people use the word *fake* when discussing breast augmentation. They say it as if the breasts themselves were lies, forgeries, as if someone were being hoodwinked. Yet there is very little deception in the matter of implants, since most of the time the whole story is right there for you to look at. In point of fact, you're supposed to look. For men that's the best part. Most men have lived some portion of their lives surreptitiously regarding cleavage, stealing glances from across the tenth-grade-English classroom, from behind a magazine, from the end of the bar. I don't know a single heterosexual guy who doesn't rubberneck when it comes to this part of a woman's body. I've seen preachers, therapists, pharmacists, and university presidents eyeball a woman with great cleavage, often cleavage obviously built on the back of great implants. You don't have to be an evolutionary biologist to know that men are visually stimulated. So the tacit invitation to have a look at a woman's breasts is, in itself, a wonderful thing. And whether what one is looking at is a miracle of technology or the real deal seems less than the point. The compact is clear: A woman with breast augmentation asks to be regarded. It really isn't about size; it's about attitude. Her attitude. That's a provocation most men welcome.

Good implants look more than real; they look miraculous and animated—firm, elevated, shaped. They seem unimported, wholly of the woman. The word you want to use is *incredible*. Cheap implants, on the other hand, look painful and cartoonlike. They make the breast look flipped up, appended. The skin is stretched too tight, giving every inch of the grape the tactile feedback of a grapefruit. The word here? *Unbearable*. I know men

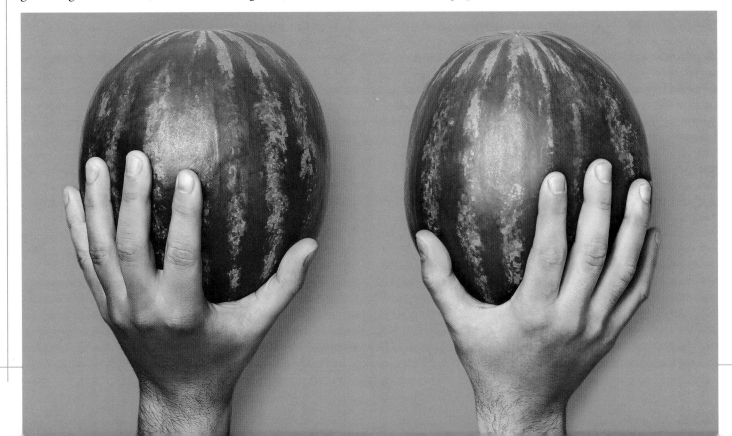

who claim they don't care, either way—they just love them big. Size queens. There's no arguing subtlety with guys like that.

Encountering an augmented breast for the first time is a bit like sitting in a very expensive car before a test-drive. It's unfamiliar and more than a little exciting. It's different from your normal ride. Things have been tricked up. It may be bigger than you're used to, and certain places are firmer, appear newer, seem to offer a different kind of function. You can't help responding to the features—the DVD player in the console, the fancy steering wheel, the huge speakers. You shake your head; it is, after all, just a car. Still, you feel lured.

But when you get intimate with the augmented breast, two things are certain: You can always feel the implant, and feeling it will always lead you to the conscious realization that someone pimped this breast. Any guy who has ever had so much as a lap dance will tell you that implants are an undeniably different tactile experience. The truth is in the touch.

I once dated an airline gate agent who'd moved to a C cup after years as an A. I had seen pictures of her—before pictures—and I have to admit that as I sat there, with the after picture in the flesh, it seemed to me she had made a reasonable choice. She was wildly proud of her new breasts and took her shirt off the first night we dated just to show me, long before we even kissed. "More is more," she told me as we sat thigh-to-thigh on her couch. We were 30 minutes from our first meal together, and there she was with her shirt off, her shoulders square, her back firm and upright. She asked me if I liked her posture. "My doctor said good posture is just as important as the implants." He had a point.

She admitted even then that the implants came at some cost. She spoke like a sage. "I didn't go to church for four weeks after I had the surgery," she said. "But people always forget who you were. They only remember what you are." She was, she told me, completely used to the change within a few months of the surgery. However, in the coming weeks, she introduced me to a series of breast-related routines that indicated otherwise. She didn't like any weight on her chest, not even my arm around her shoulder at the movies, because she could feel the implants. She couldn't sleep on her left side easily, though she asked me to favor her left breast during sex. She held a hand to one breast when she rolled over.

Look, I'm like any guy. I've always thought a woman's breasts were a tremendous pleasure, both publicly and privately. A real gift. But while I loved the way this woman looked, within weeks the presence of her implants dominated everything intimate between us, so much so that I started to feel they were like a really annoying pet. Like a really needy toy poodle, an indulgence that was running the household. Late in the game, in the days before we cut it off, she told me I could skip the nipples during foreplay. She tried to reassure me. The implants, she told me, had changed the sensation. "It's not bad exactly," she said. "It just feels a little grinding." I had to agree.

I can report that my friends are all over the map on the subject of implants. I have a college friend who hates them because they killed the pleasure of strip clubs for him. "I remember when breasts were soft. Now it's like someone stuck a big wet washcloth in there," he says. "When the music gets going, it feels like a kickboxing class." Other guys love the whole phenomenon, the very sight of augmented breasts, the very idea of them. Sleeping with a woman who has implants is a special accomplishment for these guys, though I've never heard any of them report much in the way of advantage or disadvantage, any real amplitude in the giving or receiving of pleasure. When I called one of them just now to ask for his thoughts on the matter, he was sanguine. "Implants are like women," he said. "Every one is different." I feel compelled to add that they actually pay this guy to teach at the university level.

For many men, the self-consciousness of breast implants is a remarkable, and I think legitimate, turn-on. To them it feels like an offering. "You can't deny the power of it," a buddy told me of sleeping with his girlfriend now that she's had augmentation. He deeply appreciates the change, though he never asked for it or even felt unhappy with the real thing. The implants, he says, solved something for her, not him. "She did this thing. She decided to make this change. It filled something up in her." I laughed at the pun, but he shook his head. "We don't even joke about it because it's that real. It made things better for her somehow. And you know, that's just better for both of us."

I asked if he could tell the difference—meaning could he feel the implants themselves? "Sure," he said. "It's not the same. Not at all. The great part is *she's* the same woman, but she's, well, she's just more."

I got that straightaway. It wasn't size or volume at issue. It was a question of appetite, his and hers. In this, the very best case I could imagine, the implants brought together the lodestars of great sex, or maybe desire itself—wanting more and being more, all in the same moment. Very real. Very, very real. ◖

What Women Feel

"**If someone pinched my nipple, I wouldn't know it,**" says Maggie, 37, whose jump from a "very small" A cup to a large C seven years ago left her with numb breasts and "dead" areas on her back. Bruce Cunningham, MD, president of the American Society of Plastic Surgeons, says numbness after implant surgery is often a function of size: The larger the implant, the more likely "you'll encroach upon a nerve." Regardless of size, implants make themselves felt. FDA stats show that five years after surgery, 10 percent of patients have hypersensitive nipples and 10 percent have no nipple sensation at all (bad news if they're like the 82 percent of women who, according to a recent study, are aroused by nipple stimulation). Even patients whose side effects are limited to temporary numbness may endure the assault of battered nerve endings firing back to life: burning (as one law student said, "like a match lit inside my breast"), shooting pains, and can't-quite-scratch-it itchiness. Yet women like Maggie, who used to wear a shirt during sex, aren't complaining. "The implants were the ultimate confidence booster," she says. "I've loved them from day one."

Talking & Listening

How to Get Through to a Man

If he bristles when you try to comfort him, tunes out when you want him to do something, and refuses to admit when you're right, W. BRUCE CAMERON— that famous traitor to his sex—lets you in on a few proven strategies. You may call it manipulation—we call it applied psychology.

As a man, I can assure you that despite outward appearances, we are highly evolved communicators, capable of deep, meaningful conversations—as long as the topic is basketball. Otherwise we're somewhat nervous about the idea of talking to you, for fear that the discussion will involve either (a) feelings or (b) words. Frankly, we'd rather you just made us a sandwich.

If you're faced with the challenge of trying to verbally comfort, nag, seduce, fight with, or compliment a man, here are some ways to make it a less frustrating experience.

"YOU'RE SO STRONG."

Let's say a man you care about is suffering through a personal crisis, such as a setback at work. Your instinct is to soothe him, yet he reacts to your overtures by turning sullen and withdrawn, even angry. Baffled by this inexplicable hostility, you may decide that the best way to express your compassion is to bake him a pie—and then throw it in his face.

The problem stems from the fact that as boys, we learn that any sign of vulnerability will be mercilessly punished by our peers. Through this Darwinian process, the strongest boys become the leaders of the playground, while the weak ones are forced to take refuge inside the school library and go on to make all the money. Standard words of comfort make us feel like you're saying, "Your pain is showing," which is the same as saying, "You are a sissy who can't play dodgeball."

To comfort a man, highlight his power. If you say, "You're handling this with such strength," he'll get the message that you care about his troubles—but not that you think he's a weakling. Admire him for being tough under the circumstances—that's what he needs to hear.

"LET ME GET YOUR POWER DRILL."

Suppose you want a man to do something for you, and you've asked him, oh, a thousand times. He's promised he would, which is what's so frustrating—if he flatly refused, at least you'd understand why he isn't taking action. He seems to be getting increasingly irritated with each gentle reminder and eventually accuses you of nagging him.

A nag is a broken-down horse, which is appropriate because what you're telling your man is straight from the horse's mouth, while his excuses probably sound like they're coming from the other end. But you don't want to be a nag—you just want him to keep his word.

The catch is that no matter how nicely you ask him to do something, he's going to hear it as an order—and since when are you the five-star general of him? Remember, he is a fully independent adult, capable of taking care of himself, who just needs you to make dinner and do his laundry. He doesn't want you to remind him about what he needs to do, even though he keeps forgetting.

Giving a compliment is like giving a gift: Make it about what he wants.

The solution lies in the fact that men are very status conscious—in other words, *he* wants to be the five-star general. Don't ask him to do a specific task ("Fix the drip in the shower") but to be in charge of solving the problem ("The leak in the shower is driving me crazy"). Offer to help him ("Tell me what tools you need, and I'll go get them for you").

Men love to show women their tools.

If he's still not acting, consider going to him in distress ("I took the shower head off, and the drip is worse"). Now he's not only the general but also a war hero, coming to your rescue and breaking a gasket so you have to call a plumber.

Anytime you can make a man feel more like a general than a private, he'll be motivated to do what *you* want.

"WANNA DANCE?"

What do you say to a man to seduce him? First determine if he has that one element necessary in a man to make him seducible: a pulse. Next recognize that nothing you ever say will be as effective as nudity, which men feel is appropriate in all circumstances, even an orthodontist appointment.

You say you can't get his
attention? Finally, there
are ways to make him
face the music (and you).

It's been said that men do most of their thinking with their "little brain" instead of their "big brain," which is ridiculous: Men don't have a "big brain." We pretty much evaluate everything that ever happens in the world, from stock market fluctuations to sudden changes in continental drift, according to whether or not it will somehow lead to us having sexual intercourse. Most of the time we think, *Yes, it will*. This means that the following words can be very seductive to a man: *massage oil, skimpy lingerie, septic tank.*

Of course, you don't want to just turn him on—you want to lure him into flirtation, teasing, and mystery. You'd like to ignite a shivering spark of electricity between the two of you with words and suggestive glances, whereas he would just as soon get the electricity by plugging directly into the socket.

The best way to seduce a man the first time is to let him know you're interested—but not easy—with the word *maybe*. Maybe you should get together, maybe you'll have a drink with him, maybe you'd like to see his place. There's enough *yes* in *maybe* to keep a man from feeling rejected and enough *no* to keep him challenged. If it's a long-term relationship, the approach is different, but you'll do well if you still think of it as a dance. Get him to snuggle, kiss, and play—but once you are there, let him take the lead.

Telling him you think he's sexy and you want to sit in his lap is far more effective than saying you want to make love, because whether it's a date or your 30th anniversary, a man likes to think it's his idea.

no matter how ridiculously false, with the observation that he is absolutely correct...but you still want what you want. In boxing this is called rope-a-dope, and even if you don't know what the rope part means, the dope part sounds pretty applicable. Basically, you're accepting punishment (in the form of pretending to agree that, yes, your mother is Satan) in order to wear him down so that he'll give in on what you really want (and she's coming to visit for a month).

This is called win-win—except you did and he didn't.

"WHAT A MANLY SWEATER!"

Men like receiving compliments because they think it means that you are going to have sex with them. This can make complimenting a man awkward, no matter how straightforward you are about your intentions.

You: That's a nice watch, and I would never sleep with you under any circumstances.

Him: Thanks! (Thinking, *Hey, she wants to sleep with me!*)

He'll reach this same conclusion if you (a) say "good morning" to him, (b) smile at him, or (c) ignore him, so you might as well go ahead and compliment him if you want. And maybe you *are* sleeping with him or would consider it, so what are the best ways to get your message of appreciation across?

Simply put, we want to hear words that sound masculine. You can understand why telling us "You did the hard thing" or "I admire the thrust of your argument" makes us feel pretty good,

> We pretty much evaluate everything that ever happens in the world, from stock market fluctuations to sudden changes in continental drift, according to whether or not it will somehow lead to us having sexual intercourse.

"YOU'RE 100 PERCENT CORRECT."

My father once told me something very wise about fighting with my mother: "Son," he said, "a fight is just a form of negotiation—with broken china."

The best way to negotiate with someone is to know what you want and to know what the other person wants. The same is true when it comes to fighting with a man.

Do you know what you want? Because I already know what he wants, and it doesn't matter what you're arguing about—he just wants to be right. He wants you to acknowledge that he is correct about all his facts, including the ones he just made up. This is his weakness; you can use it like judo, turning his own momentum against him.

Saying two little words, "You're right," is the verbal equivalent of darting a raging elephant with animal tranquilizers. It gives him what he wants, reducing tensions and leaving the way open for you to get what you want. Try it: "You're right, but I still want to go to the party." Meet every protest and argument he makes,

while praising us for being "open" or "receptive" sounds sort of, well, feminine, can't you? Telling us you think our sweater is "handsome" is a way of saying we're manly, while a "cute" sweater sounds like something worn by a female schnauzer. Women seem thrilled when you compliment their shoes, while men would rather hear that our feet are impressively large. (I think you get the thrust of my penetrating analysis.)

Giving a compliment is like giving a gift: Don't make it about what *you* would want, make it about what *he* wants. And what he wants is to hear that you think he's a man. (Though if you'll sleep with him, he'd be willing to skip the conversation altogether.)

Despite the difficulties, my recommendation is to keep talking to men, even about those feelings you're so fond of, but with the few simple changes I've identified. You'll discover that much of the time, you'll get the response you're looking for.

If not, just hit us in the face with a pie. ◖

Before Your Next Fight, Read This!

He hadn't done the dishes. She was livid. He was livid that she was livid. Which gave expert negotiator DANIEL SHAPIRO, PhD, the perfect opportunity to practice what he preaches: turning an adversary into a partner. (Thank you, Aunt Margaret.)

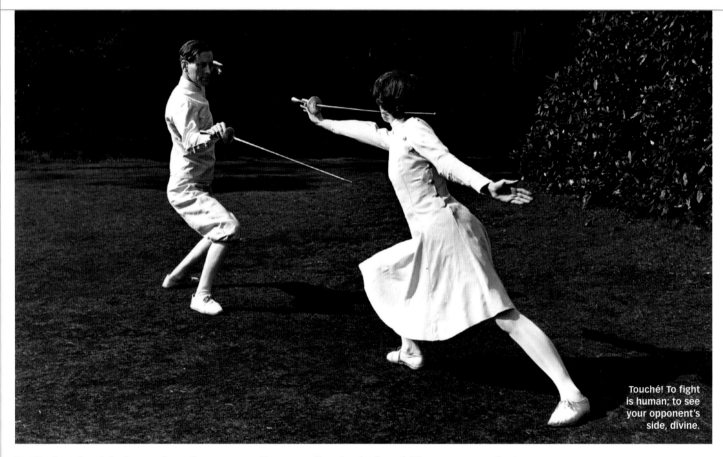

Touché! To fight is human; to see your opponent's side, divine.

I t's eight o'clock on a Saturday morning, I was up all night doing taxes, and I've had only four hours of sleep when my wife, having decided this would be a good time to torture me, wakes me with an angry accusation: "You didn't do the dishes!"

I put a pillow over my head.

"You said you were going to do them!"

"I'm trying to sleep, Mia."

Mia doesn't care. "How come I have to do all the work around here?"

I hold the pillow tighter. "Can't this wait?"

"No."

Now *I'm* angry. The woman I love, the woman who's such a good mother to our son, Noah, the woman who picks up my dirty socks and accommodates my almost daily craving for Chinese food, is out to get me. And there's no way I'm going to let her. If I apologize, I'll feel weak. If I say I'll do the dishes, I'll feel as

though I'm agreeing to be her servant.

Yet even as my anger builds, somewhere in the back of my mind I know that the real problem isn't a bunch of dirty plates. It's how we're treating each other. *I'm right. You're wrong. And I'm going to argue until you admit it.* We've started behaving like adversaries. And the longer we fight, the more defensive we'll get and the more we'll lash out—until a spat about dishes turns into a heated referendum about which one of us deserves to live.

Issues like these creep up in everyone's life. At work, a colleague fails to include you in a meeting you wanted to attend. At a party, a friend blurts out a secret you thought was in the vault. On its own, the small stuff is just that—small. But if you're not careful, it can turn into a big problem that tears at the fabric of your relationships. I know this because I've spent the past 15 years researching the role of emotions in conflict situations, and because I've had lots of experience as a consultant to disputing political leaders. Unfortunately, all my knowledge doesn't make me any less human. Like every husband on earth, I fight with my wife.

Luckily, my work has given me insight into dealing—constructively—with fights. The key insight is that solving the big problem first prevents the small problems from snowballing. Though that may sound backward—and impossible to pull off in the heat of battle—it's not. Here's how it works.

As Mia and I exchange insults, friendly conversation seems miles away. But before I criticize her for attacking me, I focus on a sign in my mind that reads TURN AN ADVERSARY INTO A PARTNER.

This is important because it will change the way I'm acting toward Mia. As her adversary, I want to defeat her. As her partner, I want to listen to her—really listen. The trouble is, it's hard to listen when all the circuits in my brain are telling me, "She's wrong! I'm right!"

I need to regain my emotional balance, but I can't do that while Mia's giving me the evil eye. So I fall back on a plan I've made in advance. Step 1: I suggest taking a 15-minute break to cool off and figure out how to move forward.

"Fine." Mia walks out. I can tell she was sorely tempted to slam the door behind her.

I sit up in bed so I don't fall back asleep. My anger, on the other hand, stays right where it is. How dare she accuse me of not helping around the house? And what gives her the right to wake me so early on a Saturday morning?

In a way, it feels good to travel down this road of blame. But knowing that the further I go, the worse things will be for my marriage, I recall step 2 of my plan—channeling my aunt Margaret, a 60-year-old lawyer from Pittsburgh. You may not have an Aunt Margaret, but chances are you have someone like her: a compassionate person with a knack for listening without judging. If Aunt Margaret were here, she'd tell me to take a deep breath and explain the situation. And then she'd gently try to steer me toward seeing Mia's point of view.

What's brilliant about Aunt Margaret's approach is that it has my interests at heart. Once Mia feels heard, she'll be much more likely to listen to me. So, reluctantly, I resolve to try to imagine—just for a moment—that I'm my wife.

In my professional life, I frequently teach this role reversal tactic. In class students pair up and actually speak as though they are the other person; though some students at first feel silly, they soon come to understand the powerful difference between describing what "he" or "she" is doing and how "I" feels.

If I were to become Mia right now, I'd say, "I wake up at the crack of dawn to Noah crying. I feed him, drop him off at day care, and then put on my social-worker hat. After work, I pick up Noah, come home, bathe him, eat with Dan, and—a lot of the time—do the dishes and clean up around the house. I know Dan has a busy schedule, *but so do I.*"

Seeing Mia's side makes me feel uncomfortable, less entitled—and that's a good sign. I keep going. I see that I've left her with two bad choices: Do the dishes herself or nag me. She wants to

be supported, but instead she's trapped. Now I'm really starting to squirm—because my sense of empathy is waking up. I never meant for my wife to feel unsupported.

It feels as though a weight has been lifted from me. I think I understand Mia's viewpoint, which makes all those venomous thoughts about how mean she is start to disappear. But happy days aren't here again—yet. Mia is still angry. And telling her "I get it!" won't be enough. Step 3: I have to communicate my new understanding.

In the family room, Mia sits on the couch, reading. She doesn't look up. Her anger is palpable. Normally, this would be enough to retrigger my own anger. Today, though, I come prepared. I interpret her behavior not as a desire to attack but rather as a need for support.

"Look," I say. "We can spend all day today arguing over the dishes. Or we can talk this out."

She nods.

I say, "I've thought about how things might look from your perspective."

"Really?" Mia says sarcastically. "So what am I feeling?"

Now I'm in danger, but I take the risk. "I started thinking about how much you're doing every day. Between taking care of Noah and working and keeping up with the house, it's a lot. If I were in your shoes, I'd feel overwhelmed."

"Of course it's overwhelming! Why should all the work be left to me?"

My heart skips a beat. My hostility surges back. Not only did I spend last night doing both our taxes but I also cleaned the basement the night before. I'm about to defend my position, to tell her all the reasons I'm right and she's wrong, when it occurs to me that she's come prepared with a list of her own. Arguing like this will put us back in the roles of adversaries—exactly where we don't want to be.

Here's where a crucial truth comes in handy: There *is* power in one. Even if Mia initially resists my invitation to talk through our fight, I don't need to react in kind. I can say and do things to turn both of us into partners. All it takes is persistence in trying to understand her point of view so that she feels appreciated. For some people—me included—this can be an exciting challenge.

I look Mia in the eyes and ask, "What are you hoping for right now?" I'm not attacking, and immediately her anger loses some steam. Her face softens. "I feel like I don't have a second to myself—between work, taking care of Noah, cleaning the house." As I listen, we both become more engaged. The tone of our conversation slowly shifts. We're becoming partners again.

Once our emotions are working with us, not against us, we can figure out any number of ways to deal with the mess in the kitchen sink. We can also address the deeper issue: making sure Mia has some time to herself. And the next time I leave a chore undone, she'll wonder what came up and probably ask me about it. I, on the other hand, will do my best not to put her in that situation. Not because clean dishes are the most crucial thing in life, but because we never want to dish out more than our relationship can take. ◘

Seeing Mia's side makes me squirm— and that's good.

Help! Mayday! SOS!

Having trouble with your computer? Your pile of bills? Your life? Help is out there if you know how—and how often—to ask. MARTHA BECK explains.

My friend Wes* has a brilliant mind, a wicked sense of humor, and a fairly involved case of cerebral palsy. When he and his wife, Sue,* bought their first house, Wes insisted it be as thoroughly modified for special needs as was his bachelor apartment. Sue argued that she could always do things for Wes that he couldn't do for himself. "No," he told her firmly. "One day we're going to have an argument, and on that day, I'll get hungry. I need to be able to make dinner for myself without asking you for help."

Wes's physical constraints have made him highly sensitive to the way helping and being helped shapes relationships. Like him, most of us resist asking for something even when we need it. We have our pride. When a tired driver causes an accident or a lonely teen becomes homicidal or a depressed mom neglects her children, their failing to reach for aid isn't noble; it's criminally stupid. So how do we walk the tightrope between self-sufficiency and need? When and how should we ask for help? I'd argue that the solution is to follow Wes's example and answer such questions before the need arises.

Asking for help is psychologically risky because it triggers a mechanism in the human psyche called the norm of reciprocity. If you give me something—money, advice, time—I must give something to you that we tacitly agree is of roughly equal value. Otherwise we won't sustain an amicable bond for long. Only the churlish keep score overtly, of course, but even generous people get uneasy when one party in a relationship takes and takes and takes without giving anything in return. Sociologist Alvin Gouldner called the norm of reciprocity a "plastic filler, capable of being poured into the shifting crevices of social structures and serving as a kind of all-purpose moral cement."

This means that the more I ask of you, the more everyone will expect me to repay you—and what I can't repay in goods and services, I'll typically surrender in power and control. Children need constant attention and support from their parents, so society gives parents near-total control over them. The same used to be true for wives and husbands, slaves and masters, serfs and lords. Powerful people often infantilized, repressed, and deliberately enfeebled those they were "helping" in order to maintain dominance. For their part, the powerless struggled like hell not to ask for anything, since this drove them deeper into the position of weakness (hence Wes's remodeling project).

There's one type of situation where the norm of reciprocity breaks down, where some even deeper instinct kicks in. Call it empathy, codependency, or grace: When humans see true need,

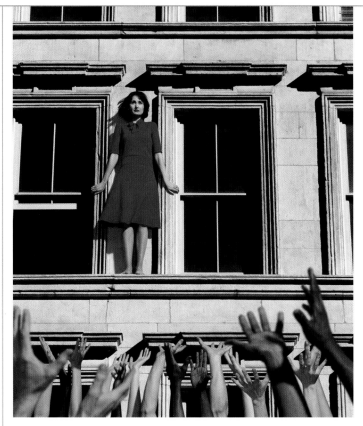

Call it empathy or grace: When humans see real need, they extend a hand.

we frequently offer help without expectation of repayment. For example, last week I stopped on a busy freeway to catch a very scared Boston terrier, call the number on its ID tag, and return it to its owner. I think I got more unalloyed pleasure from this simple event than from my own wedding. It felt fabulous to do a favor when it was really needed, no strings attached.

The problem with the purely helpful side of human nature is that people, unlike dogs, take advantage of it. I once met an aspiring writer—a doll-faced woman I'll call Gloria—who had lost whole chapters of her half-finished novel because she didn't know how to back up her computer files. Thinking this was a lost-puppy situation, I hired a babysitter, went to Gloria's house, showed her how to save a file (point this, click that), and sat beside her while she repeated the procedure for each of 20 chapters. Early the next morning, my phone rang. "I wrote a new chapter!" Gloria chirruped. "Come over and show me how to

* Name has been changed.

216

back up the file!" I'm not sure what became of Gloria; I sort of lost touch with her after that.

I mean seconds after.

Now, I don't think Gloria was an evil manipulator. I think she felt genuinely incapable of saving the file—but my gut told me it was learned helplessness, not real need, and the norm of reciprocity inspired me to drop that potential friendship like a bad habit.

My point: We should ask for help guilelessly, confident in human graciousness—but only if it's absolutely necessary. If we abuse the privilege, we risk becoming pariahs. So how do I make this crucial judgment under pressure? How do I know if I am about to get smushed on the freeway of life because I failed to seek aid or become ditched by people who are sick of my manipulative begging? For answers, I turned to someone whose job it is to stay in the sweet spot of need.

It's hard to imagine a more vulnerable population than the residents of the Neonatal Intensive Care Unit at Cedars-Sinai Medical Center. I'm visiting the NICU with parent liaison Dorothy Williams, who introduces me to the patients, most of whom weigh less than my mocha Frappuccino. No chubby cherubs here: These babies combine the heartbreaking scrawniness of the extremely old with the total inexperience of the extremely young. I'm moved to tears, partly by their fragility and partly by the complicated machines and devoted professionals around each tiny person, attesting to human determination to help the truly helpless.

"It's the parents I focus on," says Dorothy. "They're exhausted, they're in shock, they have to take care of other kids and jobs and mortgages."

I ask her if most parents tell her when they need help.

"Oh," Dorothy says, "they always tell you—even when they won't tell you." I tell her that I'm not quite following.

At this point, one of her coworkers says, "Well, I know it's time to help when they start asking how. 'How do I comfort my newborn?' 'How do I talk to my relatives?' 'How will we pay for this?' The more they ask how, the more they need help, and the more able they are to receive it." Dorothy nods.

For me, this is a minor epiphany. The phrases I've always associated with asking for help are passwords of pathos: "Please, sir, I want some more." "Would you mind...?" "If it's not too much trouble..." These supplications ooze helplessness and mark the moment we turn over control to someone else. The word *how* is different. It's an active term, one that bridges the gap from powerless to empowered. I use it right away. "How," I say, "do I help people ask for help?"

And just like that, Dorothy helps me figure it out. Here's the strategy that emerges from her kind assistance.

HOW TO GET HELP (A PRIMER)

1. **FRAME ALL YOUR PROBLEMS AS HOW-TO QUESTIONS.** Simply begging for aid when you feel overwhelmed is likely to make honest folks back away, while exploiters smell blood in the water. Instead, you might do better to phrase all your problems as "how" questions: "How do I break through the glass ceiling in this company?" "How should I go about changing this flat tire?" "How can I help cure AIDS?" Whether your problem is tiny or monumental, asking "How...?" means you're a capable person in the process of becoming even more capable—not a charity case or a manipulator's mark.

2. **LOCATE SOURCES OF INFORMATION AND INSIGHT.** The more specific your how-to questions, the more quickly they'll lead to useful strategies or solutions from individuals, books, TV shows, Web sites, and a thousand sources you won't even notice until your attention is primed. The more actively you pursue the knowledge and skills to extricate yourself from a mess, the more new sources you'll locate. As *New York Times* columnist Thomas Friedman (among others) has pointed out, the accessibility of information has exploded so dramatically over the past few decades that humble individuals can now solve problems and perform feats once reserved for a few elite experts.

3. **TAKE FISHING LESSONS.** To paraphrase the adage: If you wheedle a fish from someone, you'll eat for a day; if you wheedle advice from a great fisherman, you'll eat for a lifetime. The key here is that you're soliciting help that won't diminish the resources of the other person. Each person's supply of "fish" (funding, energy, time) is limited, but fishing know-how can be replicated infinitely, at negligible cost. Even if you're going with a money problem to your filthy-rich uncle, ask for education, not a handout. "Please give me money" is a self-disempowering request. "Please show me how to resolve this financial muddle" is a self-empowering one, even if Uncle Buckmeister also pitches in with a cash donation (which he's much more likely to do for a determined problem-solver than a simple beggar).

4. **RECEIVE WITH GRATITUDE, NOT GRASPING.** If you honestly set out to learn how to untangle your own snafus, you'll find that even people who shy away from raw neediness start offering advice. Whether you've asked for it or not, help that's given freely is part of grace, meaning that the only response necessary to satisfy the norm of reciprocity is gratitude. And what I mean by gratitude is not "Thanks...and what else can you do for me?" Grasping at help like a drowning swimmer tends to scare away the resources you've already got, as well as potential assistance.

5. **PAY IT FORWARD.** Once you start pushing the limitations of your own abilities and learning to solve your own dilemmas, you'll find that many people, like Dorothy Williams at the NICU, are actually out there looking for you, wanting to be of use to you. You're going to end up receiving support both material and intangible, much of which you couldn't repay if you wanted to (who could pay back the gifts of a great teacher?).

At this point, the norm of reciprocity will express itself in you as a spontaneous desire (not obligation) to help others. You'll come to understand that asking for aid doesn't need to be dangerous. By playing an active part in your own deliverance, you'll get the most helpful thing of all: the realization that anyone—angry spouse, lost pet, struggling novelist, tiny newborn, grieving parent, or you at your very worst—is always well within the reach of grace. **O**

Stand Back from the Rope!

No matter how close you are to another person, sooner or later you'll move too far into their space or they'll crowd you—and there'll be a sudden chill in the air. Therapist JEFFREY B. RUBIN, PhD, helps people figure out how to be intimate without being intrusive.

Harry had a long day, and now he's excited about seeing his wife, Deanna. During the car ride home, he fantasizes about kissing her when he walks in the door. She greets him when he arrives, and he bends to meet her lips—but Deanna turns her face away and he gets her cheek instead. Harry has become intimate with the side of her face since their baby was born eight months ago, and he's not happy.

When they get into bed that evening, Harry feels guilty. He knows that he sniped at Deanna during dinner and wishes he could repair the damage. So he makes a sexual advance, which she rebuffs. They each sleep badly. At breakfast they argue over trivia. The baby, picking up on the tension, is crying as Harry leaves for work. Later that morning, Deanna calls me and makes an appointment for couples therapy.

During our first session, Deanna focuses on Harry's hostility, expressing her dismay at his unprovoked attacks. When she stops, Harry says, "I'm tired of getting a cold shoulder from you. I don't deserve it." Then he says to me, "She doesn't love me," with tears in his eyes. Deanna is shocked.

"Of course I love you," she says.

"Then why do you push me away?" Harry asks.

"How do I push you away? Aren't I always there for you?"

"When I come home from work at night, you act like my sister," Harry says. "I just want a kiss between a husband and a wife, on the lips."

"That's not all you want," she says.

"Is that a crime? Would you be happy if I weren't interested in you that way?"

"No. It's not that I don't love you. You aren't the problem."

"Of course I am," Harry says. "I'm the one you don't want to kiss."

"How do you feel when Harry walks in the door?" I ask Deanna.

"Excited to see him," she says.

"And then what?" I ask.

"I just seem to shut down," she says. "His advances feel like too much."

"Do you feel pressure?" I ask.

"Yes!"

"What's the pressure?"

> Your feelings are your reality. Neither you nor the other person is inherently right or wrong.

"Having to perform—having to put out, no matter how I feel," she says.

"Great," Harry says. "It's inspiring to know your wife is so excited about seeing you."

"Deanna's refusal of a kiss sounds like a form of self-protection," I say to Harry. "She thinks you'll want more, which she may not be able to give at that time."

Deanna is nodding. "And if I say no to making love," she says, "I'll be hurting your feelings, so I don't even want to start. I avoid kissing you. And the tragedy is you're a great kisser."

Harry looks pleased.

"Don't not give him a kiss," I say to Deanna. "And you," I say to Harry, "don't go any further than a kiss unless Deanna gives you a go-ahead signal. That way she can express the physical affection she feels without withdrawing. Until she tells you differently, Harry, a kiss is just a kiss."

Deanna grabs Harry's hand, and they both smile. "Is this permission to go ahead?" Harry asks. Deanna kisses him on the lips. We all laugh.

Deanna and Harry's story illustrates a universal truth: Avoiding one problem can sometimes create a worse one. Her fear of where a kiss would lead cut off any physical affection and left them both feeling isolated. Recognizing Deanna's misguided tactic led to a genuine resolution: negotiating boundaries that respected both Harry's need for closeness and hers for space.

Eileen could barely speak. On the way to her session with me, she'd gotten a call from her daughter, Laura, who was single, in her late 20s, and living three hours away. Laura was calling from a pre-op appointment—she had a lump in her breast that was to be removed the next week. She was upset and said that she wished Eileen had been there with her.

"I feel absolutely horrible," Eileen said to me. "I should have gone." Divorced from a highly critical man when Laura was 10, Eileen had essentially raised Laura on her own. Mother and daughter had once been very close. And as a retired nurse, Eileen could have offered Laura valuable information and support.

But I knew it wasn't that simple. Just the week before, Eileen had suggested she go to the pre-op meeting, and Laura had insisted she was "making way too much of this whole thing."

Eileen didn't want to intrude on Laura, who had struggled to be autonomous since adolescence. Advice and even questions often made Laura feel judged, controlled, suffocated.

"I know I can be overbearing," Eileen says to me, "but Laura has a hair-trigger reaction to me and a long history of pushing people away. She says 'I'm fine' so fast that it's hard to tell if she means it or if she's afraid of asking for too much or losing herself. I'm damned if I do and damned if I don't. I bend over backward not to interfere, and then she feels abandoned."

"What if you connected without being intrusive?" I say.

"How do I do that?" Eileen asks.

"First you have to accept that when you offer advice, it's just an offering and you can't be attached to whether or not she takes it. You can also say to her: 'We have a dilemma. If I follow your wishes and back off, you'll feel less intruded on, but later you may feel alone. If I get more involved, you may feel suffocated. What do you think we should do?'"

"I think that will help," Eileen says, "because it respects her boundaries and gives her a choice. But I have to be willing to accept whatever she says, even if it's 'Back off, Mom.'"

Eileen came in two weeks later to report that she and her daughter had had a good visit and the lump was benign. "I stayed within range but let her call the shots," Eileen says. "It still doesn't feel easy, but I'm getting the hang of it."

Lily and Jim are in my office because she's afraid they're growing apart. He works hard at a corporate job; she takes care of their three children. "I feel abandoned," Lily says. "He's staying up later and later, sometimes until after I've fallen asleep. We've always been close. But now we can't talk in bed because he's dawdling in the bathroom or puttering around on the computer, as if he's avoiding me. He isn't getting enough sleep, and he has circles under his eyes."

"Nighttime is a nightmare," Jim says to her. "What you call talking is really me being a sitting duck for your harangues." Turning to me, he says, "How would you like it if, just as you're leaving the day behind, you're confronted by your spouse, who feels that now is a fine time to discuss finances, new construction projects, family visits, or worst of all, differences in parenting styles?"

"But there's never a good time to talk about this stuff," Lily says. "Morning is a rush hour, and you don't want to talk when you get home. On the weekends, you don't want to deal with anything you have to use your brain for. Bedtime is the only time you're available."

"But I can't handle the heaviness before bed, honey," Jim says more gently. "I just want to go to sleep, maybe cuddle a little. I've started to dread the end of the day."

"Lily," I say, "there's a great temptation to discuss all your concerns as you're going to bed because you finally have a captive audience. But it's not a good time for Jim—and it's not good for you, either, because you still aren't heard if he's

tired and resentful. And, Jim, you have to show Lily good faith and prove to her that you'll take her concerns seriously at a specific, agreed-upon time."

So often we have the right impulse but the wrong solution. In our efforts to take care of ourselves, we set boundaries inappropriately, walling ourselves off from the people we care about. Appropriate boundaries, rather than alienating others, make it easier for us to connect in a satisfying way. For instance, once Deanna could regulate her physical intimacy with Harry, she could be affectionate without feeling so vulnerable.

The first step in a healthy negotiation is to figure out what the real conflict is. Ordinarily, the negative interaction happens so quickly that it's difficult to determine who's doing what to whom. Each person has to recognize his or her own reactions and needs. Many people feel entitled to their feelings only when they're in crisis mode. But Jim doesn't have to wait to speak to Lily until he becomes sick from lack of sleep. And Eileen shouldn't wait till she's frantic with guilt before discussing her wish to be on hand for her daughter. Your feelings are your reality. Neither you nor the other person is inherently right or wrong.

The second step I suggest is for each person to express his or her needs clearly and directly, without blame or rancor. For instance, Eileen might simply tell Laura, "I'd like to be closer to you," and leave out "You're a cold fish." Laura could say to her mother, "I know you love me, but I need more space."

Third, it's essential to understand the other person's feelings and take them seriously. I make it clear that this does not mean automatically agreeing with or accommodating the other person but compassionately, empathetically listening.

When each person understands the other's motivations, it's time to revisit the original conflict. The most useful attitude is, here's what I need, tell me what you need, and let's figure out how we can both feel respected and nurtured without either of us overstepping the other's boundaries.

People who find mutually gratifying solutions to their problems—instead of indirect, patchwork ones that create greater difficulties—discover possibilities for intimacy they never imagined and free up hidden reservoirs of energy that enable them to live with greater creativity and passion. ◑

Brain to Brain: How to Get Anyone to Agree with You

Hey, everyone's entitled to their opinion. But if you want to bring someone around to yours, Harvard psychologist Howard Gardner has a strategy. BY DAWN RAFFEL

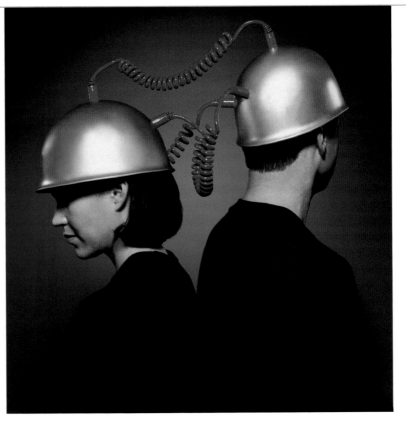

Many's the time I've argued passionately about art, politics, cultural phenomena, and, while we're at it, the proper way to hang a roll of toilet paper—and more often than not, my point never penetrates the other person's thick (in my opinion) cranium. For that matter, I rarely budge from my own position, even when presented with a battery of facts. ("Well, I was right in a different context" has sprung from my lips.)

So what does it really take to persuade someone? In pursuit of answers, I tracked down Howard Gardner, a Harvard cognitive psychologist, MacArthur "genius" fellow, and author of almost two dozen books. His most recent, *Changing Minds,* explores how we can do just that.

As it turns out, the hardest mind to pry open might be your own. "If you ask most people, 'Are you flexible or rigid?' they'll tell you they're flexible," he says. "The analogy is, if you ask people whether their sense of humor is better than average, almost everybody says yes. Of course, half of them are going to be wrong," he notes with characteristic bemusement. "All of us have areas of what I call fundamentalism. We tend to use that word with reference to religion, but there's fundamentalism—a commitment not to alter our opinions—in every sphere." From the war in Iraq to abortion to how to manage money, we find ourselves at loggerheads with others, not listening, just waiting for a pause so we can voice our rebuttal.

Gardner says we need to ask ourselves what fixed notions we're clinging to and whether they still make sense for us. "My ex-mother-in-law will never invest in stocks," he says. "She'll give you a hundred reasons. The question is, Is she open to the fact that over the past 50 years, stocks have always been the investments that yield the most, as long as you don't buy and sell all the time?"

Keeping your mind limber requires you to cultivate, if not a taste, at least a tolerance for things you'd just as soon turn up your

> "The real trick is not to rehearse your speech a hundred times until you get it perfect. It's to take the perspective of the other person."

nose at. "I subscribe to all kinds of publications that cut across the political and scientific spectrum," he says. "I know if I read only stuff I agree with, I'm not going to learn anything." But he also suggests looking for relatively balanced arguments. "Nobody watches a Michael Moore film or listens to Rush Limbaugh in order to have their mind changed," he says. "You watch or listen either because you want to have your prejudice confirmed or because you enjoy getting angry."

Gardner highly recommends leaving the comforts of home and talking to people from very different backgrounds. "One interesting fact is that totalitarian leaders almost invariably have not traveled," he says. "Hitler didn't travel. Stalin didn't travel.

Saddam Hussein never traveled. I think they didn't want to have their orthodoxy challenged."

When it comes to changing someone else's mind, Gardner says, "the biggest mistake people make is not understanding the other's fundamentalism, or resistances. Our entrenched habits of mind have been relatively serviceable, or we'd have abandoned them. So the important thing is to draw the other person out. I like to say, 'Listen charismatically.' " By this Gardner means pay careful attention and pick up on unspoken cues. "Try to put into your own words tentatively, not threateningly, what you think the other person's concerns are," he says. "Most people will appreciate your efforts if you say, 'It seems to me you're saying such and such.' Then they can answer, 'Well, no, that's not exactly what I'm saying.' "

What never works is a direct assault on another's point of view. "When you go in with all guns blazing—*you're wrong, you've got to see this my way*—you're just producing defensiveness," he says. Even the most eloquent argument is likely to fail if you don't have enough insight into the person you're trying to sway. "The real trick is not to rehearse your speech a hundred times until you get it perfect"—and how often have we all done that, winning imagined debates in our heads—"but to take the perspective of the other person." Once you understand someone's resistance, you might decide not to address it directly: "Sometimes it's better not to talk about the 300-pound gorilla," Gardner says.

Very persuasive people often choose an agreeable point of entry instead: The other day, a colleague told Gardner, "I want to convince my wife to go to New Zealand." Rather than trying to counter, say, an aversion to an arduous flight, he offered two less-direct strategies: "The first was to find lots of links between New Zealand and what she likes to do in other parts of her life. If she enjoys scuba diving or loves a certain kind of food, that's one entry point," he says. The second was a method Gardner calls embodiment—in essence, becoming the change you want to see. "I said, 'Pick something you've been resistant to and show her that you're willing to try it. If you've refused to socialize with certain people, start to do it. Demonstrate the kind of flexibility you hope she'll emulate.'

"Another technique I've used with a lot of success is to meet up with someone in a different place," Gardner says. A change of context—which breaks one pattern—can stimulate fresh thinking across the board. "I might plan to take a walk or have a cup of coffee with the person whose mind I want to change. I've actually arranged to sit next to somebody on a plane because I knew I could have uninterrupted time and do a lot of listening."

The older we get, and the longer our neural networks have been in place, the more set in our beliefs we're apt to become. Gardner's antidote is to try to occasionally think like a teenager (minus the hormonal meltdowns). "In adolescence, kids begin to consider how the world could be different from the way they've thought about it before," he says. "They have imaginative powers; they can think of utopias and dystopias. Something they considered absolute suddenly becomes one of a number of options. You ask, 'What are the possibilities?'" he says. "You open a wider panorama." **◑**

How to Win the Fight

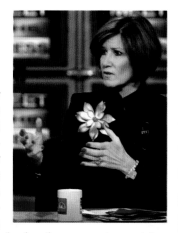

THE WIFE: MARY MATALIN, *Republican party strategist, editor in chief of conservative publisher Threshold Editions, married to James Carville*

There are four mandatory rules for winning, and all are easier said than done. First and foremost: Pick your fights carefully. I learned faster with my kids than with my husband that some hills are just not worth trying to take. With kids, brushing teeth is a necessary battle; matching hair bows is not. With husbands, respect is requisite; shared politics is not. Second: Understand your objective. What is your goal and why? Are you trying to make your husband like you or do what you need? Third: Know your enemy. Military leaders premise engagements on this concept, but spouses often walk blithely into the line of fire. Fourth: Prepare. If you are prepared, you will be in the right fight, with clear goals, so you can anticipate counterarguments. And remember: There is no shame in losing, only in not trying.

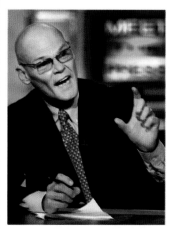

THE HUSBAND: JAMES CARVILLE, *Democratic party consultant, CNN contributor, married to Mary Matalin*

If any man has ever won a marital argument, I haven't met him. I'm 0 for 5,211 in my marriage, and I'm sure to lose 5,212, thanks to a theory I like to call SCR: surrender, capitulation, and retreat. I've read all the marital advice—you know, confront your issues, discuss them. My advice is just leave 'em go. I know couples who've been having the same discussion for 35 years. It ain't worth it. Women know how to fight better. I think part of it is—to put it delicately—biological, but you're going to be a lot happier just agreeing and doing what you're told. These days the only fight my wife and I have is when she'll say to me, "You're just agreeing with me to agree with me!" And most of the time it's true. But I'm a happily married man. It'll be 13 years this month. What can I say? **◑**

Who *Is* That Masked Man?

He's your husband, father, brother, son, neighbor—the guy who keeps up a barrier of small talk and superficialities. If you'd like to make some actual contact, PHILLIP C. McGRAW, PHD, has strategies for opening the male.

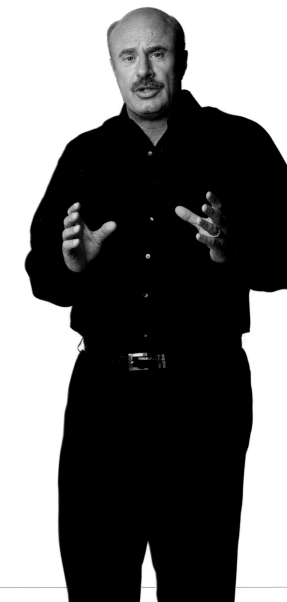

A woman in her 30s recently asked me for advice about how, after decades of shooting the breeze with her dad about baseball—and not much else—she could make their relationship more meaningful. She told me she'd tried once, asking him if he'd been afraid of dying in Vietnam. His silence and the look on his face made it clear he had no idea why on earth she'd want him to talk about his war experience. She let the subject go, because even asking the question had felt unnatural and forced.

This is a common scene. A woman cares deeply about a man—her husband, brother, father, uncle, neighbor, or friend—but patterns of superficial behavior and speech have developed over time and have become cemented in their daily interaction. Any attempt to change the pattern rings false, even though the emotion behind it is authentic. It doesn't help matters that men aren't good at talking about feelings—we're conditioned to believe that showing emotion is a sign of weakness. With all of this in the air, how do you redefine a relationship with any man in your life so that it's more fulfilling?

> When you say, "Can we talk?" what a man hears is "You are sentenced to life."

KEEP IT SHORT

When you say, "Can we talk?" what a man hears is "You are sentenced to life." He'll feel that there's no escape, and the minutes will go by like hours. Tell him: "I want to talk to you for 30 minutes, and then I've got to run." He'll think, *Heck, I can do anything for 30 minutes,* and he'll be more likely to stay engaged if you show him that there's an end in sight.

EMPOWER HIM

Men often put up their guard because they feel unsafe. You might start out with: "You're not doing anything wrong, but I want to talk to you about what I need. And the reason I need it is because you're important to me." That way you're stating your feelings while also complimenting and empowering him. He's got something you want, and he can feel good about doing what he can to give it to you.

KEEP THE FOCUS ON YOU—NOT HIM

You want to be careful that you don't come across as critical. If you start the conversation with "We never talk about anything that matters" or "You don't really want to know me," you're not likely to get the result you want. Instead you might say, "I think our relationship is missing some crucial elements, at least in terms of my needs." Notice we're trying to make your needs clearer to him—even though that's only half the battle.

There's a reason for taking this approach. If he thinks you actually mean that you're going to push and probe until you feel closer to him and really know who he is, you'll see the walls of defensiveness go up around him. You've got to ease him into the situation. By engaging him with openness, candor, and vulnerability, the principle of reciprocity should kick in and he'll be more likely to respond in the same way.

JUST ASK

Men don't have a lot of emotional intelligence. You would hope that if you say something like "Our superficiality is hurting me," a man would immediately conclude, "Well, then I need to be more genuine, feeling, empathetic, and forthcoming." But most men won't make that leap. You have to spell out what you want. Try posing narrow questions that require disclosure. Don't say, "What do you really think of me?" Rather, you might say to your father, "Tell me how you felt the day I graduated from college" or "What was it like for you in Vietnam? You never told me, and I've always wondered." Don't expect him to read the subtext; be precise about exactly what you need.

WORK THROUGH THE AWKWARDNESS

If both of you are thinking, *This isn't us; this isn't how we talk,* don't be coy about it. Say to him, "Dad, I don't really know how to do this without it feeling forced. What I do know is that I really need this. So if I seem different, or if it feels as though I'm putting us on the couch, can we just work through it anyway? I'm willing to muddle through because it's important to me." Don't be smooth or try to disguise the awkwardness. The more uncomfortable the conversation feels, the more you need to speak to that weirdness. If you don't know how to step up and begin, try writing your thoughts in a letter or e-mail. That will give each of you the opportunity to do some prep work before launching straight into emotional territory. You can follow up by saying, "Thank you for reading my note; it means a lot to me. I don't know exactly what to do, but I want to start by telling you how I feel and by telling you more about me."

> You don't have to pull up a chair in front of your dad's recliner and say, "Let's share our feelings."

HAVE A SENSE OF HUMOR

Your goal is to get where you're going; it doesn't matter what route you take. If you get his attention with a little humor and y'all have a good laugh, you might waltz past obstacles that have gotten you off track before. Try saying something like "If I get too goofy or touchy-feely for you, tap twice on the table with your left hand." It's okay to break the tension and make light of the process.

BRING A TO-DO LIST

If you think you might go into brain lock once you start talking, come up with a list of ten things you want to share about yourself. Tell him: "I actually wrote down some things that I think you should know about me." If it feels right, after you explain what you want him to know, you can turn those thoughts into questions about him. It may sound corny or contrived, but men like to fix things and solve problems. If he knows there's an agenda, it gives him something solid to work from.

TAKE A HIKE

You don't have to pull up a chair in front of your dad's recliner and say, "Let's share our feelings." That could make him feel self-conscious, and he'll clam up. Suggest a trip to the park, or start the discussion as you're driving to a ball game. A guy will tell you more while he's walking along kicking a rock or fiddling with a stick—situations where he doesn't feel stared at. By moving your chat to a neutral environment, you make it more of a sideshow than the main attraction—in fact, just shifting the setting might be enough to motivate him to take the first foray into a more thoughtful exchange.

EASE HIM INTO IT

Don't focus the first conversation on something tragic or hard to discuss, like saying to your brother, "We never talked about Mom's open-casket funeral and how that made you feel." Start with subjects that aren't quite so fraught. Ask his perspective on an issue you're dealing with at work that he might have some insight into. Maybe you can ask him for some advice on parenting a temperamental toddler. Once you've established a link, you'll both find it easier to move from less-weighty subjects to feelings about a parent's death.

Breaking out of your usual pattern may take time, but it is possible to start communicating on a whole new level. You can create a connection that has you talking about your fears, hopes, and dreams. Don't expect tears or an outpouring of emotion. That's not how we operate. You will need to be patient and pick your moment carefully. If you watch the World Series together every year, you know better than to start opening up in the ninth inning. But don't give up. If it feels scary, unnatural, or just not worth it, stick to your guns and take the risk. You're likely to discover a world of depth, sharing, and love. 🄾

Family

Great Moments in Mothering

What if there were an Oscar for Outstanding Performance by a Mother in the Line of Duty? Here are two stories.

HOW TO STEAL A SHOW

ELIZABETH GILBERT

When I was in the third grade, our class put on a play called *The Lemonade Stand.* Which told the story of, well, a lemonade stand. Which featured three little girls spending a lot of time waiting for something to happen. Which may sound like an avant-garde Samuel Beckett production but was actually just one of those generic plays written for third-graders, wherein all 25 kids in the class get to say at least one line. Except for the three female leads, who, naturally, get to be onstage, selling lemonade, and speaking the whole time.

Now, I don't want to boast, but I was a formidable performer back in the third grade. My older sister and I had already produced *dozens* of plays in our living room, and my voice was capable of projecting powerfully across the school auditorium (and everywhere else, I'm afraid), so there was no question in my mind that I was a natural choice for one of the leading roles. Nonetheless, show business is a cruel mistress and I did not get cast as one of the starring lemonade girls. What I got instead was the part of Mrs. Fields—the only adult character in the play. Surely this made sense to Mrs. Domino (the director of this production) because I was about 11 inches taller than everyone else my age. Fine, except that Mrs. Fields was one of the smallest roles. Mrs. Fields had exactly *two* lines.

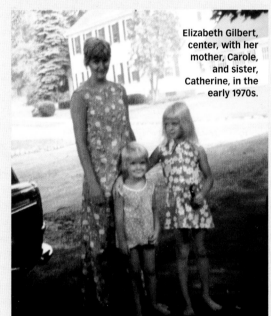

Elizabeth Gilbert, center, with her mother, Carole, and sister, Catherine, in the early 1970s.

The three leads went to the three cutest girls in the class—a triumvirate of ballet students with ponytails, whom I could thenceforth see only as one three-headed, giggle-spewing, Garanimals-wearing monster.

Was I angry?

No—I was *shattered.* And in my sorrow, I did something so completely out of character that I still can't really believe it myself: I walked up to Mrs. Domino and basically told her where she could stick her stupid play. And then I quit the stupid play. And then I sobbed for approximately the next seven hours.

This is where my mother comes in. Such moments of high distress are true tests of parenting. My mother is not a saint or a paragon; she's just a woman who, like many mothers, tried to do her best with her kids, sometimes failing, sometimes succeeding. But this was the moment of my life where she succeeded perhaps most brilliantly, where she really did it right.

First of all—what she didn't do: She didn't charge into the principal's office demanding that her daughter be given a better part, nor did she congratulate me on having quit the play, saying, "Yeah, screw Mrs. Domino." She never indicated that the three-headed monster shouldn't have been given the starring role, nor did she allow my letdown to feed her own insecurities, worrying that her child (therefore, she herself) was a failure. And, of course, she'd never have dreamed of scorning my sorrow with a comment like "Buck up, kiddo—crap happens. Now go get Mommy another beer."

What she did do was to assemble an extraordinary step-by-step program of loving reconstruction. First came solace. I sobbed, she soothed. But—in childhood grief, as with the adult variety—solace is beneficial for only so long. Which is why my mother finally wiped my nose and asked, "Don't you *want* to be in the play, sweetheart?"

I did! But I wanted to be one of the three starring lemonade girls! Or nothing!

Yes, she agreed, naturally. But given the reality that I couldn't be a lemonade girl, wouldn't I feel left out to be the only child who wasn't in the play at all?

I hadn't thought of that. I hadn't imagined what it would feel like to watch as everyone else had fun putting on a play.

"Sometimes the smallest parts are the most unforgettable," she went on. "What if you and I made sure Mrs. Fields was really memorable?"

As my mother laid out her cunning plan, I could almost feel the tears crawling back up my cheeks. But first, my mother said, I had to apologize to Mrs. Domino for having called her a stupid stupid-head, and humbly ask for my part back. I agreed, shamefaced. The next morning, though, when I made my nervous apology to Mrs. Domino, she was like, "What? Oh, yeah, no problem." It was as if she had no recollection of my massive personal drama.

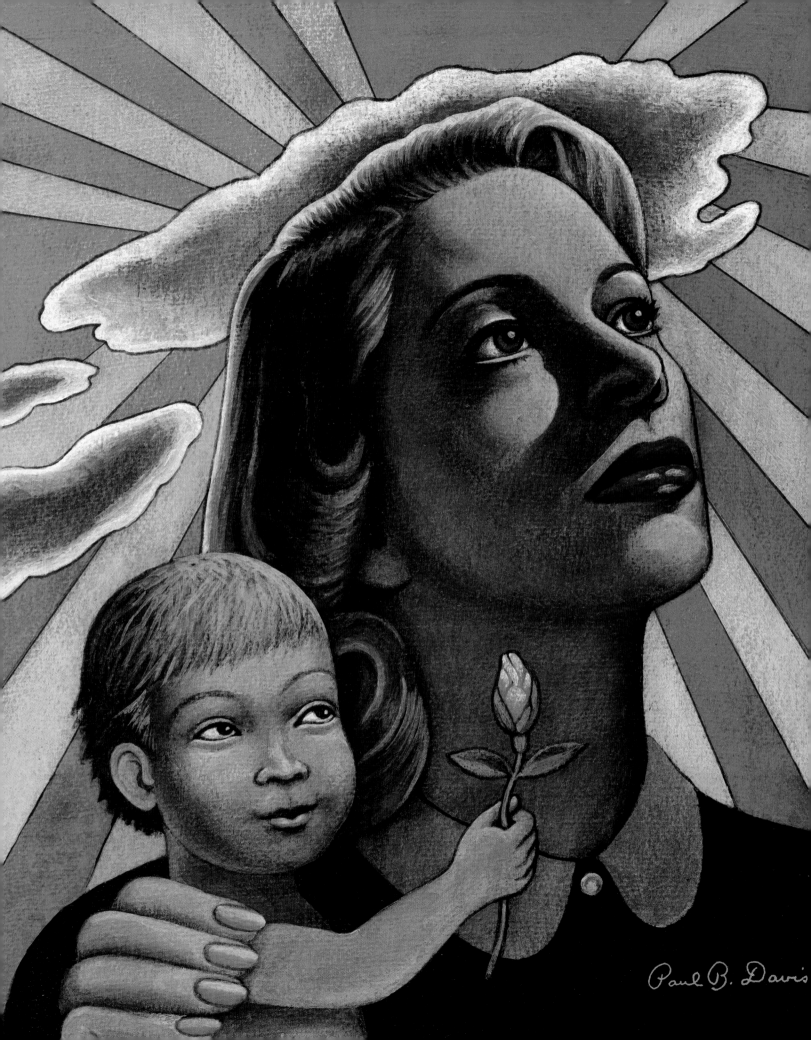

Paul B. Davis

(Thus handing me yet another important life lesson: Nobody's really paying that much attention to your massive personal dramas.)

Over the next month, my mother threw herself into helping me create a Mrs. Fields who would never be forgotten. Or at least that's how it felt to me. Looking back on it now, mind you, it occurs to me that she probably had other things going on besides her 8-year-old daughter's play. She had, for instance, a small family farm to run, a nursing job to maintain, another daughter to raise, and a marriage to attend to. But I didn't notice any of that. Because somehow, in those four weeks, she made me feel as though she had nothing better to do than run my two boring lines with me constantly, as though we were rehearsing Ophelia for the Royal Shakespeare Company. We experimented with accents, motivations, and fancy walking styles. Best of all, at a local thrift shop, we found an awesome Mrs. Fields costume—a vibrant pink vintage ball gown with matching high heels, purse, and sun hat. (A particularly noticeable getup, given that no other kids were wearing costumes.)

Opening day: The play droned to life. Bored parents fanned themselves in the audience, straining to hear mumbled lines. When I exploded onto the stage, as confident as (and dressed rather like) a drag queen, I could feel the crowd pop awake. Towering over the cast, I sashayed toward the lemonade stand and drawled languidly, "May ah have an oatmeal *cookie* and a glass of lemon*ade*?" (The honeyed Southern accent had been my mother's brilliant, last-minute suggestion.)

The audience hollered with laughter. Still in character, I drawled my next and final line ("*Thank yoooouuu!*") to the three dumbfounded stars and began my exit. But—not so fast. The audience was still laughing, still loving this 8-year-old Blanche DuBois. And that's when I had a clarion revelation: *They still need me!* This is when I made the charitable decision to give the crowd just a little more Mrs. Fields. Instead of heading for the wings, I swished back to center stage, dropped an imaginary quarter on the lemonade stand, and ad-libbed, "Keep the change, *sugar.*"

At which point, you know—the show pretty much had to be canceled on account of audience riot.

Afterward I stood in the school hallway, collecting compliments as though they were bouquets of roses. It had been a mighty victory, and, with Mom standing quietly beside me, I knew it had been her victory, too. My mother had grown up poor and underestimated, always cast into roles smaller than she was worth. Having succeeded in life despite being told she wasn't bright enough to go to nursing school, or sophisticated enough to be a naval officer's wife, she well knew the pleasure of exceeding people's expectations. So it was probably a culminating joy for both of us when the principal shook my mother's hand and said, "You should take this kid to Hollywood."

Final moment of perfect parenting? She didn't.

No, there would be no more stage mothering from Carole Gilbert. Instead Mom let me revel in exactly one hour of triumph, then took me home for an afternoon of household chores. The most significant part of the day was over, anyhow. Not the thunderous applause part, but the part where a mother had conveyed successfully to her young daughter these five critical survival lessons of life:

1. Make the most of whatever you are dealt.
2. If you are given only one opportunity to speak, be certain your voice is heard.
3. Have a ball.
4. Perfect your character relentlessly. And most important—
5. If life gives you lemons, don't settle for simply making lemonade—make a glorious scene at a lemonade stand.

A TALENT TO AMAZE

ANNE FADIMAN

Good mothers are supposed to feed sick children steaming chicken soup, coax medicine down their throats, and swaddle them in quilts. Whenever I had a cold, my mother did all the above, in addition to uncomplainingly scooping up the mounds of moist Kleenexes that had missed the wastebasket. (Basketball was always my worst sport.) But she also believed firmly in the therapeutic properties of nature.

We lived on a largish property in then-rural Connecticut, the sort of place where my brother and I could be permitted, without fear of prying neighborly eyes, to dance naked on the back lawn before a rain, when the sky had turned what we called thunderstorm green. It was also the sort of place that harbored such a ravishing array of wildlife—pheasants, foxes, pileated woodpeckers—that we might as well have lived on the African veld. Once, when I was 5 or 6 or 7, I caught a flu-y cold, or perhaps it was a cold-y flu, in the middle of winter. I was too sick to read, too sick even to watch *Captain Kangaroo.* My mother bustled up to my bedroom and announced we were going outside.

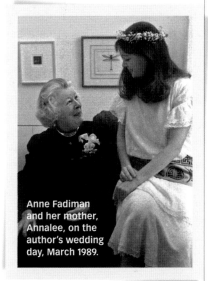

Anne Fadiman and her mother, Annalee, on the author's wedding day, March 1989.

Outside?

She was already dressed in a wool jacket and boots. She wrapped me in several blankets, hoisted me against her shoulder, and stomped out through the snow. We could see our breath condense in the freezing air. After a minute or so, she stopped in front of a blue spruce. There, in a low branch not ten feet from us, was a baby owl, its incompletely fledged feathers fluffed against the cold.

We watched it together, in silence, for a minute or so, and then my mother carried me back to bed. I wish I could say my fever broke instantly, but I doubt that was true. I can say, however, that during the next 40 years, until my mother's death, a single four-word sentence, spoken by either of us, conjured up all that was best about childhood. It was: "Remember the baby owl?" ◑

Band of Brothers

Nobody understands men like a woman who grew up with seven cool, teasing male siblings. Ask SARAH BROOM.

Here is the thing: I can barely remember ever considering men to be great mysteries. There were far too many of them messing around in my life for that. I was born into a clan of men, seven brothers in all. They measure all shades of a brown rainbow and for every tall and lanky one there is an opposite. One fishes, one cooks, another guards prisoners. They're mine. And whenever I imagine them, they are always in one room. When I put myself in there with them, I have this warm feeling of being surrounded.

I am the youngest of 12 children. Since I knew I wasn't always being paid sole attention to, I learned how to fight my way into things. So when my sister closest in age moved away, I was left in sweaty New Orleans to try to run happily around town with my brothers. I was nosy and into everything, including the boys' upstairs room where there was porn all over the walls. They would cringe to know that I know this.

Now, as a grown woman, so much of the way I see men has everything to do with these brothers. They are the ease I feel when men outnumber me in a room. They are the knowing nod I give girlfriends who, as adults, are just realizing the kinds of male things I first knew as a kid. My brothers were really the ones who showed me other kinds of intimacy, too. The way we express love and closeness is different from the way I might with my women friends (or my four sisters, for that matter). Through my brothers I see the power in lulls, in silence. A quiet room is not threatening to them; it is time together. Instead of so much talk, we get closer through shared experience, like second-line dancing to brass bands in hole-in-the-wall places or eating boiled crawfish out in the sun. This is how I see them get closer to each other, too. And time together for them means ignoring whatever else is going on in the world. My elbow scar will never let me forget this. I was a small child playing hopscotch when a boy neighbor dared me to put my arm through the glass window of the den of our house. I know it was the den because right there on TV the New Orleans Saints were losing a football game and I remember my brothers cheering them on. I know I showed them the bloody elbow. One of the brothers, I can't remember who, glanced at me and said, "Wipe that up, girl." And so I took a sheet off someone's twin bed and soaked up the blood. What I knew then was this: Major things can happen, and I still might not get their full attention.

For they are vastly different men. The ways in which they love and relate to women vary, though they all lend women great power in their lives. A woman could get them to do all kinds of magic, especially when it came down to not hurting her feelings. I've seen them disappear in seconds as teenagers when a probing girlfriend showed up at the door. Back then, I lied to a few on some of their behalfs (sorry, ladies). "He's not here," I'd say over the phone as a brother mouthed the words. My brother Carl can lower his voice to a girly whisper to sweet-talk a woman. He seems to know exactly what women want, though this has nothing to do with whether he'll do it. From all this listening and watching, I developed a repertoire of the charming and conniving stories men tell women: "I heard every word you said...." "I like a woman who can do her own thing...." "She's nothing compared to you...." This must be why, by date two, I let a man know about all these brothers. What I want them to hear is: "I've already heard that story—and that one, too."

By the time I was in elementary school, most of my brothers were grown men: happily married, or divorced, or loving women who didn't love back. Tucked into their periodic comments on their relationships were their own ideas about how a woman should carry herself in the world. I was to be dignified. And they were often more honest than my sisters. They'd ask, "Why is your hair sticking up?" about a new haircut that I called stylish. They stayed honest with me because I never shot them down. I'd joke back, talk about how their clothes didn't match, how their hairline was backing away from their forehead. We'd laugh a loud one. And that is how we get along, how we stand each other.

I love who I am around them, so I look for pieces of them in men of a certain age and demographic. The other day, I was walking home when I noticed three neighborhood men circling my Harlem, New York, stoop. One of them was Duke, an elderly and halfway-homeless-looking ladies' man. I saw him swigging from a bottle he'd pulled out of a jacket pocket. Here is when I understand something else about myself: Having had all these men in my life, I see the particular man behind the obvious. I never bought into the supermasculine myth, because I saw these men, up close, with so much complexity. Saw them sappy sweet and macho and teary-eyed. So when Duke pokes my shoulder in play, I remember my chef brother, Michael, the way he often draws me to the nook of his arm even though I am 5'11" and taller than him. He says, "Baby girl, you just like us, like the boys." I give him a sideways look with a grin and say, "Oh yeah huh." And that, right there, is the truth of it all. ◐

Raising New Orleans celebratory umbrellas, Sarah and her brothers let the good times roll. *Clockwise from top left:* Carl, Michael, Darryl, Troy, Eddie, Byron, and Simon.

RELATIONSHIPS

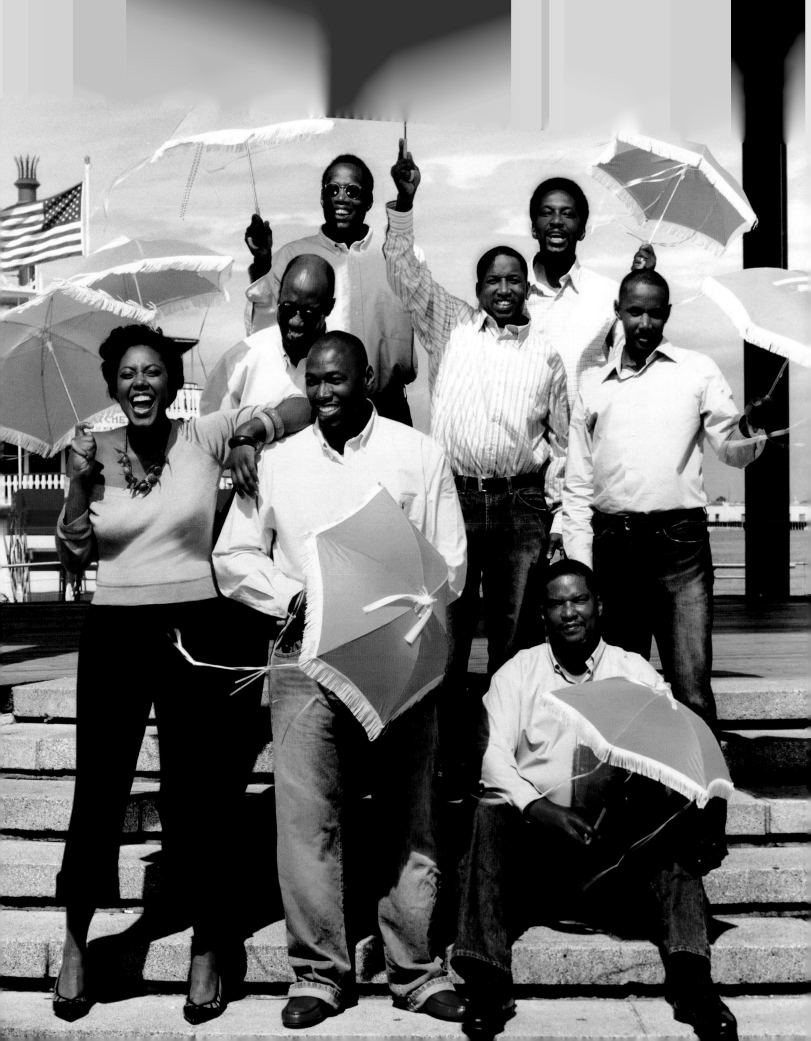

Meet the Parent

What does it take to raise a child on your own? Nerves of steel, nonstop energy, and a thing for short, bald people. LISA KOGAN writes one for her baby.

The love of my life is shorter than I am, does not have quite as much hair as I'd like, could never be considered a scintillating conversationalist. You're probably thinking this is one of those situations where a whole lot of money or great sex figures prominently. Nope. We generally grab a bite to eat, watch a video, do a little reading, and call it a night. I suppose when I thought about the future, I imagined a Vera Wang wedding gown (serious décolletage, hold the train) in ivory, followed by a fabulous husband and a whip-smart, funny, delicious baby girl. Given that I never did get that fabulous husband, the ivory Vera Wang seemed like an unnecessary extravagance, but one out of three—especially when the one turns out to be that whip-smart, funny, delicious baby girl—ain't bad. There's no getting around it, Julia Claire Labusch is the love of my life.

That said, let me add that we are fortunate, as she's also the love of her father's life. My sweetheart and I have been together for nearly 12 years, but he lives in Europe and can visit only every couple of months. It's more than a lot of single mothers get—and it's nowhere near enough. So each morning I rise up out of the mire of my own narcissism and set some parenting goals. Sometimes they're lofty: She will attend the ballet, eat organic blueberries, learn to speak Malay, and be enveloped in a blanket of unconditional love. Other days my goals are a bit more basic: Please, God, let me just raise this kid so she doesn't end up in a Texas bell tower with a high-powered rifle and a grudge.

Whoever said "One is the loneliest number that you'll ever do" never spent six hours in a steam-filled bathroom with a croupy 2-year-old. But it's not the 3 A.M. fever, the supermarket tantrum, the left front wheel coming off our stroller as I cross Second Avenue, or even the knowledge that this little person has only me for her sole support and emotional nourishment, that makes bringing up a baby on my own so...what's the word? Challenging? Exhausting? Nerve-racking? Heartbreaking? All of the above. The time I most wish I weren't flying solo is early Sunday morning when I'm making breakfast and this little monkey girl is having a long, deeply passionate phone conversation with a recording that repeats, "If you'd like to make a call, please hang up and dial again." That's when I crave a witness, someone as besotted with her as I am, a person who, like me, just can't believe that something went so completely right. And I remember the feeling two Aprils ago, when this flawless infant was placed in my arms. I guess they weighed her, because somehow I knew I was holding 7 pounds 0.5 ounces. I should have thought of something poetic to say. I should not have let the moment pass. She was, after all, the only miracle I had ever experienced. But the only thing I could do was cry.

I cried because she smelled so good. I cried because I could see my family in her face. I cried because all around me were mothers and fathers and newborns and shared joy. I cried because I knew in five days my boyfriend needed to leave and I'd be left alone with her. I cried because I was terrified to be left alone with her. I cried because I know that nature isn't stupid—two people coming together to care for a third is an excellent plan. After I cried, I slept. After I slept, I worried, I ached, and I slept some more.

When I woke up, Julia was brought to me and the curtains were drawn, partitioning me and my girl from the rest of the world. I counted toes and marveled at their delicate nails. Her tiny body revealed that where she had been attached to me, an umbilical cord had clearly been cut, allowing us to separate. Here was someone squishy and pink who needed me for survival, and I needed her back for the same reason. I'd never loved anyone so fiercely before. And so it began. The holding on for dear life, and the learning to let go, the push me, pull you, the particularly intense hothouse of single parenting.

I have spent two years now trying to get through each day with a modicum of grace and humor. I get regular visits from unmarried friends closing in on 40 who have the same look of raw yearning that I used to have. They pour themselves a glass of Merlot, curl up on my sofa, and tell me that they never really considered the possibility of *not* having a baby. "You come to a point in life where you can do without a Saturday-night date or a bigger apartment or even a fabulous coffee table for the smaller apartment," said one friend, sipping her wine and trying not to cry, "but you cannot do without a child." I nod my understanding as I attempt to keep Julia from stuffing little Cheddar Goldfish into the VCR. "It's a complicated issue," I say, knowing that they're looking for something magical and soothing and enlightening, and knowing that those words don't actually exist. "It depends on how much money, love, and time you have to spend. It depends on whether or not you can find other ways to fulfill your instinct to nurture. It depends on both how selfish and how selfless you're capable of being."

Invariably, my friends will squeeze Julia's drumstick thighs, make raspberry sounds on her tummy, and inhale the back of her neck. We walk them to the door and head for our copy of *Angelina Ballerina* as I remind myself that I'm unbelievably blessed, pray not to screw it up, and wish somebody would give me the answers. Of course, in my less sleep-deprived moments I realize that no single person—and no couple, either—has all the answers. And that not being exactly sure how to raise a daughter on my own, not having all those answers, brings me more in touch with the voice in the back of my head that whispers, *Maybe, in the end, everything will be all right.* I said *maybe.* ◑

Talking Sex with Maud

Do daughters talk to their mothers about sex anymore? If the mothers are lucky, yes.
TRISH DEITCH on the birds, the bees, the teenager, and the pact.

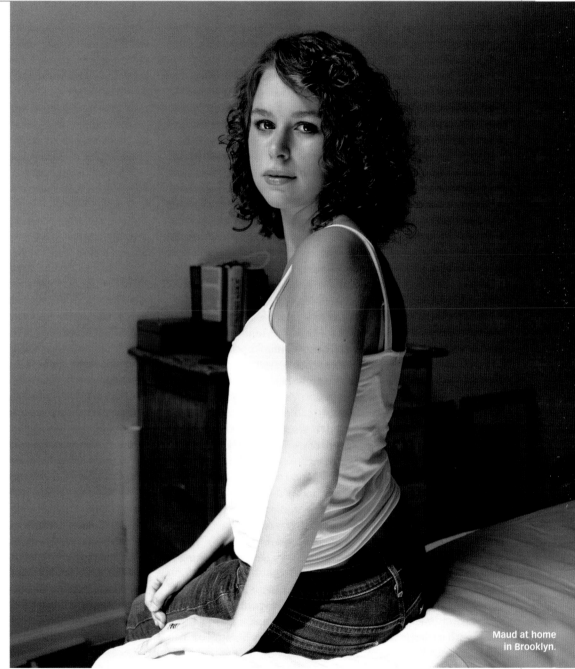

Maud at home in Brooklyn.

It never occurred to me that I'd have to talk to my teenage daughter about sex. At her insistence, we'd had the initial "Where do babies come from?" session when she was 5. ("But how?" she'd shouted, frustrated by my tight-ass lack of detail. "How does the sperm get *in* there to fertilize the egg?!") And after the mandatory New York City sex-ed course that left her fifth-grade classmates weepy with its descriptions of anal and oral sex, I figured she probably knew more than I.

The bottom line is, I don't like talking to anyone about sex; it seems such a private and dangerous subject. But two summers ago, a few weeks before Maud, at 17, was due to spend several months in proximity to the boy she'd loved from afar since she was 12, a magazine asked me to review a book called *Everything You Never Wanted Your Kids to Know About Sex (But Were Afraid They'd Ask)*. The gist of the book is that teenagers want their parents' advice about sex; they're interested in our experience and our thoughts, and they'd like to tell us about theirs.

I assumed that Maud would be an exception. She's a private person—the kind of kid who, at 8 or 9, hid, from teasing passersby, most of the books she read—from *Harriet the Spy* to her beloved illustrated primer on social etiquette. To this day, she finds public displays of affection undignified and rude, and she was never the kind to confide in me about matters of romance; the most intimate thing she told me about the boys she hung around with was that they smelled. Still, on the advice of the book, I felt I had to ask her: Do you want to talk about sex?

She was walking past the living room when I called out to her from the couch. I didn't look up from the magazine I was flipping through—just called out and kept on flipping.

It's Never Too Late to Have an Okay Childhood

Your mother was absent, your father angry (or was it the other way around?). You think that's all behind you...but until you mourn the disappointments and losses of your childhood, chances are you'll continue to be controlled by those same family patterns. Therapist ROBERT KAREN, PhD, on why the remembrance of painful things past can set you joyously free.

Soon after I became a father, I was haunted by the fear that I would lose my son. The fear was not that one of us would contract a terminal disease or that we would be separated by earthquake or war, but rather that we would stop loving each other. Power struggles, bitterness, and hatred would tear us apart, and we would become enemies.

Why was I so certain of this? You could say it was written into my psychology, a remnant of the heartache etched in me as a result of my boyhood relationship with my father.

My father used to say that he liked children till they reached the end of the age of innocence. I knew what he meant. Until age 3 or so, they adore you and hang on your words. Then they start having ideas of their own, and it's the beginning of the end. My father never got over his own childhood injuries (including having lived with a father who never spoke to him), injuries that often left him feeling powerless and uncared about. No one ever doted on him when he was growing up, and he still longed for it. He couldn't enjoy my challenges or independence; he couldn't tolerate my anger. He didn't have the kind of resilience and security that come from having been well loved. When he got angry, he went to a dark place and stayed there.

My father loved me, and in later years the love between us was affirmed. But growing up, much of the time, I couldn't feel it. Power struggles had turned us into antagonists who could flare up at each other over nothing. If I had not been able to face and deal with the legacy of that relationship, I would surely have repeated much of it with my son.

The childhood we never had—that is to say, all the love and understanding and help we needed but didn't get—is haunting. It haunts our relationships with those we love the most, and it undermines our capacity to deal with emotional hardships. Not solely because we were wounded as children—all children get wounded—but because as children we rarely get to mourn the most difficult hurts and losses.

> My father didn't have the resilience that comes from being loved. When he got angry, he went to a dark place and stayed there.

Let's take a closer look at this idea of mourning, which is so widely misunderstood. Ideally, mourning is not just suffering. It is productive suffering. Mourning is about processing the hurt, about expanding the self, about growing and moving on—without having been crippled or diminished by the loss. Mourning is complicated. It takes time. It takes creativity. Anger and depression may be part of the mix, but ultimately, mourning is completed under the auspices of love. Especially in childhood, it requires the loving assistance of others, which is gradually converted into a loving concern for the self. If we learn to mourn as children, it serves us for the rest of our lives. If we don't, all losses come to feel unmanageable, self-love is elusive, and every sorrow becomes a cause for depression.

People can learn to mourn as adults. That is one of the fundamentals of successful psychotherapy. In therapy, mourning begins when we open forbidden internal territory to the therapist's caring. But it's not easy to give up the defenses that have shielded us from pain. Or to drop patterns of relating that pay secret homage to the past. These are part of what Wilhelm Reich called character armor. Caring threatens to pierce that armor, to interfere with our comfortable misery. Long ago Freud referred to psychoanalysis as a cure through love. But he knew that, even when offered with the greatest sensitivity and tact, love could be stubbornly resisted.

Alicia, the mother of a newborn boy, is in a lousy, postpartum funk that takes her into a dark part of her psychology. She finds herself without feeling for her baby. When I question her about what she expects her relationship with him to be like, she imagines him growing up to align himself with her husband, her brother, and her brother-in-law, creating a male cabal that cuts her out. Although she suspects there's something irrational about it, she already sees the baby as ungrateful, as preferring others, like her younger sister, and crying whenever she herself approaches.

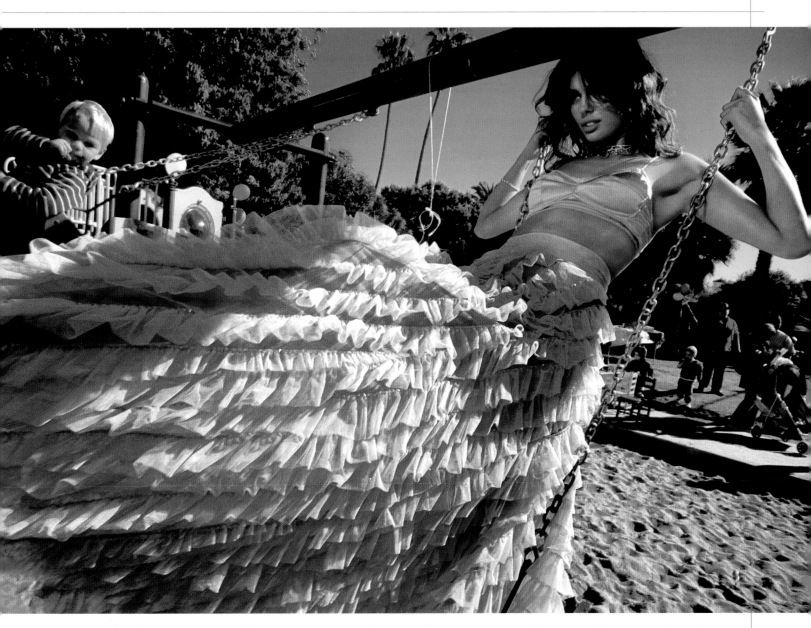

Interestingly, Alicia's perceptions of her newborn are similar in certain respects to the way her mother perceived her, while in other respects they represent the way her mother *was* with her. Her mother was an envious person who felt oppressed, burdened, and bitter about having to give of herself, and who was very critical of her little girl, whom she constantly accused of being overly demanding, impossible to please, and ungrateful. The mother not only saw Alicia as the agent of a persecuting, depriving world, but she projected onto her daughter many of the bad feelings she had about herself.

Not surprisingly, Alicia came to believe these accusations. As an adult, she complains angrily about her mother, but psychologically speaking, she still clings to her, longs for her, and does imaginary battle with her almost every day of her life. Indeed, it often seems that no one else quite matters. Being stuck on a parent in this way is a common symptom of unmourned trauma. It usually includes some emulation of the disliked parental qualities and a refusal to let love in from others. Like her mother, Alicia,

too, is prone to envy and bitterness. She resents those she perceives as having more and does not want to bless anyone with her gratitude.

This issue of gratitude, so central to feelings of loving and giving, arose in one of our recent sessions. She was complaining about feeling unappreciated and unloved by the baby and others, when we had the following exchange:

R.K.: *Do you feel* I've *been giving to you?*

A.: Yes, Bob, you've given me a lot of insights over the years.

R.K.: *How about I've also fought like hell for you?*

A.: Yes, yes, that's true.

R.K.: *And yet I get no acknowledgment.*

A.: Hmm.

R.K.: *Sometimes I feel as if you suck me dry and then walk away as if you've gotten nothing.*

This statement may seem odd coming from a therapist, but it represents an important part of the therapist's job: to mirror for the patient the kinds of feelings she induces in others, in this case that one must give, give, give, and yet all one gives is useless. My observation hits its mark, and Alicia starts grumbling—first, that she doesn't see what I'm getting at; then that she doesn't know what to do about it; and, finally, that she feels guilty and bad. But it's not the kind of guilty or bad that does me any good; indeed, it's meant to make *me* feel guilty and bad. Her complaint is really a temper tantrum disguised as confusion.

In the end, Alicia argues that she doesn't see us as having a real relationship anyway—so what difference does all this make? When I remind her that we've known each other for a long time, that of course we have a relationship, and that it's natural for us to be affected by each other, she protests:

A.: I always thought of you as a therapist and not needing anything back from me.

R.K.: *But that's how you treat everyone—like a functionary. You feel horribly deprived and everyone is measured by how much he can give you. But you don't give back.*

A.: Yeah, my husband says that about me, too.

R.K.: *But even now you don't seem particularly concerned about it. It's just a curiosity that he and I say the same thing.*

She remembers now that her husband had given her a card that morning and a little present to try to lift her spirits. But she'd thought, *Damn it, after everything I've been through lately, why couldn't he get me a nice piece of jewelry!* It was a good insight, and she wasn't fighting me off anymore, but neither was she at the point of feeling regret.

R.K.: *How do you think he feels when you thank him with a fake smile and never say another word?*

She becomes reflective and her tone changes:

A.: It's got to be hard for him. He's been really putting out, and I know he wants so much for me to appreciate him.

For the first time today, she speaks with genuine sorrow about how she has behaved. She has momentarily left the blighted realm of Alicia and Mother and entered a more soulful, more loving place, where her deepest feelings matter and where what she does with others has consequence. It's at moments like these when she is most emotionally available that she becomes a person you'd really want to be close to.

Alicia's moment of sorrow fades quickly. The world for her remains in many respects her mother's world, one in which she has to ward off assaults and grab whatever she can from people who don't really care and don't want to give; it's not a place where mutual warmth and concern pay off. But such feelings, of regret and concern for others, if taken seriously and returned to repeatedly—and if coupled with a recognition that others care about her as well—can eventually tap into the hidden reservoir of tears within her. This would make possible a better life for her with her son, her husband, her sister, and me, not only because she would be more empathic toward us but because she would allow us to feel more for her.

But perhaps most crucial, permitting herself feelings of regret and concern might be the beginning of a more caring relationship with herself. Instead of holding on to her mother's view that she was an impossible child, Alicia might find that she wants to cry for that child. Eventually, she might find herself able to both take in and give herself the understanding and love that were too scarce when she was growing up.

Childhood is full of losses. The worst is the loss of a parent because of death, abandonment, or some other cause. But there are smaller losses as well. We lose the paradise of our mother's breast, the status of fussed-over baby, the privileged position of only child, the fantasy that we will marry Mom or Dad when we grow up, the security of our intact family if our parents separate. If we're lucky, we get lots of help with such losses so that they don't leave us scarred. We're reassured that we're loved, we learn that life is good even if it isn't perfect, and this enables us to be more realistic about life, more tolerant, and more forgiving of ourselves and others.

But when a child has problems with a difficult parent—involving feelings of neglect, rejection, or betrayal—the need for help is especially great. When a girl's mother has a terrible temper and is prone to fits of blaming and threats, a sensitive father (or grandmother or older sibling) can be a huge ally. He can not only try to straighten the mother out but can help the wretched girl sort out what's going on. Through him she can understand that it's not her fault (as children are prone to believe), that Mom has a problem, that Mom still loves her, and, despite the girl's own hurt and fury, she still loves her mom. Her father can hold her and reassure her and go through the tempest of her emotions with her. With that kind of loving ally, she can be introduced to a more satisfying mode of relating. There are other critically important lessons as well: that love can withstand fury, hatred, even brutality. That forgiveness is possible. And that she can care for herself—and get caring for herself—when in pain.

But most children suffering the stresses of parental failure don't have anyone to play that supportive role. The second parent is usually not much help, either blaming the child or offering platitudes or denying that there is a problem at all. The relatives are out of reach. And a therapist is not consulted. So the child has no choice but to feel bad and unlovable, and also terribly guilty. She's so full of anger that she mistakenly believes she has committed the gravest crime in the universe: She no longer loves her mother. She either acts out and becomes a behavior problem, hating herself and the world, or she puts the whole thing out of her mind even as it gets hardened into her psyche.

In other words, as children, instead of mourning our losses, we may get all tangled up in them. They remain inside us in raw, unprocessed form and haunt us with depression or obsessive efforts to avoid depression. Meanwhile the parents who hurt us become the most prominent beings in our psyches, even if we've ruled them out of our lives and moved to the other side of the planet to avoid them. The natural process of separation, which is a part of a healthy growing up—and which enables a child to feel secure in a parent's love while moving on to other realms and relationships—gets derailed. Sometimes in our longing to have the love and support we missed as kids, we stubbornly refuse to grow up. Unconsciously, we imagine that our immaturity will be rewarded with the magical appearance of the perfect parent in the form of a lover or a boss, a friend or a child. But, inevitably, in an unreturned call or a tone of voice, we find our hurtful parent instead. We elicit or imagine the slighting responses we expect, and we replay our past with all the important figures in our lives.

Alan, an extraordinarily accomplished man, with one foot in industry and another in the arts, recently broke up with an abusive girlfriend, the latest in a series. Even now, months after they've separated, she showers him with invective. He comes to me, beaten down by her complaints, his head hanging, feeling guilty as charged, wanting to make amends, give her money, and so forth. I encourage him to recognize why he lets himself live in this forlorn place. Why does he seek punishment from women? What does he gain from martyring himself to them? Why is making a female sourpuss smile the greatest pleasure he knows? These questions bring us back to the causative pain, the pain he suffered with parents who barely noticed him—except, in his mother's case, to yell and find fault.

To win his parents' admiration, Alan became a superachiever, and to cope with his mother's anger, he became supercompliant. He felt a powerful need to make things right for a mother whom he believed he'd somehow wronged. Why else would she be so hostile and tormented all the time? If he could fix her life, she'd forgive him, love him, exalt him. In his adult romances, he accepts all blame, pays all bills, accedes to irrational demands, tamps down his anger, and becomes self-hating and depressed when his earnest efforts only garner more abuse.

Looking in the rearview mirror of failed relationships, Alan sees his ex-girlfriends the way he saw his mother, as "wonderful and perfect," while he's the "miserable guy who ruined their lives."

Alan, who sometimes would prefer that I simply give him advice, has asked me several times, "Why do I have to remember the past?" And my response has generally been to up the ante: You have to do more than remember—you have to re-feel; you have to suffer the pain again. Emotionally speaking, there's something of the orphan in Alan. That orphan boy has been locked out and disowned—like a wounded, raging *enfant terrible* that Alan has kept in the woodshed because he's ashamed of him, hates him, doesn't want to see him. But that boy needs to be acknowledged. For Alan to let his heart break for that forgotten part of himself—guilty, confused, indicted, swollen with unrequited love, wanting to hurt back—would bring about a revolution in self-love.

Re-owning unwanted parts of ourselves brings us face-to-face with emotions we fear and dislike and forces us to find a way to absorb them creatively into a broadened identity. In Alan's case, anger is one such emotion. Because his mother never allowed him his anger as a child and he has not allowed it to himself as an adult, it's foreign, it's volcanic, it's untamed by the wisdom of good models and thought-through experience. Just to let himself

Sometimes in our longing to have the love and support we missed as kids, we stubbornly refuse to grow up.

know that he is an angry man, to feel entitled to his anger, would be an important step in the rehabilitation of the cut-off parts of himself. Indeed, at this point in Alan's development, walking around in an angry state would not only be a whole lot better than masochistic submission but also an indication that mourning has begun to take hold.

Any move toward mourning on Alan's part—remembering, resuffering, letting in caring and feeling it for himself—would inevitably include a pause in his obsessive quest to achieve, to be admired, to gallantly win the love of a rejecting woman. Which means that mourning would play another crucial role in his life—as an antidote to his workaholism and romantic obsession, qualities that might otherwise end up making him a remote parent much like his dad.

We know from research that children can be securely or insecurely attached to a parent. The securely attached child is confident of the parent's love, feels freer, as a result, to explore the world, and is better able to make intimate connections with others. The insecurely attached child is either clingy or avoidant, is more likely to be a bully or a victim with peers, carries within her bad feelings about herself, and is frequently either desperate or cynical about love.

Mary Main, a psychologist at the University of California at Berkeley who studies the quality of parent-child attachment, showed that one of the aspects that distinguishes parents of children who are securely attached to them is their ability to talk coherently about their emotional lives, including the sorrows and losses they've suffered. They convey a sense that they can acknowledge a tragedy and move on—without having repressed or forgotten the experience. In fact, their memories were the most rich and detailed of all the parents.

Most parents of insecure children lack this capacity. They either are still preoccupied and emotionally enmeshed with the parents who disappointed them or they flatly deny any problems. Both types are alike in their lack of mourning—displaying either an inability to deal with hurts that were remembered and relived on a daily basis or an unwillingness to think about them at all.

Much of modern life is built around avoiding pain, and we have more things to divert us from our unwanted feelings than mankind ever imagined. But as Main's research shows, attending to the very feelings we so much want to escape holds the promise of a better emotional life.

Mourning should not be confused with an obsessive holding on to a pain that never heals. In healthy mourning, we do heal, if not always completely. We are able to recover—even from the deaths of people we love—without losing the sense that the world is a good place, that the lost person is still within us in a good way, and that new love can come into our lives. In the end, it's through mourning, which deepens our relationship with ourselves, that we are able to deepen our connections to others. ◗

My Family on the Other Side of Town

She'd never met her father. Then one day MICHELLE BURFORD worked up the nerve to call him. The result: conversation (stilted), understanding (finally), and an extraordinary sisterly connection she came *thisclose* to missing.

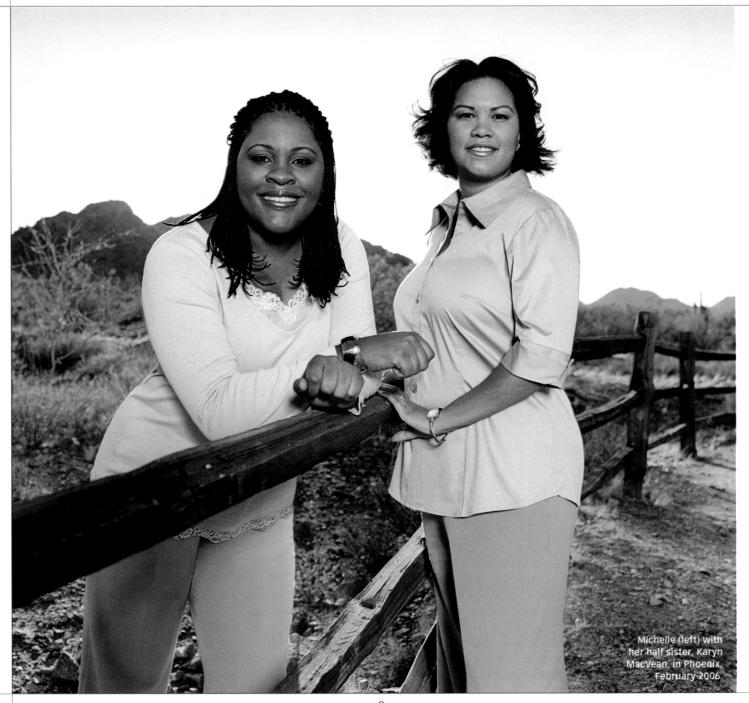

Michelle (left) with her half sister, Karyn MacVean, in Phoenix, February 2006

I discovered my father through a circle of whisperers: my aunt, my grandmother, and my mother, clustered around an oak table on a Sunday afternoon in 1981, the year I was 9. My aunt, who'd flown into Phoenix from Los Angeles the day before, had already traded that morning's Baptist church heels and pearls for a housecoat, and was tearing into a plate of collards and a round of scuttlebutt. "She looks just like him," my aunt said when I was presumably out of earshot. "Has she met him yet?"

I hadn't. I had been told that I'd once spent time in my father's presence as a toddler, but I had no memory of his face. After years of eavesdropping on a mother who was understandably reluctant to dredge up difficult memories and wanted to guard me from pain, I knew that he'd remarried and moved across town to Glendale. Once, my mother referred to him as "the spittin' image of that gospel singer Larnelle Harris." When I was 7, I had overheard a family member mention my dad's other daughter, Karyn. Still, in the hours after midnight as I lay atop my bunk examining the cover of the Harris album with a miniature flashlight clutched in my hand, I forgot about Karyn and fantasized that I was Dad's only girl. His lone beloved daughter. The child he'd one day reunite with.

During the summer I turned 17, my day dream took flight. "Are you Mike Burford's daughter?" the salon stylist asked as she eyed the ticket that bore my full name. I was terrified. My photo had just made *The Arizona Republic* because I'd been named Phoenix Young Woman of the Year, in recognition of stellar grades and community service. The next morning on TV, I was to be honored by the mayor. To tame my frizzies, Mom had dropped me at the $9-a-head beauty school for an assembly-line hairdo. "Uh, yes," I finally stammered to the stylist once the shock of hearing my father's name aloud dissipated. "I am Michelle Burford, Mike's daughter." This was the last piece of truth I uttered that afternoon. As Pat the beautician snipped my ends and gushed about my father, I pretended I'd always known him, only because I longed to gather any detail I could about this man she called a friend. "I cut your dad's hair at my other salon across town," Pat said. "He talks about you all the time." I froze. Though I'd always imagined my father had been following my life from afar, this revelation somehow frightened me.

Which is probably why I waited another three summers to call him. On break during my junior year of college, I flipped through the Phoenix Yellow Pages in search of the salon where I'd met Pat. "I've never known my father," I confessed once I tracked her down. "I want to." A day later, Pat gave me his number.

The first time I heard his voice on the answering machine, I snapped down the receiver and wept. "This is Mike, JoAnn, Karyn, and Michael" is how I remembered my father had another family: a wife, a daughter, and a son. The next afternoon, I called twice more before my father picked up.

"This is Michelle," I said with zero pause between each word. "Michelle Burford."

Silence.

"I know," my father said finally. "Pat told me you called her."

Two days later, he arrived to pick me up for dinner. Nothing about our meeting resembled my fantasy. No dad and girl running toward each other across a field of tulips. No lingering hug and irrepressible tears. No hours spent retracing 20 missed years. Just one incredibly nervous girl and one play-it-cool man trying to make the moment less awkward. Seconds after I opened the front door, I mumbled hello before lowering my gaze to my sandals, then grabbed my purse and practically knocked him over as I hurried toward the passenger seat of his car. On our way to the restaurant, we rode along to the sound of jazz. "How are you?" he asked in an attempt to melt the iceberg I'd placed between us. "Good," I shot back, looking away. I wanted to say more. I wanted to know: Where have you been all my life? Yet all I could do was set a new personal record in nail chewing.

Thirty minutes later at a restaurant in Glendale, I sat across from my dad; across from his wife, JoAnn, an elegantly dressed Mexican woman with irreproachable manners; across from my then-15-year-old half sister, who shared my last name and my father and, it seemed, little else. As the next two hours snaked along, I could not have said more than a few complete sentences to this row of Burfords I was stunned to be sitting near.

Karyn was as gracious and refined as her mother and attempted polite conversation across the chasm that separated our worlds. For two sisters who grew up in the same city, our realities couldn't have been more different. Karyn attended one of Arizona's premier private high schools; though my mother and stepdad encouraged me to excel, I went to a school more renowned for its ills than for its academic rigor. Karyn spent her childhood in the "other" box—a racial hybrid in a sea of white faces, a girl refuting a question she still despises: "What are you, exactly?" Across town, I lived in the city's largest enclave of blacks.

Mostly, it was my father who talked, and I—who had two decades of questions lodged in my throat—cannot remember a single word he said. I pushed risotto from one rim of the plate to the other. Each time my father looked away, I stole a glance at

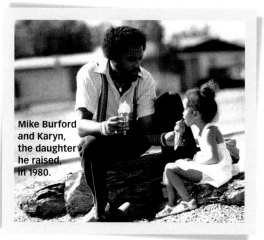

Mike Burford and Karyn, the daughter he raised, in 1980.

For the only time in my memory, I looked at both the man and the woman who'd given me life. I will never forget that moment.

the man whose face and comportment were so eerily like my own. My aunt was right: I was undeniably his daughter.

At summer's end, before I returned to college in Los Angeles, my father schlepped from Glendale to Phoenix for our second visit. The first time he'd arrived to pick me up, my mother had chosen to let me meet him alone. This time she was home. And this time when I dashed for the door, she got there first. "Hello, Mike," she said as I appeared around a corner. A second later, I stood in the triangle I'd been born into: My mother, my father, and me, staring at one another in silence. For the only time in my memory, I looked at both the man and the woman who'd given me life. I will never forget that moment.

In the years that followed, he called often. And each time, I found myself dreading the five-minute "How's the weather?" conversation because it felt meaningless, a way to elude the pain of 20 years lost. For months at a time, I avoided him. I seldom returned his calls or acknowledged his birthday cards because I knew our connection was built on a shaky foundation of unspeakables, but I didn't have the courage to march the truth out onto the scaffold and stand there with it.

I can't tell you where my chutzpah came from, but one afternoon when I spotted my father's name on caller ID, I gathered the nerve to take our connection deeper. "I can't remember the last time it was so hot here," Dad began. "Why didn't you ever call me?" I interrupted. Long pause. Followed by a sentence that changed the direction of our friendship: "I should've called you, Michelle. There's no excuse." He went on to say that he hadn't wanted to barge into the new family my mother had made for me. Any other explanation—a lie like "I loved you, but I just couldn't find you"—would have made me put down the receiver forever. I didn't always like my father's answers, but that day I promised myself that I'd hear him. Not because he wanted me to listen, but because I needed to face the history I was born into.

Ten years after I found my father, I sat across from him again—this time from chair to hospital bed, palm to palm. That night and in the year before colon cancer claimed his life, he and I finally made it around to the biggies—like why he and my mother split. Like how his proudest moments and his biggest humiliations had changed him. I cried. I forgave. I asked to be forgiven for all the times I'd shut him out in the years after our meeting. I left his room that night knowing I might never see him alive again. I did not.

In the space left by my father's death, I discovered Karyn. For a decade, we had been acquaintances, delivering the double-cheek kiss and the two-minute catch-up every few months. But as with so many people I've dismissed with a glance—certain that too much makes us different to bother nurturing similarity—I never really saw her. Instead, I pegged her as a wavy-haired, privileged girl who had zilch to share with me. I was wrong.

"You sit like Dad," Karyn said when she visited me for the first time in Harlem, about a year and a half after our father's death. We'd strolled through Central Park for two hours, and we were taking a break on a wooden bench. There we posed our stored-up questions. (She: "What does your mom look like?" Me: "What was it like growing up with Dad?") We exchanged the file of details that gal pals often keep on each other (hideous hairstyles, first kisses, best lipsticks, jerk boyfriends). I sat. I heard. I revealed. And later that evening, I cried because I'd nearly allowed my judgments to eclipse a connection of such magnificence.

I've set out looking for my father twice: First on the cover of a gospel album, next in the praises of a chatty beautician. On a park bench in Harlem one fall day, I glimpsed him through a gift he gave me—an extraordinary woman he left behind. **O**

Lisa Kogan Tells All

Our chronically unmarried columnist got the distinct feeling there was more than one turkey at the Thanksgiving dinner. Now she's noodling around with a few new traditions.

I spent ten Thanksgivings volunteering in a Harlem soup kitchen because—hell, I'll just say it—I'm one of the few women of my generation who look really good in a hairnet. Also, I love to cook. I love turning nothing into something. I love the smell of garlic and lemon and ginger and onion. I love how blissed-out a tableful of people get over a crumbly cornbread stuffing or a perfectly dressed salad or a sweet potato–bourbon pie made from scratch. Oh, and there's one more reason I went out of my way to spend every holiday surrounded by a group of strangers: I couldn't bear to be with my family.

It's not that I don't love them—I do. They are a decent, God-fearing lot who would walk a mile out of their way to help if they thought you were in trouble. They recycle, they vote, they pay taxes, they e-mail the warning signs of a stroke. They are pillars of their communities, credits to their race, sugar and spice and everything nice, the cat's pajamas, the monkey's espadrilles. They'll meet your plane, they'll walk your dog, they'll remember your birthday, they'll save you a drumstick. But here's where my family and I parted company: They were all married with children, and for the first 42 years of my life, I was neither.

One of these things is not like the others. One of these things just doesn't belong, goes the lyric to my favorite *Sesame Street* tune. Who'd have guessed that Big Bird would end up killing me softly with his song, but it's true—while I hardly qualify as the family's black sheep, in the race for odd duck I've broken away from the pack and am currently maintaining a significant lead.

Now, if you've read my column before, you know I have a boyfriend (that would be Johannes) and we have a 3-year-old daughter (the lovely and amazing Julia Claire). But I would remind you that the boyfriend lives in Europe and, as I just mentioned, the daughter wasn't born till I was in my 40s. I've looked at life from both sides now, but with Johannes off raising his son in Zurich eight months of the year, I continue to live with one foot planted firmly in the land of the single woman. And I'm here to tell you that it's hard out here for me and a whole lot of other bachelor girls in their 30s and 40s.

I'm not entirely sure why I never married. I've been accused of being too picky, too career oriented, too selfish, too difficult. If too picky means that I happen to be partial to men who chew with their mouths closed, then by all means, color me picky. As for the rest, frankly I've always found myself to be utterly delightful (or at least no more ambitious, selfish, difficult than any of my married friends). Still, in the interest of fairness, I invite those with opposing viewpoints to go ahead and vent away in *their* columns.

So what did happen? Is it possible that, like the dizzy comic-strip women in those Roy Lichtenstein paintings, I simply got too caught up in the little psychodramas of everyday living? Here's a thought: Maybe I was so busy dealing with all my family's and friends' weddings that I didn't have time for one of my own. I checked registries and bought the silver seafood forks, the ice cream makers, the Tiffany corncob holders, the lacy black camisoles for three dozen bridal showers where I drank Prosecco and made nice to the groom's aunt from St. Paul. I walked down the aisle in satin pumps dyed Kit Kat–bar brown to match the strapless taffeta dresses I was assured I'd wear again and again. I sat through the toasts to couplehood, the questions about when it would be my turn, the casual mention that "it's perfectly okay to be gay...you know...if anybody happens to be." I smiled gamely as the band played "Someone to Watch over Me." I made a point of being in the ladies' room during the bouquet toss, I threw sachets of politically correct birdseed, and I went home and waited for the baby showers to begin.

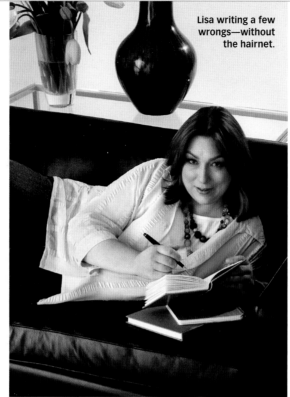

Lisa writing a few wrongs—without the hairnet.

Evidently, nothing leads to pregnancy faster than chowing down on a scoop of homemade ice cream and an ear of corn while dressed in a lacy camisole, because it wasn't long before I was buying the newlyweds a car seat, a crib set, a soft yellow squeaky thing that played "Twinkle, Twinkle, Little Star," and listening to brand-new mothers extolling the virtues of a good epidural. Legend has it that my friend Brenda found herself licking the anesthesiologist's fingers during the birth of baby number three, but I'll save that for my Valentine's Day column on unrelenting pain. Meanwhile, back at the Thanksgiving column, my list of cousins was growing. The holidays became about sippy cups and I became "the kid with the interesting job."

The only someone to watch over me was me, and everybody knew it. Conversational gambits at holiday dinners were confined to safe subjects guaranteed not to draw any attention to the fact that I'd never be on the receiving end of a silver seafood fork. Allow me to elaborate:

Uncle Sol: "Say, did you know that Dalmations tend to be hard of hearing?"

Me: "Umm, no."

Uncle Sol: "It's true."

Me: "Okay."

Uncle Sol: "So [*long pause*], how's your bicycle doing?"

Me: "Pretty good...yours?"

Uncle Sol: "Great."

Me: "Great."

They tried, I tried, we all tried, and the harder we tried, the more strained it got, until one day, I had a baby of my own, and suddenly my relationship with Johannes was deemed legitimate and motherhood took me from screwup to grown-up in the eyes of the people whose respect I craved most.

That was a few years and a million somebody elses ago. Jules is in preschool now—and (as we go to press) still single, though she has been seeing one Mr. Bennett Orenstein, who is not only potty trained but was recently awarded a medal for swimming with his face in the water.

I know that someday soon my girl will come home with a construction-paper Pilgrim hat and a pipe-cleaner turkey and they will become the centerpiece for our own Thanksgiving dinner, complete with our own traditions. We will invite all our friends who, thanks to divorces and long distances and family dynamics, find themselves free that night. We'll raise our glasses and drink to being who we want to be. And then we'll sit down to a large platter brimming with fettuccine Alfredo and all the trimmings. Once an odd duck, always an odd duck. ◖

90 Is Not the New 50

Young at heart will get you only so far. BARBARA GRAHAM reports.

It's a cold, stormy night in late November when I collect my mother at the hospital. Rain lashes sideways as I help her out of the car and up the walk toward my house. Once she's safely inside, I'll run back to grab the walker and the supplies I was given as we were leaving. But for now all I can think about is getting her inside without incident. Without another fall. She is 90 and rocky on her feet. A few days earlier she blacked out; I found her on the floor of the guest room coming to, her head in a pool of blood. After the paramedics whisked her away, she was admitted to the hospital with a bleed in her brain, a subarachnoid cerebral hemorrhage. According to the attending neurosurgeon, it was a "subtle" bleed. She can spell *world* backward and aces the rest of the cognitive tests. She is pronounced "lucky."

But she doesn't feel lucky. As I struggle to unlock the front door while keeping a firm grip on her and the umbrella, she chides herself for her unsteady gait. "I'm so clumsy," she says with despair.

"You're not clumsy," I say. "You're old."

The words just come out, unpremeditated. My mother is startled, and so am I. She looks at me as though I have accused her of committing an unspeakable crime—and in a way, I suppose I have. But then we both laugh. It's true: She *is* old. The colossal elephant in the room has finally been named.

Years ago she made me swear that I would keep her birth date out of her obituary. This was when she still believed that aging meant nothing more unpleasant than moving to Florida and having fewer opportunities to show off her mink coat. It didn't occur to her or my father that someday one of them would likely wind up alone, in deteriorating health, a thousand miles from their children and grandchildren. Life seemed to stretch out before them—an endless round of golf games and cocktail parties, spiced up by the occasional cruise. She often joked that she would live forever because she was "too mean to die."

We have not had an easy time of it, Irene and I—no cozy mother-daughter camaraderie, no affectionate natural bond.

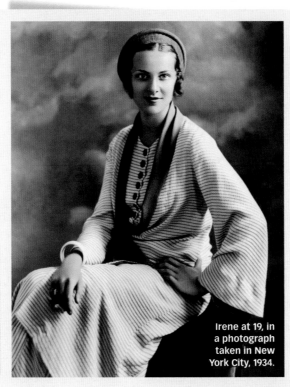

Irene at 19, in a photograph taken in New York City, 1934.

Growing up, I often felt as though we were mismatched, like two landmasses that don't fit together—say, Greenland and New Jersey. I always imagined that she would have been happier with a daughter more like her: glamorous, stylish, a celebrated hostess and arbiter of good taste. She is, among intimates, a famously harsh judge of other people's looks. During my high school years, she asked almost daily if I was sure I didn't want a nose job. I rejected the whole package and shacked up with a stoned cowboy, living in hippie outposts from Boulder to British Columbia. Whenever we settled in one place long enough to have a phone, I kept the number unlisted so she couldn't call. But now, as her only daughter, I am also her designated caretaker. She is old, and death is no longer just a nasty rumor.

"Spell *world* backward." This challenge has been posed at least two dozen times: by residents, interns, and medical students in the hospital; by the visiting nurse who came to assess whether Irene needs home healthcare (she does); by the physical therapist and the guy who rigged up the medical alert button she now wears around her neck. I can tell by her crumpled expression as she conceals the device beneath her sweater that she is shamed by the accessory. She'd prefer a little something from Tiffany—and who wouldn't?

Before her ill-fated trip to visit my husband and me in Washington, D.C., Irene was self-sufficient. She had survived the loss of my father—her husband of 63 years—as well as the passing of a gentleman caller. She lived alone in her Florida condo and refused to consider the possibility of moving to a retirement home closer to me.

"I manage," she'd insist, holding up her hand like a school crossing guard to halt me whenever I broached the matter. "I get along." And so she did. She drove, went to movies and dinner with friends, kept her regular appointment at the beauty parlor, and did her own grocery shopping and cooking. All this despite the fact that she'd fallen a few times and often leaned against walls and furniture to keep herself from tipping over. Never mind that a broken hip could spell disaster for her as it had for her mother; when I suggested a cane or walker, she'd shrug and say, "I'm too vain."

At 90 this former belle of Pittsburgh was still trading on her girlish good looks. Even with no makeup, even with a black eye and nine stitches in her left temple, she looked like a wilted beauty queen. She flirted with the doctors and was the talk of the hospital. Without exception, everyone who examined her (and asked her to spell *world* backward) did a double take upon finding out how old she was.

I may have shied away from using the word *old,* but for years I had poked fun at Irene for refusing to admit her age. "You're an elder," I'd point out. "It's nothing to be ashamed of. Just think of how revered you'd be in Native American cultures."

"So you think I should move to a tepee?" she'd snap.

Yet it wasn't just vanity that made her feel the way she did. Ours is arguably the most unforgiving country on earth in which to age. One glance at the titles on the best-seller list or the headlines in magazines says it all: SIXTY IS THE NEW 30; GROW YOUNGER, LIVE LONGER; STOP AGING NOW! Sooner or later, some "expert" is bound to declare that "80 Is the New Pink." As a society, we're engaged in a massive cover-up; age is treated like a preventable disease and death its avoidable outcome.

In her book, *The Denial of Aging,* Harvard professor Muriel Gillick, MD, writes, "Denial is sometimes a good thing; it can help us cope with intolerable truths. In the case of aging, however, widespread belief in perpetual youth or eternal life has pernicious consequences." In our desperate pretense that aging can be eradicated by modern medicine, positive thinking, diet, exercise, vitamins, or crossword puzzles—all of which can influence our quality of life, none of which can stave off our inevitable decline—we set ourselves up to spend our final years feeling defective, weak, and guilty for having failed. But the real failure is our refusal to accept that we're mortal—human—with all the joy, pain, hope, and loss that condition brings.

"Spell *world* backward." Though she now rolls her eyes whenever a well-meaning member of the helping professions issues the request, Irene's own world has shrunk precipitously. Since our return to Florida a few weeks after her fall, she has not cooked a meal or left her apartment alone. Some of the people in her circle still call, others drop by, others send food but can't seem to find time to visit, and a few stay away completely. One woman, a neighbor and former close friend, breezes past my mother in the lobby of their condominium as if she weren't even there. No doubt the woman worries that my mother's affliction—old age unmasked—might be contagious. Almost overnight, Irene has become a stark reminder of what lies in store for her more robust friends. Perhaps they cling

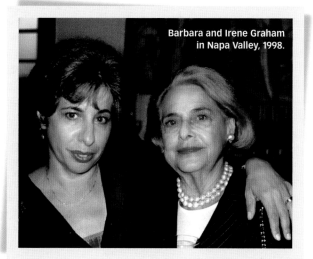

Barbara and Irene Graham in Napa Valley, 1998.

to the magical belief that if they look away they'll be spared. I can imagine this because I'm frightened for myself, too.

Still, I try to remain upbeat as I prepare to say goodbye. Now that she's set up with a health aide and a spiffy new walker, I'm flying home to Washington.

"Here's everything," I say, handing her a sheet of paper with a list of important names and numbers.

"You're so good," Irene says in a shaky voice.

"You're good, too." I take her bony hands in mine. This may be the first adult exchange we've ever had without a hint of defensiveness (me), criticism (her), disappointment at our failed connection (both of us).

"I'm no good," she protests, weeping. I know she is referring to her bruised, vulnerable body, the indignity of needing help, the loss of autonomy and control. I wish I could kiss away my mother's shame over the truth of her life the same way I healed my son's scraped knees and elbows with a kiss when he was small. But it is her grief, her life, her choice to embrace or reject it, with all its startling limitations.

In *The Journey of Life: A Cultural History of Aging in America,* gerontologist Thomas Cole, PhD, writes that aging, "like illness and death, reveals the most fundamental conflict of the human condition: the tension between infinite ambition, dreams, and desires on the one hand, and vulnerable, limited decaying physical existence on the other." My mother is right in the eye of the storm. The day after I get back to Washington, I ask her on the phone if she's had the grab bars installed in her shower as she promised. "Don't bother me," she hisses. But the next day she admits that even though Lupe, her aide, can't cook to save her life ("Tell me, how can someone ruin a baked potato?"), she couldn't manage without her. And not long ago, I was heartened to hear Irene working out the logistics of getting to and from the ballet so that she could still thrill to the spectacle of dancers soaring, no matter that she can barely walk. Bit by bit, she is putting up less of an argument with reality and adjusting to the new normal.

I like to think that the adjustment is made less bitter by the fact that despite her mounting losses, there has been an unexpected gain: the change in our once-turbulent relationship. I have heard of this happening between mothers and daughters—a mutual mellowing, a rapprochement—but my relationship with Irene was always so fractious, I never dreamed that intimacy and tenderness could be ours.

"I don't know what I'd do without you," she says now almost daily. "And I don't know what I'd do without you," I reply, amazed that I mean it. No matter how you spell it, the world we share is touched by grace. **Ⓞ**

Please Daddy, No

We lock up adults who molest children—but what if the molester is the child's parent? All too often, an outrageous quirk of the law known as the incest loophole metes out only a slap on the wrist and sends the father (or mother) home to abuse again. Shocked? So were we. JAN GOODWIN reports.

Six-year-old Melissa Hammer dreaded getting home from elementary school. Her mother was at work, but her stepfather, who'd adopted her, would be waiting at their Oceanside, California, home, his shift as a Marine Corps communications specialist having finished early. She'd shudder as his hulking 200-pound, six-feet-one-inch frame appeared in his bedroom door. "I don't feel good; come and make me feel better," he'd say to the child as he grabbed for her, his pants off or unzipped. Then, forcing her head down, he'd make her perform oral sex on him. "Don't tell anyone," he'd insist. "If you do, you'll be in trouble. This is our secret."

And for more than a year, it was. Melissa was particularly afraid to say anything to her mother, who was pregnant and then gave birth to her younger sister, Kristina. Finally, though, she did tell her best friend's mother, who contacted the police. Melissa was taken out of school, interviewed, and fortunate enough to be believed. Jeffrey Hammer was arrested and pleaded no contest, at which point he was removed from the home.

But he did not go to jail. Instead the judge gave him probation and required the whole family to undergo therapy with Parents United International, a treatment program with more than 20 chapters across the United States that emphasizes rejoining offenders with their spouses and children.

It wasn't long before the counselor was asking Melissa, "Don't you want to be back with your dad? He was sick; now he's better. He didn't mean to do what he did. He loves you. He won't do it again." Although she resisted at first, she says, they kept pushing until she gave in. Melissa was 8 when her stepfather moved back home. No one said one word about the abuse—it was as if nothing had ever happened. But soon enough, he was grabbing at her and making her sit on his lap, his erect penis escaping from his thin shorts, which he wore without underwear. Melissa started living defensively, trying to stay out of the house as much as she could, refusing to take a shower unless her mother was home because the bathroom lock could be easily opened from the outside. There was a reprieve when her parents got divorced. But it lasted only six years; they reconciled when Melissa was in high school, and her stepfather started putting the moves on her

again, nibbling on her ear, propositioning her for sex.

Then one day, the abuse stopped. Melissa had no idea why. It was only later that she discovered the reason: At 17 she was now too old to interest him. Jeffrey Hammer had turned his lusty attention to 10-year-old Kristina.

The thought of a little girl's being sexually assaulted by her parent—an adult charged with loving her and keeping her safe— is difficult to take. But when a child reports the crime, only to be forced to continue living with her molester, that is an unconscionable breach of justice. And yet in most states, the law allows that to happen.

All across the country, legal loopholes let convicted incest offenders go home and crawl back into bed with their traumatized daughters and sons. Even in states where that's not the case, weak links in the judicial system often leave a child in the groping hands of the molesting parent. "In our culture, if you grow your own victim, you are legally protected," says Linda Davis, a licensed clinical social worker and the executive director of Survivors of Incest Anonymous (an international support organization). "If a stranger rapes a child it's, 'Call the police, jail him, and throw away the key.' But if that same man rapes his daughter, it's, 'Call the therapist, slap him on the wrist, let him go back and do it again.' "

In Huntington, West Virginia, for example, Jeffrey Scott Grass was charged with sexually abusing his daughter, Charla, but he pleaded down to a lesser charge and received only five years probation. Today, the probation completed, he is living in Georgia and has applied for lengthy, unsupervised visits with Charla, now 12. Patricia Ash, his ex-wife and the girl's mother, is outraged and afraid he might get them.

In Madras, Oregon, Vesta Johnson watched in frustration in 1993 as her husband, John Hudson, received only 90 days in jail and probation for attempting to sexually abuse her daughter. Then he failed to comply with the sex offenders program he was ordered to attend. "He boasted that he would pretend to be crazy so he wouldn't have to go to jail or pay child support, which is exactly what he did," says Vesta. Now divorced, she was horrified when she applied for John's court records in connection with this article and learned that he'd admitted to sexual offenses against

> "Incest offenders are just lazy pedophiles who don't have to go outside the home to find children to sexually abuse."

23 victims when he was in treatment. "I'm shocked," says Vesta, who is currently completing a master's in business and plans to go to law school, with hopes of using both degrees to help sex abuse victims. "I thought my daughter was the only one. I had no idea of the extent of his problem."

Jackie Lawrence, a 30-year-old divinity student in St. Louis, was 12 when her father was charged with sexually abusing her and got off with probation. During the court-ordered counseling that followed, she remembers being made to apologize to him for breaking up the family. "This was a man who for three years used to order me to strip naked and get into his bed on Sunday mornings. When he was finished with me, he'd tell me to get dressed for church," says Jackie. "With the charge against him, he did have to move out of our house. But he moved in with my grandparents two doors down the street and stayed there until the state realized a child molester was living with the foster children my grandparents took care of. Three years later, after he was charged with molesting his adopted sister, his probation was revoked and he went to prison. It was supposed to be for five years, but he served only half that because, we were told, the prisons are full and his crime wasn't violent in the eyes of the law."

Melissa Hammer's testimony before the Senate Public Safety Committee in 2005 was instrumental in closing the incest loophole in California. Enacted in 1981, the exemption had allowed judges to grant offenders probation instead of jail time and typically made child victims participate in the parent's attempted rehabilitation. Now many believe it injured thousands of children. Yet nearly three-quarters of states have similar laws on their books today. (The states that do not, along with California, are Arizona, Arkansas, Colorado, Connecticut, Illinois, Kansas, Maryland, Michigan, Mississippi, Montana, New Hampshire, New York, and Rhode Island.) In Utah, for example, prison sentences for the rape of a child, sodomy of a child, or rape of a child with an object can, under certain conditions, be suspended if the perpetrator is "a parent, stepparent, adoptive parent, or legal guardian of the child victim." Minnesota has an "intentional family preservation policy" along the same lines as the one amended in California. Hawaii's expedited sentencing program allows criminals who have committed felony sexual assault on children who are related by blood or "reside in the same dwelling unit" to avoid prison. In fact, Hawaiian law actually requires police officers to confer with prosecutors and then give suspects who are deemed eligible written notice that they may be exempt from ordinary prison sentences and should contact a lawyer immediately.

These laws were originally considered progressive in their efforts to protect the family unit and approach incest as a mental health issue that should be treated rather than punished. "The thinking in the eighties, advanced by Child Protective Services, was that removal of the perpetrator, most often male, meant removing the breadwinner from the home, so jailing him would be devastating to the family income," says Polly Poskin, executive director of the Illinois Coalition against Sexual Assault, a statewide network of 34 community crisis centers. "It was also felt that children shouldn't be made to testify against a parent." But Poskin and many other experts now argue that these principles are outdated and dangerously flawed, with grave consequences to the youngest Americans. "The long-standing practice of treating incest as an 'offense against the family' and not a serious offense against the person allows child sex abuse to be minimized and prosecuted lightly, if at all," says Grier Weeks, executive director of the National Association to Protect Children, a registered lobby dedicated to overturning these laws.

What's most contested about the exemption laws is the assumption that adults who molest their children can be rehabilitated. Many experts don't believe treatment typically works. After witnessing what happened to offenders under the Illinois incest exemption law, Poskin—who actually helped write it in 1983—pushed to overturn the same law in 2003. "We didn't see a reduction in recidivism," she says. "In those 20 years, a lot of children were probably harmed. We now know that if an offender is put back into the home, it is highly likely he will offend again." A 12-year study conducted by the Washington State Department of Corrections showed that about one in five sex offenders who avoided jail under that state's exemption law had their suspended sentences revoked: The primary reason was "willful violation," which included committing new offenses, possessing pornography, violating "no contact" orders, being caught luring children, or engaging in unauthorized relationships. Nevertheless, that law, Washington's Special Sex Offender Sentencing Alternative, remains in place.

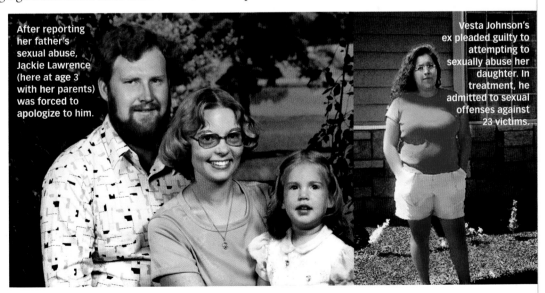

After reporting her father's sexual abuse, Jackie Lawrence (here at age 3 with her parents) was forced to apologize to him.

Vesta Johnson's ex pleaded guilty to attempting to sexually abuse her daughter. In treatment, he admitted to sexual offenses against 23 victims.

Deborah Johnson, PhD, a clinical psychologist who heads Parents United International, the program that failed the Hammers despite its claim of a less than 1 percent reported reoffense rate, voices the philosophy of many in the treatment and social services fields. "Incest is the most treatable offense on the books," she says. "Most incest offenders are not pedophiles. Fixated offenders are predatory toward children, but these [pedophiles] are in the minority. The majority of incest cases are what we call regressed offenders, people who, for example, under stress, turn to kids. When you've had a crappy day at work and your boss yelled at you, and your little 5-year-old pats you on the cheek and says how much she loves you, if you have really bad esteem—and if your boundaries are poor and you confuse sex with affection—it's not a huge leap to incest."

Her point, she continues, is that "incest is not an act of sex; it's about power and control. You can't tell me you have good sex with a 3-year-old." Many leading child abuse experts, however, call this logic tragically misguided. "It's time people realized that incest offenders are just lazy pedophiles who don't have to go outside the home to find children to sexually abuse," says Peg Snyder, a clinical and forensic psychologist who served on the Indiana governor's Child Protection Task Force.

One of the country's most respected authorities on child sexual abuse, Bruce Perry, MD, PhD, senior fellow at the nonprofit ChildTrauma Academy in Houston, agrees. People who molest their own children, he says, "do it because it's a sexual preference. You could put me in therapy every day for the next 20 years and I'd still want to have sex with women. When you place incest offenders back in the home with their children, they'll just be a lot more careful about being caught the next time. The kids, too, then often become compliant. They tried reporting it, and it didn't work. Now, for their own safety, they are likely to be much less resistant and much less likely to disclose a reoffense."

Leona Mae Page, 35, knows exactly what he means. She was stunned, then heartsick, when a detective contacted her five years ago and asked her to testify in an incest case against her father. "All I could think was, *Oh, no, not again, not again,*" recalls Leona, who lives in Connecticut. She was 3, she says, when her father, DeWitt Page, began sexual abuse that lasted nearly ten years. DeWitt never went to jail: The only restriction put on him when the incest was disclosed during his divorce from Leona's mother was that visits be supervised for a few years. Once that stopped, he went back to molesting her. And now the 60-year-old computer programmer was being charged with sexually abusing two other child relatives—a 3-year-old girl and 5-year-old boy.

Once again, the case never went to trial. The parents and prosecutors decided that it was not in the best interests of DeWitt's latest young targets to have them testify. A video of the 3-year-old girl describing to a female police officer in detail being digitally penetrated was not admissible because the defense lawyer wouldn't be able to cross-examine a tape. "It's always been about protecting his rights, never the rights of his victims," says Leona. Consequently, her father ended up receiving a one-year suspended sentence on reduced charges, plus three years probation, and had to register as a sex offender.

A month after that verdict, photographs of naked children were found on his computer. He pleaded guilty to violating probation. Yet despite the prior one-year suspended sentence, he got only three months of time. "He finally went to jail, but for having something inappropriate on his computer, not for the real abuse of children in his life. And even then, only for 90 days," says Leona angrily. "It doesn't make sense. You see stickers on gas pumps that warn you'll get three months imprisonment if you don't pay for the gas." Yet, while a petty thief gets locked up, she points out, a repeat sexual abuser of young, vulnerable victims goes unpunished. "It's criminal that the system has allowed my father continual access to children. Although he's a registered sex offender, he is walking around free. But the harm my father did to us will be with us forever."

Leona, who has been through ten years of therapy trying to recover from the impact—bulimia, problems with jobs and body image—is still haunted by the time when she was 13 and her mother was hospitalized. "My father applied for temporary custody, and it was given to him. When I was called to the school office and told he was coming to fetch me, I vomited out of terror." Leona got on the phone to her mother's lawyer, who intervened,

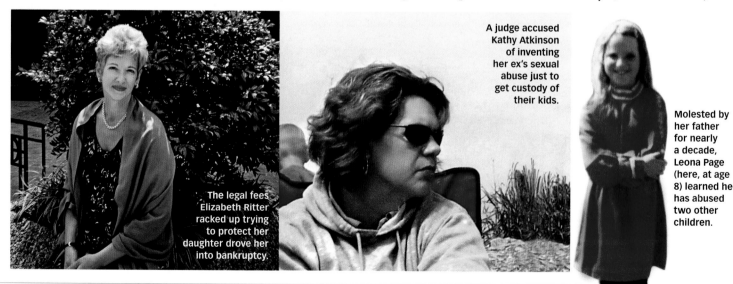

The legal fees Elizabeth Ritter racked up trying to protect her daughter drove her into bankruptcy.

A judge accused Kathy Atkinson of inventing her ex's sexual abuse just to get custody of their kids.

Molested by her father for nearly a decade, Leona Page (here, at age 8) learned he has abused two other children.

and she was able to stay with the parents of a friend. "The experts say that pedophiles continue to offend," says Leona. "I believe that, right now, men like my father are either offending, thinking about doing it, or lying about having done it."

Even in the states that do not have exclusion laws, incest offenders rarely do jail time: Only 4 percent of cases reported go before a jury; the vast majority are plea bargained, resulting in probation, suspended sentencing, or short sentences, according to lobbyist Grier Weeks. Poskin considers the legal system's indifference a gender issue. (According to the latest statistics, more than 94 percent of sexual assaults on children 17 and younger are committed by men.) "Primarily, it is men who commit incest, and primarily, it is men who make the decision to investigate, prosecute, and sentence," she says. "Women and girls are usually the victims."

Professional ignorance also victimizes children, says forensic psychologist Peg Snyder. She specializes in training therapists and law enforcement in Indiana on child sex offenders, although such education is not always required. "I rarely see judges take a training course," she says. "Yet all too often, it is judges who minimize incest. You'll hear them say, 'Well, there was no penetration; it was just a little touching, so it's no big deal.' The lack of understanding by those making decisions of the harm caused by incest to a child victim is appalling."

Prosecutors, too, often display a remarkable myopia about the issue, even when the evidence is clear. Snyder cites a case in which an ER physician confirmed that a 3-year-old boy's anus had been stretched way beyond what was normal. "The prosecutor admitted that he believed the father had abused the child and his 2-year-old sister but didn't think the children were in danger any longer," says Snyder. "His 'logic' was based on the fact that because the father had been warned, he would be careful not to continue the sexual abuse. Unfortunately, the father did continue abusing the children, and five years later, the boy is a stammering, fearful, and depressed child, and his sister is catatonic and mute, dissociating as a way to cope."

It wasn't until 1974, Snyder points out, that the government passed the first child sexual abuse law, the federal Child Abuse Prevention and Treatment Act. As late as the 1980s, the notion that children were the aggressors in incest was still popular, and that perpetrators, generally of low intelligence, were unable to resist. Even today, adds Snyder, "offenders often say they were seduced by the child and the sex was consensual, so it must have been the child's fault."

Nothing could be further from the truth, according to child abuse expert Bruce Perry. "And to make children live with their molesters is devastating," he says. "It is tremendously difficult for children to disclose incest in the first place, because they know it will cause significant pain to the family, and they are likely to be ostracized by family members. Then, when the system treats the abuse as a minor traffic violation, it is a secondary betrayal by those in positions of power and authority. Yet we know that incest is more intrusive, more emotionally violent and destructive than a sexual assault from a stranger."

A major obstacle for parents trying to rescue a daughter or son from incest can be the guardian ad litem (a Latin term meaning "for the lawsuit"), known as a GAL. Judges appoint GALs, often attorneys, to look after a child's best interests. Their actions supersede the rights of the parents, who must pick up the tab for their services, and the courts give considerable weight to their reports.

Donald Lerch was devastated after a GAL recommended, and a judge agreed in 2001, that his 5-year-old son continue living with his ex-wife, Paula, who was about to marry Larry Phillip Slack, a convicted child sex offender. Larry never told Paula about his criminal history, but "after she began dating him, she asked me, for the heck of it, to run a background check on him," says Donald, a federal police officer from Warfordsburg, Pennsylvania, just across the border from Larry Slack's Maryland home. "I found he'd been charged in 1993 on two counts of child sexual abuse. At first we both thought maybe I'd typed in the wrong name. After all, this guy was active in the church and seemed very nice. But I double-checked, and sure enough, it was the same man. I was very concerned, and Paula was also. Later that night, though, she called to tell me Slack had explained that he'd babysat a neighbor's son on several occasions and this young man came forward and made some false allegations. He said that to avoid the embarrassment of a trial, he pleaded guilty just to make it go away."

Still suspicious, Donald went to the courthouse to look at the records and learned that Larry had been indicted on one count of child abuse and one count of third-degree sexual offense, but was able to plead down to only one count of child abuse, for which he received a suspended sentence of 15 years and five years supervised probation. In psychological evaluations made at the time, Larry admitted he was a victim of incest when he was 8 and remained sexually fixated on young boys. Aware of his attraction to males, he was careful to always have a girlfriend. He claimed he had abused only three victims over six years. One year after his probation ended, he began to date Paula, who had physical custody of her and Donald's then 5-year-old son.

All this information was made available to Patricia Patton, the GAL. In her report, she characterized Larry Slack as a pedophile "in remission" and noted one expert's concern that he didn't tell his church he was a convicted sex abuse offender when he volunteered for their children's program, which exposed him to a "population of potential victims." Still she recommended that the boy stay in his mother's home. Quoting from another expert's psychological evaluation, she wrote in the report that Slack knew he would be sentenced to 30 years if he reoffended, and he was

> "I believe that men like my father are either offending, thinking about doing it, or lying about having done it."

a member of a "conservative, Christian religious [community] that would likely ostracize him completely were he to resume...criminal sexual behavior." In light of these and other factors, the court decided Larry Slack was not a high risk. Patton did request that an existing restraining order remain in place so he would never be alone with the boy, although one might wonder how that would be possible considering the two were about to begin living together full-time.

In an impassioned 11-page letter, Donald wrote to Judge Frederick Wright III of Hagerstown, Maryland, after the decision: "You gave Mr. Slack the benefit of the doubt. But what about my son? Doesn't he deserve the same consideration? What if you are wrong? What could you do for my child? Say you were sorry? It would not change his experience. It would not give him back his childhood innocence."

In 2006, Larry Slack was charged with 28 counts involving Paula and Donald's son and the child's playmate, a neighboring boy. He pleaded guilty to two of the counts concerning Donald's son, which reportedly included oral sex and anal sodomy, acts that began a month after Slack's marriage to Paula, when the judge had set the restraining order to expire.

Judge Wright has refused to comment on the case, as has Paula. But Patricia Patton, the GAL, agreed to explain her actions. "I have advocated that sex offenders with a similar history to this case be placed with children," she said. "In my experience, a record of a single sex abuse event in seven years is not by any means on the serious end of the scale." Patton added: "At the time, Slack was a sex offender. But he had no history of committing incest." Experts note, however, that child sex offenders often woo vulnerable women to get access to their children.

When asked how a restraining order could be effective if the man and child are living in the same house, Patton replied, "Either the mom would be supervising at all times, or there would have to be a rotation of family members, or you have to get motion sensors"—although it's hard to imagine motion sensors detecting an adult sexually abusing a child. While this is uncommon in cases of child abuse, she says, "It is certainly not unheard of."

Norris West, a spokesman for the Maryland Department of Social Services, for which Patton is a contractor, originally told *O* magazine, "We are not at liberty to discuss this case or the GAL.... Despite what a judge thinks is the best decision, some terrible things happen." Two days later, he was having second thoughts. Calling back, he added, "It is never appropriate, under any circumstances, for a child to be placed in the home of a convicted pedophile. It should not have happened, and we will do everything in our power to make sure it doesn't happen"—a promise that comes too late for Donald Lerch's son.

Elizabeth Ritter filed a malpractice suit against her child's GAL on behalf of her daughter. The Chevy Chase, Maryland, mother, who is an attorney, charged that because of his favoritism toward her ex-husband, the GAL blocked expert testimony from being presented in a case over visitation rights that sexual abuse may have occurred. This omission, she believes, resulted in significant harm to her now 11-year-old daughter. (Although the local Department of Health and Human Services found an indication of sexual abuse by her ex-husband in an earlier case, an administrative law judge and appellate court rejected the finding, citing no credible evidence.) "What's frightening is that these individuals can exhibit blatant biases and wield such extraordinary powers over the lives of our children," says Ritter, who got stuck paying for almost all the GAL's services because her ex had little income at the time (her case against the GAL is still pending). As a parent, she had no control over the GAL, "but his legal fees were about $30,000, plus at least another $20,000 in medical and psychological assessments and therapies the GAL initiated, including a mental health evaluation for my ex-husband for which I was billed. This was in addition to my own legal fees, which came to about $110,000. All of which drove me into bankruptcy."

When judges appoint GALs, it's often as payback for past political favors, says attorney and former prosecutor Randy Burton, founder of Justice for Children, a national organization that advocates for abused minors who have been failed by child protection services and the courts. "It's a classic case of cronyism. A judge appoints a child guardian he knows—his former finance manager, or former law partner—and in turn, the GAL follows the way a judge rules. They are not zealously unbiased or independent. They should be there for the interests of the child, but they frequently are not. When I was a prosecutor, I saw this happen all the time."

The American Bar Association feels that lawyers should not be GALs. "Attorneys should be representing the child, not acting as friends of the court," says Linda Rio Reichmann, former project director of the ABA's child custody and adoption pro bono project. To make matters worse, many states offer GALs partial or full immunity, which protects them legally from civil litigation.

"We've had multiple GALs, and they have been hell-bent on my daughter's visiting her father, a man I've subsequently discovered had a criminal record before I met him," says a frustrated mother in Ashtabula, Ohio. At this point, if her daughter, now 13, refuses to visit her father, the court has threatened to place her in foster care—a decision made even though his chosen psychologist was among the many experts, including Child Protective Services, who confirmed that he is likely to have molested her. "When she's been taken to meet with him, she hasn't gotten out of the car; she lost ten pounds, and her grades dropped," says her mother. "She's terrified of this man. It's been awful and heartbreaking living through this. And the financial burden is horrific. So far our legal fees have totaled $54,000, wiping out our savings and our children's college fund."

The judge stated that it was okay to discipline a child so hard you could leave marks on her.

Another roadblock women face in trying to protect their children is parental alienation syndrome (PAS), a defense trotted out regularly by offenders accusing the mother of inventing the incest charge to win a custody case. PAS is also used by judges as a way of dismissing these cases. "Parental alienation syndrome is a cancer on family court. It is a bogus, pro-pedophilic fraud concocted by Dr. Richard Gardner," says Richard Ducote, the last attorney to cross-examine Gardner in court before he committed suicide in 2003. Gardner, whose work seldom appeared in medical journals—it was mainly self-published—made no bones about his bias. "What I am against is the excessively moralistic and punitive reaction that many members of our society have toward pedophiles...," he wrote in his book *Sex Abuse Hysteria,* "going far beyond what I consider to be the gravity of the crime."

Ducote, the author of several child welfare laws, says PAS "has not been accepted by any reputable scientific organization considering it, including the American Psychological Association. Yet Gardner and his theory have done untold damage to sexually and physically abused children and their protective parents. I'm appalled at what I see going on every day in courts."

Kathy Atkinson, head of a day-care center in Shrewsbury, Pennsylvania, had the kind of degrading legal experience Ducote is talking about. Convinced her ex-husband was sexually abusing her daughter and physically abusing her son during visitations (he was never charged), she was lambasted repeatedly by Judge J. Norris Byrnes of the Circuit Court for Baltimore County, Maryland, who referred to her concerns as a case of PAS. As to the argument that the syndrome is junk science, he said, "Of course it is not, but it suits her to think that." When police testimony supported her accusations and the Department of Social Services requested a "no contact, stay away" order, Judge Byrnes denied the order, and disregarded the testimony of the social worker and detective.

"There ought to be an obsessive mother syndrome," Byrnes told the court. "There's no real physical evidence [of abuse]. So all of it comes out of the mouth of a 5-year-old.... I'm worried that Mrs. Atkinson is causing irreparable harm between those kids, her, and their father." During a meeting in his chambers he disagreed with Kathy, saying that it was okay to discipline a child so hard you could leave marks on her. She went on to file a complaint against Byrnes with the state commission on judicial disability. Citing insufficient evidence, they declined to sanction the judge. He retired shortly thereafter.

In most cases, it's the judicial system that allows incest to fester, but parents are often complicit. In Florida, Meredith Taylor (who asked us to change her name) chose to continue living with her husband after she learned that he was abusing her 13-year-old daughter. The girl had told a school friend, who reported the abuse to a guidance counselor; the police were brought in, and the girl was removed from her home. Meredith's husband, the child's stepfather, only had to go to counseling. "I thought of divorcing him. But this was my third husband, and I didn't want it to be one more failed marriage," says Meredith.

"It's no fun to be out on your own. I'm sure my daughter thinks of it as a betrayal. But I chose to be supportive of my husband.

"I learned that child sex offenders usually never quit and that other things happen. I wouldn't expect an adult woman to be forced to live with her rapist. But it's not as important for a child because she can recover from any situation faster than an adult, and because a child may think of it as loving and caring. Scientific evidence says incest destroys a child's life. But children may think of it as a way of showing love. My daughter didn't know her own dad. She needed love so bad. And he [the current husband] took advantage of it."

Today, that same man, still married to Meredith, babysits her grandchildren by her other kids and volunteers at their preschool. "For a long time, I was very concerned," she says. "I saw how his grandbabies captured his mind." Yet she leaves them in his care.

Whoever it is—GAL, judge, lawmaker, mother, "the people responsible for placing children back with their sex offenders are, at the very least, criminally negligent in any subsequent sexual abuse," says Randy Burton of Justice for Children. "The concept of family preservation in incest cases is completely bankrupt. All it does is create a circle of abuse. If we do not protect these kids and we keep reunifying them with their abusers, the results are plain. It is well documented that a significant number of prison inmates were abused as children." A 1996 report from the Department of Justice estimated that rape and sexual abuse of children costs the United States about $23 billion every year in medical and other expenses.

By the time Jeffrey Hammer finally stopped sexually abusing Melissa at age 17, the horror had started for her little sister, Kristina. One day Kristina came home from the beach with a sunburn, and he removed her shirt, rubbed lotion on her back and front, then twisted her nipples. After she caught head lice at school, he made her completely undress to shampoo her hair, exposed his penis, and told her to open her mouth. As he forced her head down, though, Kristina freaked out. Escaping from his hold, she ran from the bathroom. He warned her not to say anything because he would go to jail.

But she did. And when her brother told the police what was going on, the prior conviction regarding Melissa came up. On October 6, 2000, Jeffrey Hammer was found guilty. Eventually, he was sentenced to 105 years in jail. By then it was 16 years after Melissa's stepfather had first abused her, and 14 years after the system permitted him to continue doing so and to target her sister as well. "That man made my life a misery. Then he was sent back home to live with us and was able to abuse my little sister," says Melissa, now 25. "When my stepfather started abusing me again, I told Child Protective Services, who visited us once a month while my stepfather was on probation. Nothing happened. I felt so betrayed."

For a society that prides itself on its love for children, our handling of incest is a dangerous hypocrisy. A child molested by a stranger can run home for help and comfort. A child sexually abused by a parent cannot. And that tragedy will repeat itself again and again until we stop looking the other way. ◖

Friends

Oprah and Gayle, Uncensored

After 30 years of four-times-a-day phone calls, Oprah and Gayle sit down for a nice, long, startlingly honest chat—about their friendship, those tabloid rumors (who could forget that night in the Bahamas? Not the bellboy), what Oprah really thought at Gayle's wedding, and why they are still "more or less the same people." LISA KOGAN listens in.

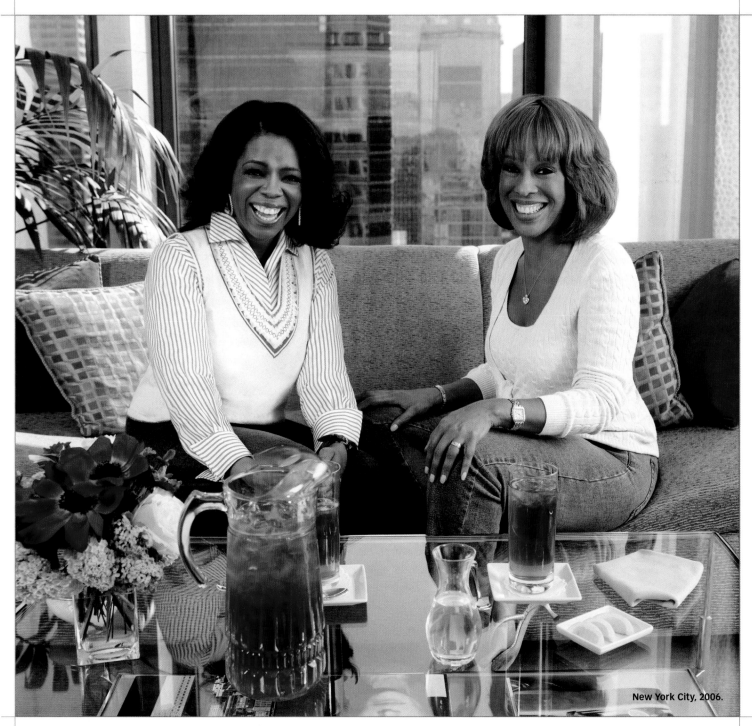

New York City, 2006.

When the photographer begins clicking away, Oprah Winfrey and her best friend, Gayle King, will be impeccably cooperative. They'll pose, they'll percolate, they'll shine. They've been shot before.

But for just a moment on a gorgeous day in New York City, these two women who've spent 30 years in constant conversation, who've stuck together through fame and fortune, kids and dogs, marriage and divorce, miniskirts and shoulder pads, are happy to be quiet together.

"What?" Oprah asks as Gayle plucks at a wisp of her pal's hair. "I miss the curls," Gayle answers. This is not news. "Gayle doesn't like my hair, but that's okay 'cause I do," Oprah tells me.

"So, that's allowed?" I venture. "It's fine to criticize each other's looks?"

"Sure," Gayle says. "I tried growing out my bangs a few months ago, and Oprah hated it."

"Yeah, that was bad," Oprah says, "but then I thought, *Hey, I don't have to sleep with her.* Now, if we were sleeping together, it'd be like [*in her best Barry White voice*], 'Baby, I want the bangs....'" And on that note, the interview begins.

So I get why people have to label it—how can you be this close without it being sexual? How else can you explain a level of intimacy where someone *always* loves you, *always* respects you, admires you?

GAYLE: Wants the best for you.

OPRAH: Wants the best for you in every single situation of your life. Lifts you up. Supports you. *Always!* That's an incredibly rare thing between even the closest of friends.

GAYLE: The truth is, if we were gay, we would so tell you, because there's nothing wrong with being gay.

OPRAH: Yeah. But for people to still be asking the question, when I've said it and said it and said it, that means they think I'm a liar. And that bothers me.

GAYLE: Well, particularly given how open you've been about everything else in your life.

OPRAH: I've told nearly everything there is to tell. All my stuff is out there. People think I'd be so ashamed of being gay that I wouldn't admit it? Oh, please.

LISA: *Do the rumors bother you, Gayle?*

GAYLE: Not anymore, but I used to say, "Oprah, you have to do

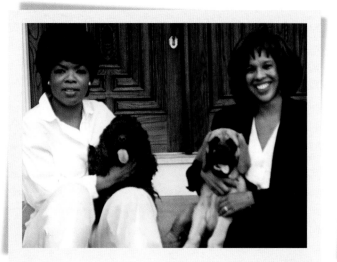

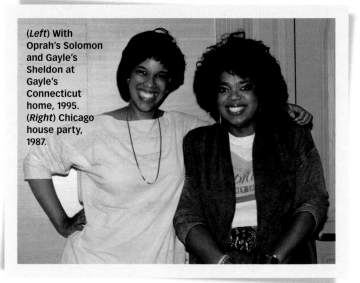

(*Left*) With Oprah's Solomon and Gayle's Sheldon at Gayle's Connecticut home, 1995. (*Right*) Chicago house party, 1987.

> "I've told nearly everything there is to tell. All my stuff is out there. People think I'd be so ashamed of being gay that I wouldn't admit it? Oh, please." — *Oprah*

LISA: *Well, let's get right to it! Every time I tell somebody, "I'm interviewing Oprah and Gayle," the response is always the same: "Oh. [Long pause] Are they...you know...together?"*

OPRAH: You're kidding. People are still saying that?

LISA: *Every single person. And I say, "No, I don't think so." And invariably, they respond with something like "You know, you're very naive."*

OPRAH: I understand why people think we're gay. There isn't a definition in our culture for this kind of bond between women.

something. It's hard enough for me to get a date on a Saturday night. You've got to go on the air and stop it!" And then you realize you really can't stop it. And, you know, somebody made a good point: "Well, every time we see you, you're together," which is true.

OPRAH: We were just down in the Bahamas—I was giving a wedding for my niece there. And we're having this big party in my suite. And who comes walking in—

GAYLE: With my suitcase.

OPRAH: With her suitcase! And I knew what all the waiters, what everybody was thinking: *They're gay. This proves it. Has to be, because Stedman isn't around.*

GAYLE: And sure enough, the tabloid headline was OPRAH'S HIDEAWAY WITH GAL PAL. Ridiculous. But that said, I have to admit, if Oprah were a man, I would marry her.

LISA: *Sorry, Gayle, I just don't buy it. Everyone knows Oprah's not tall enough for you.*

OPRAH: She has a point.

GAYLE: I do like 'em big.

OPRAH: The truth is, no matter where I am, whether Stedman is there or not, Gayle's in the other room. I mean, she's always coming in and asking, "Whatcha doin'?"

GAYLE: I really do marvel at this because if Stedman didn't accept me, it would be very difficult for us to be friends.

OPRAH: See, that would never be a question for me. If you don't like my best friend, then you don't like me. That's not negotiable. Smoking is nonnegotiable. It's just a deal breaker. Not liking my best friend—forget it! Or my dogs—you gots to go! [*Laughter*]

LISA: *Oprah, how did you feel when Gayle got married?*

OPRAH: Actually, I was a little sad. Did I ever tell you that? Mostly because I just didn't think it was going to work out.

GAYLE: You didn't? You never told me that.

OPRAH: No—it didn't feel joyful. You know how you go to weddings and they're full of joy?

GAYLE: Wait a minute! You didn't think it was going to work out *at the wedding?*

OPRAH: There are some weddings you go to and you're just filled with all this hope for the couple. And you feel that there's something special going on. I didn't feel that at yours.

GAYLE: But you were my maid of honor!

OPRAH: Yes, but it just felt kind of pitiful. I never told you because it wasn't my place to say that.

GAYLE: I wouldn't have believed you anyway.

OPRAH: No. And also because I felt like, well, maybe it's just me being jealous. Maybe I couldn't feel the joy because I was feeling like our friendship was going to change. But it didn't.

LISA: *What about when you had a baby, Gayle?*

GAYLE: Nothing really changed between us. Oprah was there. She came shortly after Kirby was born. She came shortly after Will was born. She was *there.*

OPRAH: I thought it would change just in terms of time. But my gift to her was a full-time nanny.

GAYLE: Right. The kids are 11 months apart, and Oprah goes, "I got you the perfect gift." And I'm thinking, *Oh, good. She's giving me a double stroller.* Back then double strollers were very expensive. But the gift turned out to be a nanny! She said, "I want to pay the nanny's salary for as long as you feel you need her."

OPRAH: She kept that nanny for like seven or eight years. But what I love is that even as a working-outside-the-home mom, she was always there to put her kids to bed. She said, "I want my face to be the first face my kids see when they wake up and the last thing they see at night." So it wasn't like the nanny came and—

GAYLE: Replaced me.

OPRAH: I admire a lot of things about Gayle. But when I think about the way she raised her kids, that makes me weepy.

GAYLE: Why weepy? That's so surprising to me.

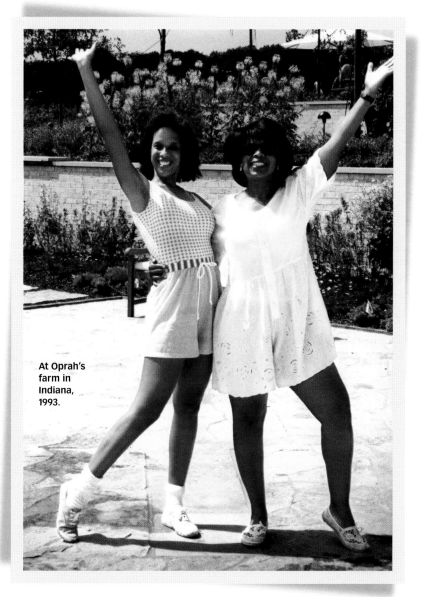

At Oprah's farm in Indiana, 1993.

OPRAH: Maybe I haven't said it to you very often, but I say it to other people all the time. Gayle is the best mother I have ever seen, heard, or read about. She was always 100 percent there for those kids—to this day. We'd be on the phone, in the middle of a conversation, and the kids would enter the room. This just happened last week, and her son's 19. She goes, "Hi, Willser. You got your Willser face on. Mommy loves you. Good morning, Bear. Hi, Kirby-Cakes." She stopped the conversation to greet them and let them know that they were seen and heard. And then she came back to the phone and carried on the conversation.

These kids have grown up with such love and support from Gayle, and also from Gayle's ex-husband.

I love the way she understood that though the marriage was not going to work, her husband still needed to have a space to maintain a strong relationship with these kids. That takes a *real* woman. It's always, always, always been about what's best for her children.

GAYLE: Years ago when Oprah was thinking of leaving the show, she said, "You should move to Chicago, and we'll incorporate you into the show. And then at the end of the year, I'll pass the baton on to you—but you'd have to move to Chicago." And I said, "I can't do that because Billy wouldn't be able to see the kids on a regular basis."

OPRAH: I said, "Do you realize what I'm offering?"

GAYLE: And I go, "Yeah, I do." But the kids were young, and I just said, "No, I can't do that."

OPRAH: That's why she's the best, and her kids are the best. Her kids are my godchildren. There are shots of me riding around on all fours with Kirby—you know, playing horsey and stuff. I remember when William first came to the farm: He was running around saying, "Auntie O, you have a pool *and* a wacuzzi? Can you afford all this?"

When he was little, little, little, I had all these antique Shaker boxes. He was stacking 'em like—

> "Nobody wants to be seen as an ATM machine."
> *—Oprah*

GAYLE: Blocks.

OPRAH: And knocking 'em over. I went, "William! Put those boxes down!" These kids weren't used to anybody raising their voice—they were never spanked or yelled at. So he was like, wacuzzi or no wacuzzi, I'm outta here. And he told his mommy, "I want to go home."

These kids made a lot of noise, and there were all kinds of bright yellow plastic things that made noise. And the TV was on and the same video was playing over and over and over. But Gayle helped me adjust.

GAYLE: I'm always kind of taken aback, Lisa, when Oprah talks about me and the kids, because I see a lot of mothers who feel about their children the way I feel about mine.

OPRAH: But they don't always have kids who turn out the way yours have. Everybody wants to raise good people, not just smart people at Ivy League schools and all that but good people. You have to be a good person to raise good people.

LISA: *Do you two talk every single day?*

GAYLE: We usually talk three or four times a day.

OPRAH: Then there's my night call. When she was on vacation with her sisters, and we hadn't had a conversation, I realized I felt far more stressed. I've never had a day's therapy, but I always had my night conversations with Gayle.

GAYLE: We talk about everything and anything.

OPRAH: What was on the show, what the person was wearing. What I really thought, what she really thought.

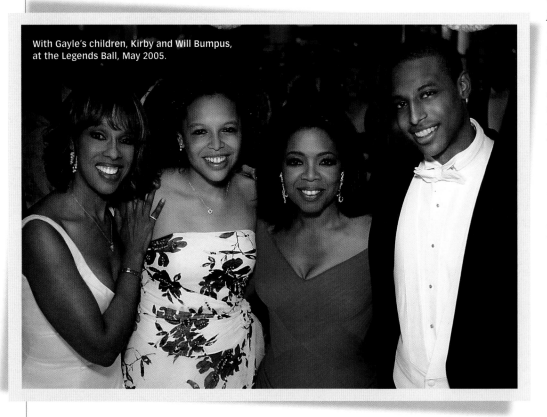

With Gayle's children, Kirby and Will Bumpus, at the Legends Ball, May 2005.

LISA: *Let me shift gears. It feels as if people are always trying to enlist my help in getting some kind of a letter to you, Oprah—and it's usually for a worthy cause. But I was thinking, Gayle, you must get that every hour of every day.*

GAYLE: Well, I know what Oprah would be interested in hearing and what she wouldn't, and, you know, I've figured out a way to politely decline. But I love that people love her so much and are so interested in communicating with her, so I never look at it as a hassle or burden.

OPRAH: She handles it. It's one of the things that's so amazing about this friendship. Gayle is more excited about my success than I am. It makes her genuinely happy. We've been friends since I was making $22,000 and she was making $12,000. We've made this journey together.

GAYLE: Not much has changed, except now she's making a stratospheric salary. [*Laughter*]

OPRAH: The first time Gayle spent the night at my house was because there was a snowstorm and she couldn't get home. She was a production assistant, and I was the 6 o'clock anchor in Baltimore.

GAYLE: Anchors and PAs do not socialize—the newsroom hierarchy.

OPRAH: But I said, "You can stay at my house." The next day, we went to the mall.

GAYLE: Remember Casual Corner? They had those two for $19.99 sales.

OPRAH: I ended up buying *two* sweaters.

GAYLE: I had to call my mother and say, "You know my friend Oprah? Guess what? She bought two sweaters!" I was into layaway back then, for one sweater. [*Laughter*]

OPRAH: Years later, for my 42nd birthday, we were in Miami, and I decided I was going to buy myself a birthday present. So we were on our way to the mall, and we pass a car dealership where I spot a black Bentley in the lot. I'm like, "Oh my God, that is the most beautiful car." So we pull over and I go in and buy that Bentley right on the spot. And I say to Gayle, "This is a Casual Corner moment."

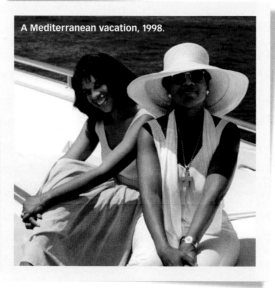

A Mediterranean vacation, 1998.

They get it all cleaned up, and it's a convertible. The top is down, and guess what? It starts to rain. It's pouring.

GAYLE: And I say, "Shouldn't we put the top up?"

OPRAH: "No. Because I want to ride in a convertible on my birthday!" Anyway, Gayle was like, "You're going to buy that right now? Shouldn't you think about this or try to negotiate a better deal?" I said, "Gayle, that's the same thing you said when I bought the two sweaters."

LISA: *What's that Paul Simon lyric? "After changes upon changes, we are more or less the same."*

OPRAH: The scale got larger. I mean, you need a moment of silence every time I write a check for my income taxes.

GAYLE: I can't even wrap my head around all this. I knew she was talented, certainly, but who would've thought that it would get this big?

OPRAH: One of my favorite moments was about ten, 12 years ago when we were in Racine, Wisconsin. We're caught in a traffic jam because everyone was headed to the concert hall where I was speaking, and Gayle says, "Where are all these people going?" We pull up to the venue, and Gayle goes, "What's going on here?"

GAYLE: The cops were lined up, double rows.

OPRAH: Gayle's going, "Who's here? Who's here?" I go, "I am, you nitwit!"

GAYLE: "You mean all these people are coming to see you?" I could not believe it. That was the first time it hit me.

LISA: *Gayle, when you started at the magazine, did either of you worry that working for Oprah might change the dynamic between you?*

GAYLE: I wasn't worried. I don't think Oprah was, either. But people did say, "Oh God, you should *never* work with your friend."

OPRAH: But that's how I know people don't understand this relationship, because other people's definition of "friend" isn't what ours is. Just the other day, I was doing a show about when your best friend is sleeping with your husband. The ultimate betrayal. Well, that is not possible in this relationship.

GAYLE: What I know for sure: I will never sleep with Stedman.

OPRAH: What did you used to say, "If you ever find me in the bed with Stedman—"

GAYLE: "Don't even be mad. Just scoop me up and get me to a hospital, because you will know I'm very ill."

OPRAH: "Carry me tenderly out the door." [*Laughter*]

GAYLE: So people ask, "But how can you work for a friend?" I say it's because I know that the magazine is called *O*. The bottom line is somebody has to have the final word. Oprah's not right all the time, but her record is pretty damn good. That's not to say you can't disagree.

OPRAH: That's why Gayle's so great for me at the magazine—she's going to have almost exactly the same opinion that I do. But when she doesn't agree, she'll fight for her opinion as though there were a *G* on that magazine. We have "disagree," and we have "strongly disagree." If Gayle strongly, strongly feels something about somebody—

GAYLE: It gives her pause.

OPRAH: It gives me pause, because she's been my—she's apple pie and Chevrolet. She loves everybody. So if there's somebody she doesn't like, that will get my attention because she's truly everybody's friend—far friendlier than I am. I would not call myself a friendly person.

GAYLE: I'm very social.

OPRAH: I'm not social. Nor am I all that friendly.

GAYLE: All Oprah needs is a good book. My only request when she's building any house is, "Could I please have a TV in my bedroom?" She goes, "You're the only one who complains about not having a TV in the bedroom." I go, "Well, everybody thinks it, they just don't want to say it to you."

OPRAH: I don't have TVs in any bedroom except Gayle's. In my house, there's a Gayle wing.

GAYLE: I don't want to offend her, but I'm never afraid to be truthful with her.

LISA: *So I'm hearing about differences. What are the similarities?*

GAYLE: We became friends that first night because for the first time, I met somebody who I felt was like me. I'd never met anybody like that. Certainly not another black girl. I grew up in an all-white community. I remember getting embarrassed in fourth grade when a boy in my class named Wayne said, "If it weren't for Abraham Lincoln, you'd be my slave." I can remember that very clearly. Oprah and I had the same sensibilities. We liked the same kind of music. We thought smart—

OPRAH: Smart and articulate—

GAYLE: Was not a bad thing.

OPRAH: We were the only black girls in our schools, and I was the only black girl in my class who loved Neil Diamond. So when you're around black folks, and they say, "Who's your favorite singer—"

GAYLE: I liked Barry Manilow.

LISA: *Neil Diamond and Barry Manilow? You guys were made for each other.*

OPRAH: [*Laughter*] It's that whole being-the-odd-girl-out thing—we didn't fit in to everybody else's perception of what it's like to be a black girl.

GAYLE: But we still had a very strong sense of being black and were very proud of being black. So to meet another black girl like that was, wow! And we were the same age, we were both single, and we just immediately bonded.

OPRAH: But she was clearly upper middle class, and I was clearly from a very poor background. Gayle had a pool growing up!

GAYLE: I had a swimming pool, a maid. We grew up very, very well.

OPRAH: She had a maid. My mother was a maid. You know what I'm saying? I'd never met a black person with a maid. It was like, "Lord, really? At your house?"

GAYLE: So that's how we became friends that first night, and we've been friends ever since.

OPRAH: See, we were always together in the newsroom. I remember when they decided to fire me—

GAYLE: Not fire, demote.

OPRAH: They wanted to fire me, but they couldn't because of the contract. My $22,000 contract. [*Laughter*]

GAYLE: They had run a big campaign: "What is an Oprah?"

OPRAH: I'd been on the air, starting in September. By April they decided it wasn't working, because the anchorman—

GAYLE: Didn't like you.

OPRAH: But I didn't know it. I was so naive. The day they decided that they were going to take me off the 6 o'clock news, I said to Gayle—

GAYLE: I'm just typing away at my desk. She goes, "Get in the bathroom *now!*"

OPRAH: We'd always meet in the bathroom. We were, like, "Oh my God. Do you think Jerry Turner knows?" Of course, Jerry Turner was the main anchor who was kicking my ass out, but we didn't know that. Jerry was like, "Babe, I don't even know what happened, babe." You know, "Sorry, babe."

GAYLE: I was stunned.

OPRAH: It's like your life is over.

GAYLE: You were going to see your dad that next day.

"What I know for sure: I will never sleep with Stedman."
— *Gayle*

OPRAH: And that was the hardest thing, because I'd never failed in front of my father.

GAYLE: He was so proud of you.

OPRAH: It was devastating. But God closes a door and then opens a window. If I hadn't been removed from the news, the whole talk show thing would have never happened.

But I didn't know that then. It was like the end of the world. You are the 6 o'clock main anchor, and there's been this huge promotional campaign. But I learned from that. When I came in to Chicago, I said, "I will not have a big ad campaign. I will earn the respect and credibility of each viewer. I will not set myself up to fail."

LISA: *Gayle, has Oprah ever said anything about you on the air that inadvertently crossed the privacy line? For example, when I was pregnant, I had the show on, and—*

GAYLE: Oh, I know, I know, I know. When she said I pooped all over the table during the birth. People literally stopped me on the street after that one.

OPRAH: You know, in retrospect I might have thought a little more before saying that. But I was talking about pregnancy, what actually happens—and that's one of the things people never tell you. She goes, "Well, listen—"

GAYLE: "Next time you're talking about shitting on a table, keep my name out of it!" I was a news anchor by then: "I'm Gayle King, Eyewitness News." And I'd get people saying, "Yes, I saw you on the news—I didn't know you pooped all over." [*Laughter*]

LISA: *Let's stay on bodily functions for a second. My best friend, Brenda, and I have established the Sunny von Bülow pact: If something ever happens to one of us, whoever's still mobile has to come by every three weeks and pluck any unseemly facial hair.*

OPRAH: We don't have that pact because it would happen automatically.

GAYLE: My only instructions have been to go get her journals.

LISA: *And if something happens to you?*

GAYLE: I would just want her to be involved in my children's lives—always.

OPRAH: Which we would do. Her children are my children. There's nothing I wouldn't do for her, there's nothing she wouldn't do for me. There is a line of respect that is unspoken, on both our parts.

I remember once when Gayle came to my house: I was already making a lot of money, and she was making not a lot of money. And we discovered I had $422 in my pocket.

GAYLE: $482.

OPRAH: Okay, $482.

GAYLE: But who's counting?

OPRAH: I had $482 just sort of stuck into a coat pocket.

GAYLE: In your pants pocket. You know how sometimes you just find a five? Or a 20 is like, whoo! She pulls out $482.

OPRAH: Okay, you tell the story.

GAYLE: In 20s. And I'd gotten to Chicago on a Super Saver ticket; you know, back when you had to buy 30 days in advance for a decent price. She was living in Chicago, and I was married, and we had scrimped—I remember that once Billy and I didn't have $10 to go to the movies. He was in law school and I was the only one working.

So for her to pull out $482 was like, wow! She goes, "God, where'd this come from? You want it?" And I went, "Oh, no. No. I'm good. I'm fine." But I'm thinking, *God, that would pay the light bill, the phone bill, the gas bill.* And she just puts it back. It's probably still in that damn pocket. She was just extending a gesture, just being nice: "Oh, you want it?"

OPRAH: But years later, she said, "You remember that time you pulled out the $482?"

GAYLE: I said, "I wanted that money so bad!"

OPRAH: "I needed that money so bad, but I wouldn't take it." You know what that's like? That is incredible for somebody like me who lives in a world where everybody wants a piece of you. I mean, people feel they deserve a piece of you. Strangers think that.

GAYLE: Now I happily accept all gifts. [*Laughter*] No, but I just wouldn't have felt right.

OPRAH: She's never asked me for a dime. There is a level of mutual respect that comes from being with somebody you know doesn't want anything from you but you. There will never be an ulterior motive. I have to say, this would have been a much different relationship had that ever happened. Not that I wouldn't have done it, but in order to have a real friendship, you have to be equals.

GAYLE: That's not necessarily financial equals.

OPRAH: No, equal in respect. I can't put myself in a position where I need you to do things for me, or expect you to do things for me with any kind of strings attached.

GAYLE: Yeah, I never feel lesser than, or one down. Never.

OPRAH: But let me just say this, too. The person who has the money has to have a generous spirit. Early on, when I started to make a lot of money and we'd go shopping, I'd say, "Look, the deal is this: If you see something you really want, I'll get it. I don't want to play this, 'No, no, no, you don't have to buy that for me,' because I'm really willing to get it for you." I do that now with all my friends.

LISA: *That makes sense. Otherwise you would have all this money and nobody to enjoy it with.*

OPRAH: What you don't want is a situation where the person always expects that you're going to be the one to pay. Otherwise you're just the bank, and nobody wants to be seen as an ATM machine.

LISA: *People ache for connection.*

GAYLE: They do, they really do.

LISA: *They want someone who doesn't have an agenda, doesn't see you filtered through the prism of their own needs.*

OPRAH: Absolutely not. And so in a way, our friendship is better than a marriage or a sexual relationship. You know, there's no such thing as unconditional love in a marriage as far as I'm concerned, 'cause let me tell you, there are some conditions. [*Laughter*] So don't ask me to give you unconditional love, because there are certain things I won't tolerate. But in this friendship, there isn't an expectation because there isn't a model for something like this. There isn't a label, there isn't a definition of what this is supposed to be. It can be all that it can be, and it's extraordinary, in terms of the level I've been able to achieve, and to have Gayle by my side as happy as I am for those accomplishments.

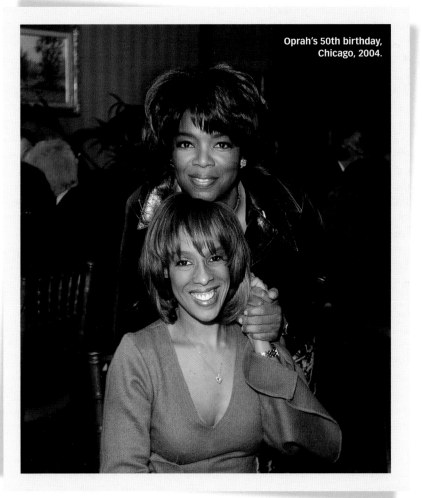

Oprah's 50th birthday, Chicago, 2004.

GAYLE: My God. Sometimes you don't even realize how big it is. You don't. Maybe I'll get some perspective years from now, when we're sitting on a porch somewhere looking back on it all.

LISA: *Do you ever think about who's going first?*

GAYLE: I think about when we get old, but I can't imagine life without Oprah. I really can't. I'll go first if I can be 90 and you can be 91.

OPRAH: Something about this relationship feels otherworldly to me, like it was designed by a power and a hand greater than my own. Whatever this friendship is, it's been a very fun ride—and we've taken it together. **O**

I Can't Believe She Did That!

What's the most stunning thing a friend ever did for you?

THE BEST REVIEW I EVER GOT

MARGO JEFFERSON

The time was the 1970s. The place was New York City, and the world was all tumult and exhilaration. Laws were changing; conventions and beliefs were, too. It was a fine thing to work against war and for the rights of women and minorities. It was exciting—no, it was thrilling—to look at your life and ask questions you'd never dared ask before.

I was lucky enough to be a young black woman in that world. I made some of the best friends of my life there.

Ingrid and I met at a party one night in the early 1970s. She was from Scandinavia, and a year behind me at Columbia's Graduate School of Journalism. We discovered we were both taking a bus to Washington, D.C., early the next morning. The occasion was a national march for women's rights. By the time we got to Washington, we were new friends, and by the time we got home that night, we were fast friends. We'd discussed our family backgrounds and our feelings about marriage and children. We'd talked about Scandinavian socialism and American capitalism. We'd compared our favorite books and our hairstyles. (My dark brown Afro billowed around my head; her straight blonde hair fell unswervingly to her shoulders.) And we had begun the first of many conversations about what it took to be a good writer.

Our professional lives began soon after. Ingrid freelanced for Swedish newspapers, at home and in New York. I took a job as a staff writer for a weekly news magazine. She was a reporter. I was a critic. We were both learning our craft.

And most of the time, I was absolutely miserable.

I was obsessed with being a perfect writer. And I was terrified that I could never live up to my own ambitions. I despaired of finding a voice that was mine alone, finding the courage to write bold, long pieces, even a book. I was ashamed of myself. Shame and despair made the work harder, of course.

I confided all this to Ingrid during those years—Ingrid, who had published poetry and translated Sylvia Plath. I don't remember what she said. I remember that she listened, that she confided her own troubles to me, and that she never stopped thinking well of me.

I left that job in the spring of 1978. Ingrid was on her way to Sweden for the summer, so we met at a restaurant to celebrate and say goodbye. And as we sat there, basking in the air of an expansive future, Ingrid handed me a big old-fashioned scrapbook bound in yellow leather. I opened it to find page after page of my own writing—almost every review and feature I had published, week after week, for five long years.

> I left the banks of childhood then, and Kathy's tears were like hands reaching for me.

I don't think I've told her to this day what it meant. But then, it took me a long time to figure that out. Ingrid had decided to treat my life with a respect I was not capable of. She had valued my work and words, ignored my foolish dream of perfection. She had known I was struggling to learn and that I could go on learning. And she had left me a record of that.

WHO NEEDED WORDS?

ELIZABETH STROUT

The place had wooden tables, their thick tops shiny from years of use, and the floors of the place were wooden, too, and shone like honey. There must have been sun coming through the high windows, because I remember light falling on the wooden table that held our cups of coffee and maybe our food. It was lunchtime, I must have ordered food, but I can't remember what it was. My friend Kathy sat across from me, waiting. We both taught at the college nearby, and earlier I had told her that something awful was happening that I needed to talk to her about.

What was happening was so painful that I had written down the words. I couldn't speak them out loud. I who was such a talkative person that I had sometimes been teased about falling asleep talking, waking up talking, talking even as I floated facedown with a snorkel in my mouth on some Caribbean blue sea, pointing out a fish to my daughter—I who had been known to "say anything"—could not now speak the words of what was happening, my terror was that deep, and so I had written the words down. Kathy's hands I can still see, spread on the table patiently, with the silver rings she wore.

I was 36, what they call a lifetime ago.

These days I often find myself thinking of the poem "Childhood Is the Kingdom Where Nobody Dies." And I think how it means that childhood is the kingdom where there is someplace still safe, and up until that day I sat across from Kathy, I was still in the kingdom where marriages were safe, where, in spite of private disappointments and difficult accommodations sometimes made, friendship still reigned, marriage still meant a safe place, where treachery might peer in a window but not come in.

Later—oh, months and months, years later—I would actually feel glad to have gone through this, to understand more fully the complications of love and accountability and sadness and healing; I would be glad later for all I had a chance to learn. But that day as I sat across from Kathy, the sunlight hitting the honey-wood table, and I pushed toward her the small piece of paper on which I had written words that made my heart crack, I was dimly aware that I was stepping into a river on whose banks I would never stand again.

And here is what I remember most: Kathy finished reading my words and, wordlessly, tears fell from her eyes. That is the gift I will always remember my friend handed to me that day. Kathy's wordless tears of empathy; a friend so generous that she wept for me. Childhood Is the Kingdom Where Nobody Dies. Where marriages are safe. I left the banks of childhood then, and Kathy's tears were like hands reaching for me, as I, stunned, afraid of drowning in the river of grown-up land, struggled to the other side. ◐

Lucy and Ethel, Behind the Scenes

Onscreen the two stars would take a pie in the face for each other any day. And off?
MADELYN PUGH DAVIS, who helped create TV's daffiest duo, spills the beans.

The first time Lucille Ball met Vivian Vance, at a script reading for *I Love Lucy,* she wasn't sure she was right for the role of Ethel Mertz. "You're too attractive," Lucy said. "I want a dumpy landlady wearing an old terry cloth robe and fuzzy slippers, with rollers in her hair." Vivian answered, "You got her. That's exactly how I look in the morning when I get out of bed." Lucy shot her a skeptical "we'll see" look. But then we read the script, and it was obvious to Lucy and everyone else that Vivian *was* the perfect Ethel. Thus began the friendship that lasted all their lives, on and off the screen.

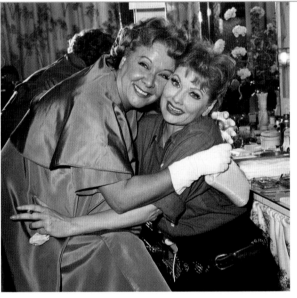

Lucille Ball and Vivian Vance behind the scenes, 1960.

Originally, when my partner, Bob Carroll Jr., and I wrote the *I Love Lucy* pilot with Jess Oppenheimer, we had no plans to include neighbors. But when it was suggested that Lucy needed a best friend, we agreed. A best friend is someone who doesn't look at you as if you're crazy when you say something like "Let's steal John Wayne's cement footprints from in front of Grauman's Theatre." And when you get into trouble with one of your ill-fated schemes and your husband says you've "got some splainin to do," a best friend is always there to help "splain."

Lucy and Ethel sometimes had arguments within the show, because let's face it, not getting along is funnier than getting along. But they always made up while crying and saying they were sorry. Lucy felt strongly that the show always had to have a happy ending.

Someone once asked Lucy if she looked at her old shows on TV. She said, "Sometimes. And when I do, I watch Viv." She had a good point. Whenever Lucy was doing one of her hilarious scenes, the camera usually cut to Ethel to catch the look of disbelief on her face, which made everything even funnier. The two

actresses had great admiration for each other's talent. Vivian respected Lucy, the fabulous comedian, and Lucy respected Vivian, the great reactor, known in comedy as a second banana.

Lucy said that when there was a scene in which she felt something more was needed, or a scene that should be played a little differently, she would talk to Viv, who was able to put her finger on the problem and come up with a good idea. She said Viv was a good script doctor.

Vivian was good at subtly handling Lucy, too. We were very lucky to write for a star who would do absolutely any stunt we thought up, if it was funny, but there was one time that she balked—the only time in the 20 years we wrote for her that she rebelled at working with an animal. It was an episode for *The Lucy Show,* and it involved an elephant. Lucy walked onto the set, caught a glimpse of this enormous creature, got a terrified look on her face, and promptly ran to her dressing room. Then word came back to us that she wasn't going to do the bit. We were in our office trying to think of something new when Vivian called. "It's okay," she said. "Lucy's going to do it." "What happened?" I asked. Vivian said, "I told her, 'If *you* don't want to do that hilarious scene, I will.'"

When Lucy did her last series, *Life with Lucy,* in which she played a grandmother, she didn't want a character to play her "best girlfriend." Vivian had died, and Lucy couldn't stand the thought of replacing her. For a long time after Vivian's death, Lucy would tear up whenever she talked about her. Everyone needs a best girlfriend she can confide in, someone who will always tell the truth and back her up. It really helps when you're doing a comedy show, and it doesn't hurt in real life, either. ◐

How to Help a Friend...

Whatever's troubling her, you want to make it better. But how?
On the next pages, JANCEE DUNN and LESLEY DORMEN round up the smartest,
kindest advice on a range of situations. But first, NANCY COMISKEY walks us
through what is said to be the toughest challenge of all.

I f there's anything I can do, just let me know." Surely you've said that to someone going through a rough time; we all have. It's the sort of well-worn, well-meaning phrase that we utter reflexively before hanging up the phone, anxious to do our friendship duty. But here's the thing: Most people in the midst of a crisis can't really get it together to tell you exactly what they need. And we friends aren't always geniuses when it comes to guessing. When psychologist Alice Chang, PhD, was diagnosed with breast cancer in 1994, some friends, perhaps thinking they were being helpful, asked stark questions such as "Aren't you afraid of dying?" Others simply stopped calling. "People don't know what to do," says Chang, "so they just disappear."

How, then, do you best help a friend who is having serious difficulties? How do you open a conversation in a sensitive manner? And what should you avoid saying at all costs? We asked the experts—and some women who have been there—how to help a friend...

...WHO'S LOST A CHILD

Six weeks after our 24-year-old daughter, Kate, was killed by an intoxicated driver, our friends Dan and Jan hauled a trailer to the house where she had lived. They spent the Saturday before Christmas helping us sort through Kate's belongings, untouched since the day she died.

They must have dreaded that day. But instead of saying, "Tell us if we can help," they said, "Tell us when we can help."

Friendship changes when a child dies. Friends either grow closer or drift apart. My husband and I are lucky: Many close and even casual friends have stood by us, making us meals, sitting with us at court hearings, spending weekends and vacations with us. Others, sadly, have not. Maybe they are unable to face what psychologists call the worst grief.

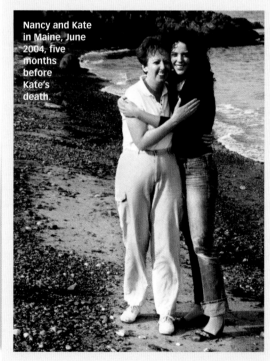

Nancy and Kate in Maine, June 2004, five months before Kate's death.

If so, I understand. Before Kate was killed, I wouldn't have known how to help a friend who had lost a child. Now I do.

The week after Kate's death, I sat on the sofa in a daze. Our house filled with so many flowers, I had nowhere to put them. Our fridge was so jammed with donated food, I couldn't find a carton of milk. I spent hours scraping out spoiled casseroles. (Weeks later, too exhausted by grief to microwave a frozen dinner, I welcomed even the simplest meal.)

Helping a grieving parent is a marathon, not a sprint, but there are some comforts you can provide right away. Go to the memorial service, no matter what you have to cancel to be there; your presence tells parents that their son or daughter won't be forgotten. Do something tangible to keep the child's memory alive: Frame a photo the parents haven't seen, plant a flowering tree. And be practical. One of our neighbors dropped off fireplace logs that could be lit with a match. Another mowed our yard.

Take some time during that first week to learn more about what the parents will be facing in the months ahead. A good place to start is the Web site of the Compassionate Friends, compassionatefriends.org, a support group for families who have lost a child. (The site explains the grieving process and offers a link to a list of recommended books.) Recognize that your friend's grief is going to get much worse and that as it does, she'll need you more than ever.

Once the funeral is over, friends often don't know what to do next. They're so afraid of saying the wrong thing that they avoid saying anything. They're terrified of reminding the parents of their loss. But we don't need reminding; we're living it, every minute of every day. My husband and I want to talk about Kate. Hearing her name is a precious gift.

So, ask often how a parent is doing, and then listen. It's okay to say, "I don't know what to say"; it acknowledges the loss and lets the parent decide where the conversation goes next. Don't try to fix things or offer religious counsel unless you know it's welcome. Don't say you hug your child every day now—that's something the parent will never be able to do again. And don't compare the parent's loss to your own loss of a mother, a friend, or even a brother. As painful as those deaths were, they are not the same. My husband—who lost both parents and a sister before Kate's death—explains it this way: "When your father died, did you wish you had died instead? Did you still wish it a year later?"

A friend who lives across the country got it just right. She took me on a long walk near the ocean, asked me how I felt, put her arms around me, and cried.

But even getting it "wrong" now and then is better than doing nothing. Every grieving parent tells of friends who disappeared before the ink dried on the sympathy cards; the phone stopped ringing, and vague references to getting together never included a date. One mother received a gift certificate for dinner—alone. Parents who have lost a child are not only the saddest people in the world but often the loneliest.

Seek out your friend's company as often as you can, suggesting specific times to get together. Keep asking, even if she says no the first time. Plan to meet for a glass of wine after work, a walk, or a game of Scrabble. Be aware that sometimes parents need to talk and sometimes they just need a break.

And know that grief for a child doesn't end after a year or even two. A mother who lost a 6-year-old says some friends seem to want her to get better "for their own sakes." But so many dreams die with a child that a parent's life can never be the same. Nearly two years after my daughter's death, I cry for Kate every day. But Dan and Jan, and many friends like them, are still here, saving our lives.

…WHO'S SERIOUSLY ILL

WHAT YOU CAN DO: Psychologist Alice Chang, coauthor of *A Survivor's Guide to Breast Cancer,* says that if a friend is ill but mobile, you should take her out to eat every week or two, because sick people are often isolated. If she's housebound, drop off some food, and bring videos and books on tape, because certain treatments impair vision. "Don't overstay your visit," she says. "Acknowledge the illness and ask what the progress is, and then talk about activities of daily living." If she's a close friend, volunteer to do laundry or clean her house, chores she may be unable to do herself. And be sensitive to the pendulum swings of her mood. Chang says, "I tell people, 'I know that the feelings are not always rational, because that's how emotions are. But it's okay.' "

WHAT YOU CAN SAY: Don't blurt out that she looks awful, but don't tell her she looks great if it's clearly not true. "Hug the person and say, 'Some days are better than others, and I hope you have more better days,' " says Chang. If her appearance has radically changed—if she's bald from chemo, for instance—don't pretend you don't notice. "Instead," Chang recommends, "say, 'You have a nicely shaped head' or 'Isn't it a lot cooler?' "

WHAT TO AVOID: Don't say, "I know how you feel." An epileptic patient once told Chang, "If I've heard it once, I've heard it a thousand times—'I had a dog with epilepsy, so I know how you feel.' " The truth is, you don't know how your friend feels, so the best approach is to invite her to tell you.

…WHO'S IN AN ABUSIVE RELATIONSHIP

WHAT YOU CAN DO: Pam Smieja, a public speaker and educator on domestic violence—and an abuse survivor herself—says that above all else, it's important to be a stable presence. A friend who is consistent, reliable, and gentle, even down to her tone of voice, is a profound source of comfort for someone dealing with an abuser's volatile moods.

If your friend is open with you about her situation, says Merry Arnold, PsyD, a Boston-area therapist who specializes in trauma including domestic abuse, "you can help her plan an escape by getting spare car keys, duplicate I.D., and a stash of cash that she can keep in her car or at your house—all things she'll need if he locks her out or she has to leave her house in a hurry." Call a 24-hour domestic abuse crisis hotline to educate yourself, then give her the number. A hotline can be more helpful than friends or family, says Smieja, because "many volunteers have been abused themselves and understand the fear and pain and chaos." Offer to let her call from your house, where she'll be safer—and give her privacy while she's on the phone. "She wouldn't want you sitting there listening," Smieja says. "It would be too shameful."

It's better to give your friend the number of a nearby domestic abuse shelter than a spare key to your house, which could jeopardize your own safety. "The address of the safe house is confidential," Smieja says. "A cop once slipped me the name and number of a shelter. I hid that sucker really well, and that's what I used when I left."

WHAT YOU CAN SAY: "If you suspect abuse, don't ask an open-ended question like 'What's going on?' " Smieja says. "Because she'll lie. I always lied. Gently touch her arm, look her in the eye, and say, 'If you need me, I'm here for you.' That will open a door. Eye contact is very, very important. If she senses you're uncomfortable, she'll never go to you."

WHAT TO AVOID: Don't ask why she doesn't just leave. "Living with an abuser is like being in a concentration camp," Smieja says. "There are consequences. My abuser copied my whole address book, waved it in front of me, and said, 'If you leave, somebody will pay.' I knew he was capable of ugly things."

Arnold agrees. "The person can leave only when she's ready. Be patient."

…WHO'S ADDICTED TO ALCOHOL

WHAT YOU CAN DO: Suggest getting together at breakfast instead of dinner, and don't drink around her. "It's okay to say, 'If you choose to drink, I'll spend time with you only when you're sober,' " says Sheila Hermes, a counselor at the Hazelden alcohol and drug rehabilitation center outside St. Paul, Minnesota. If you want to talk to her about her addiction, approach her when she's not under the influence. "When they're drinking, they'll react with defensiveness and denial," Hermes says. If she's interested in getting

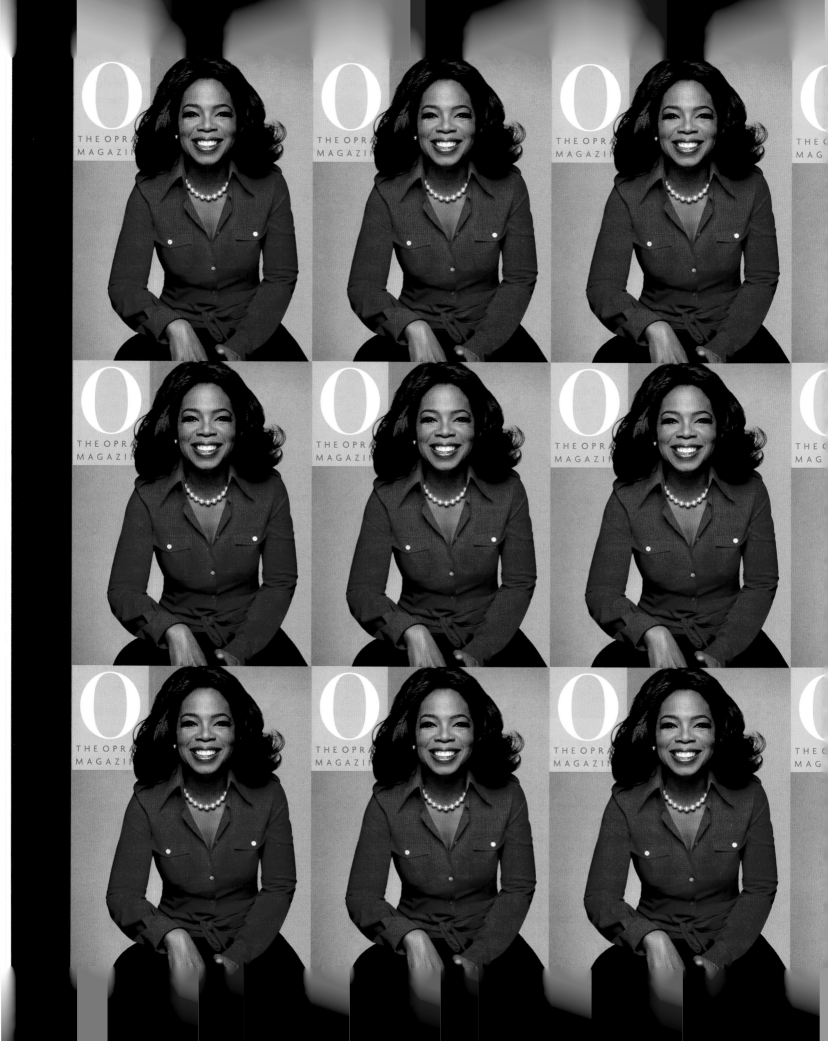

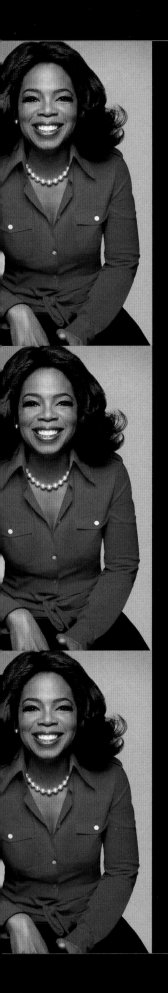

Living in the World

What you give to the world comes back to you tenfold. These stories of enlightenment, heroism, and inspiration dare you to make a difference.

Everyday Heroes

Oprah Talks to
Christiane Amanpour

She's the calm in the middle of one international storm after another, a profile in courage (and no-nonsense gutsiness) for millions of CNN viewers around the world. One of the most intrepid and admired women in all of news broadcasting opens up about her remarkable career, how she's managing motherhood and marriage, what it's like covering a war, and why she believes a thriving society must have a thriving press.

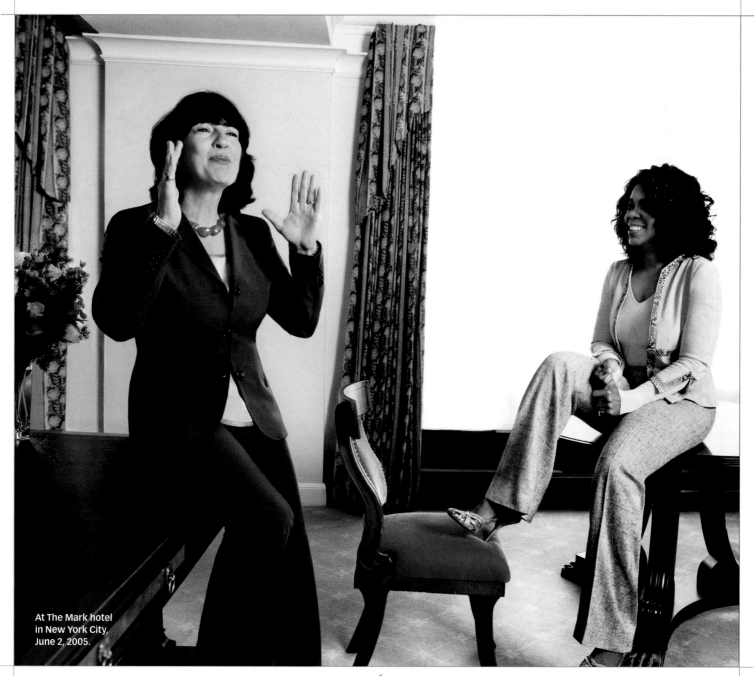

At The Mark hotel in New York City, June 2, 2005.

I don't watch a lot of television, but when I do tune in, it's usually to CNN—my connection to the rest of the world. And no matter what time of day or night it is, I'm always hoping for a story from Christiane Amanpour. I like her style: She's confident, courageous, fearless. She's a whole lotta woman.

Raised in Iran, Christiane was schooled in London (to which her family fled in 1979), then studied journalism at the University of Rhode Island. She entered our living rooms—and our national consciousness—on CNN during the Gulf War. A few years later, it was Christiane, perhaps more than anyone else, who refused to let the West ignore the atrocities in Bosnia. During nearly two decades of what she calls balls-to-the-wall reporting, she has brought clarity and context to the crises in Iraq, Darfur, the Balkans. As *The New York Times* once put it, "Where there's war, there's Amanpour."

Christiane now lives in London with her husband, Jamie Rubin (he was an assistant secretary of state in the Clinton administration), and their young son, Darius, but her need to tell the world's toughest and most compelling stories remains strong.

I met up with Christiane at The Mark hotel in New York, in June 2005, where she was already packed for a trip to Dubai. Considering that she is a globe-trotting mom on the move, she was incredibly generous with her time. As she filled me in on life on the front lines, mothering while at war, and the real meaning of risk, I saw that reporting isn't a job for her, it's a mission.

OPRAH: *When you're covering a crisis such as poverty in Africa, do you feel that your role is just to tell the story?*
CHRISTIANE: The politically correct thing to say is that it's not a journalist's role to be an advocate, to have an agenda, to agitate on behalf of any kind of political position. But in my work, basic matters of life and death are on the table—whether it's genocide in Africa and the Balkans or violations of human rights. I'm not just a stenographer or someone with a megaphone; when I

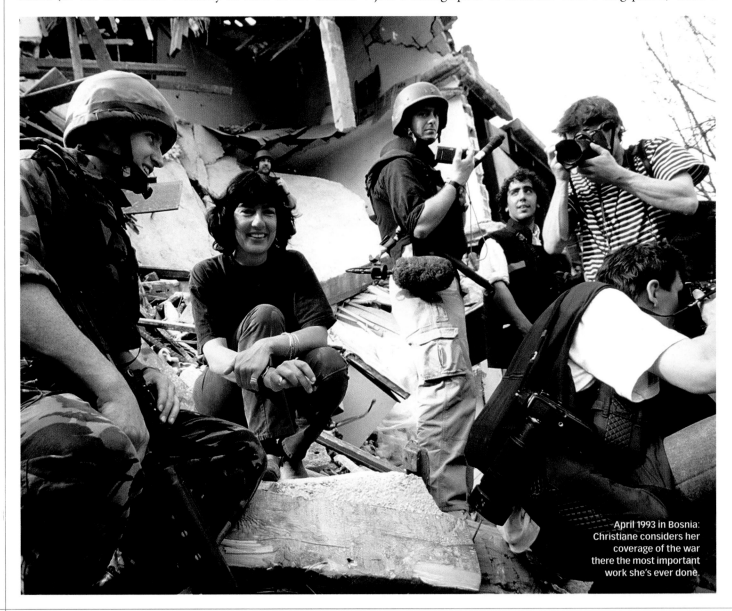

April 1993 in Bosnia: Christiane considers her coverage of the war there the most important work she's ever done.

270

report, I have to do it in context, to be aware of the moral conundrum. If I'm talking about genocide, for instance, I have to be able to draw a line between victim and aggressor. It would be irresponsible for me and CNN to tell you what the person being gang-raped says, what the rapist says—and to give each equal time and moral equivalence. I can't do that because it means being neutral in the face of unspeakable horror. When you're neutral, you're an accessory.

OPRAH: *That's right. Where are you headed next?*

CHRISTIANE: First to Dubai, then to Africa. I really believe our generation can end extreme poverty in places like Africa. If you asked most Americans how much of our budget goes to foreign aid, many would say 15 percent. Only about 0.1 percent of America's gross domestic product goes to foreign aid. Europeans are somewhere around 0.4. I think there's a lot of space for Americans to support their government in giving more aid in places where it can do a lot of good.

OPRAH: *The reason there's extreme poverty is that the world allows it.*

CHRISTIANE: True. In many parts of the poor world, there are obviously corrupt governments, and a lot of work needs to be done on that. But you can't say that we'll only help if there's a good government. Yes, we have to lobby for good government, but we also have to help the poorest of the poor. It's our responsibility. We're so rich—we have all the technology, money, power, media. This is our moment. If commitments aren't made now, they may not be made again in our lifetime. I don't believe the conventional wisdom that Americans don't care what happens in the world. Individual Americans had an incredible reaction to the tsunami—much faster than their government's reaction. Americans are a very moral and compassionate people who believe in extending a helping hand, especially when they get the full facts instead of one-minute clips.

OPRAH: *Do you have trouble getting CNN to allow you to do longer pieces?*

CHRISTIANE: Fortunately not. I just have to present a compelling case and make sure the story is valid. I'm lucky.

OPRAH: *I understand that the rest of the media wouldn't have covered the Bosnian War the way they did ten years ago had it not been for your insistence.*

CHRISTIANE: Well, look, that's a big compliment and very flattering. I consider Bosnia the most important work I've ever done. All during the war, CNN was there every day, and we weren't only covering car and suicide bombs; we did human interest stories. That made a difference. I'm absolutely convinced that had we not been there—not just CNN but every news organization there—perhaps the West might not have intervened.

OPRAH: *The news was in our face.*

CHRISTIANE: Americans are concerned with human rights. Their principles and honor couldn't tolerate it anymore. Western democracy cannot sit by forever while a genocide is perpetrated.

> "Americans are a very compassionate people who believe in extending a helping hand, especially when they get the full facts."

But let me tell you the flip side of that story—the time when we didn't shine the spotlight enough and the world did sit by.

OPRAH: *Rwanda.*

CHRISTIANE: In just three months, nearly a million people were slaughtered in Rwanda. That will forever be a badge of shame—for me personally, for our networks and news organizations, for the president, for the head of the United Nations Security Council and the Secretary-General of the UN, for the whole world.

OPRAH: *Why do you call it a shame for you personally?*

CHRISTIANE: Because I was occupied with Bosnia.

OPRAH: *That's my point. You're one person, and you were already in Bosnia.*

CHRISTIANE: I still feel it. I'm part of this sorority of journalists. As a profession, we failed.

OPRAH: *Even Bill Clinton sees it as a failure.*

CHRISTIANE: Yes. He has gone to Rwanda and apologized, and so has Kofi Annan. Every time I get an opportunity, I apologize. I still find it very emotional. We were consumed by the good-news story in South Africa, the first democratic elections, the triumph of Nelson Mandela walking out of jail after all those years of apartheid. A lot of our resources went to covering that story, as well as the O.J. Simpson trial.

OPRAH: *That's right. I just saw your eyes tear up as we were talking about Rwanda.*

CHRISTIANE: That's because of the shame.

OPRAH: *At a dinner recently, I had the honor of sitting next to Paul Kagame—the man who led the rebel forces in Rwanda and later became president. He said the horror was unimaginable—no words to explain it.*

CHRISTIANE: Taking it in is corrosive. It all happened in 100 days. People say that it was an even more rapid killing machine than the Holocaust. And it wasn't industrial. It was personal—people with machetes and clubs attacking their neighbors, their friends. Here's another big shame for the media: A radio station there was used as the propaganda arm of this genocide, constantly egging on the extremists and the militias. "Kill those Tutsi; we let them go last time; kill their children; don't let the cockroaches survive!"

OPRAH: *That's just as it was depicted in the movie* Hotel Rwanda.

CHRISTIANE: It was a constant diet of hate that we also witnessed in Bosnia.

OPRAH: *Isn't it astonishing that you can get friends to turn against friends in an instant?*

CHRISTIANE: It's brainwashing that appeals to the most base instincts in a human being.

OPRAH: *Years ago on my show, we did an experiment with a teacher who taught in a little town in Iowa in 1968, the year Dr. King was assassinated. She was trying to explain to her third graders what prejudice was, so she divided the class into two groups: those with brown eyes and those with blue. She allowed the brown-eyed children access to recess and gave them special treats, and in two days she saw the difference in terms of hate and prejudice. So we brought her in to do a similar experiment with our audience—we gave her false credentials and said that she'd discovered blue-eyed people were stupid. In just an hour, people were calling in to the show saying things like, "I always knew there was something wrong with my sister-in-law!" And then when we said, "You know what? This is just an experiment," people were infuriated.*

CHRISTIANE: Because they'd been caught. That's amazing. That's why we have to educate people and use the media responsibly.

OPRAH: *Right. I once read an article in which you said that of all the tragedies you've witnessed, Rwanda was the worst.*

CHRISTIANE: That's true. Yet Bosnia was difficult because we lived with the civilian population through years of being besieged and bombarded.

OPRAH: *How long were you there?*

CHRISTIANE: From start to end—1992 to 1996. I quickly recognized that it was an important story, and I stuck with it. We went out with the women who were trying to get water at the pump. Then a mortar would fall and all the women and children would be killed. We saw people trying to run across the airport in a desperate attempt to get a couple of apples for their children.

OPRAH: *Where were you living in the midst of it?*

CHRISTIANE: In a hotel in the center of town. I was right on the front line. No shelter, no protection, no water or heat in our hotel.

OPRAH: *Weren't you frightened?*

CHRISTIANE: At moments, yes. One morning I woke up to the incoming whistle of artillery. I was desperate to get out of my room, but I couldn't find the key to unlock the door. I thought, *Whatever happens, happens.* Then it went silent. I thought maybe I'd dreamed it. A few hours later, my colleagues and friends came banging on my door, saying, "Have you seen?" Just two doors down from me, this 105 millimeter howitzer shell came through an empty room. It could have taken off the whole floor and all of us with it, but it was faulty, so it didn't explode. Touch wood. [*Knocks on the wooden end table.*]

OPRAH: *Didn't that shake you up? If there's a Mack truck and I swerve so it doesn't hit me, I have to pull over to the side of the road to gather myself. After an artillery shell hits, do you just go have a croissant?*

CHRISTIANE: There were no croissants, but I might have done that. When you're much younger and less experienced, that's part of the whole survival drama: *Wow, we made it.*

OPRAH: *You did at least acknowledge that you could have died?*

CHRISTIANE: Of course. During my first trip to Sarajevo in June of 1992, the city was under siege. Even the zookeepers had been scared away, and the animals were starving. My camerawoman, my producer, and I went to check it out. When we got there, we did the story, and the animals did look scrawny. But we stayed just

"I love success stories, when I can show women who've beaten the odds, women who found their voices."

a little too long. The gunners on the hills figured out that we were there, and it started raining mortars. I remember kicking down the door of a building and sitting in the doorjamb. If you should sit under a doorjamb during an earthquake, I reasoned, maybe that would work in a mortar attack. All I could keep saying to my crew was, "If you die, I'm so sorry. I'm so sorry. I'm so sorry." The minute the shooting stopped, we ran out of there.

OPRAH: *Did your life flash before you?*

CHRISTIANE: No. I was too busy apologizing. Maybe it was my mechanism not to think about it. [*Knocks wood again.*]

OPRAH: *Do you sleep well at night when you're in a war-torn area?*

CHRISTIANE: Yes. But that's getting more difficult now because I'm often up round-the-clock. There's so much demand for live coverage. I know it sounds counterintuitive, but one of the great things about Bosnia is that we didn't have a live dish for a long time. When we got it, it increased the demand on reporters. What's prime time in the United States is bedtime for us abroad. So I spend a lot of time awake.

OPRAH: *Do you get punchy?*

CHRISTIANE: A bit. I've learned how to catnap in downtime.

OPRAH: *Has proper media attention been given to the genocide that's happening in Sudan right now?*

CHRISTIANE: Not enough—though columnist Nicholas Kristof at *The New York Times* stands out as an exception. We're trying to go there, but the government of Sudan has essentially shut down all media organizations for the past several months. Last summer [2004] I went there twice with my team. First we went to Chad and saw all the people being herded out. Then when we finally got visas, we went into Darfur and did a week of programming. I had an exclusive interview with the president of Sudan. They let me in at ten at night, and I had the flu and a sore throat, and it really was a surreal kind of thing. It was at a time when he was trying to make better relations with the rest of the world, so he was saying all the right things—but doing all the wrong things.

OPRAH: *Now the media is banned?*

CHRISTIANE: We can't get visas. That has a real impact on our ability to tell the story. I can't do it based only on the pictures I took last year. But every opportunity I have, I talk about it.

OPRAH: *What did you see when you were there?*

CHRISTIANE: We didn't actually see the marauding and killing, but we saw people with severe malnutrition living in camps. We heard stories of women who'd been brutalized.

OPRAH: *It's not like Rwanda?*

CHRISTIANE: There aren't thousands of corpses piled up, but it's still a very brutal assault on the people by government-backed militia.

OPRAH: *Is there a story you wanted to cover but didn't?*

CHRISTIANE: There are lots of stories. One person can't get to everything. I really love to report on women and children. Women are the backbone of so many families and societies. They are also, by and large, the oppressed members of so many parts of the world. I love success stories, when I can show women who've beaten the odds, women who found their voices. As for children, few lobby for them; they don't have their own organizations. Sure, there's UNICEF and certain nonprofits, but children have virtually no rights.

OPRAH: *No voice.*

CHRISTIANE: The next big issue I want to cover is pediatric AIDS. Some inroads have been made on adult AIDS in Africa and in other parts of the world. People have given a lot of money and berated a lot of drug companies to make affordable medicine. But what about the children's crisis? I've heard that in one year, 500,000 children die of AIDS and there are no drugs for the poorest. Drug companies are saying, "Give half the adult dose to a child." But a child's biochemistry is different from an adult's.

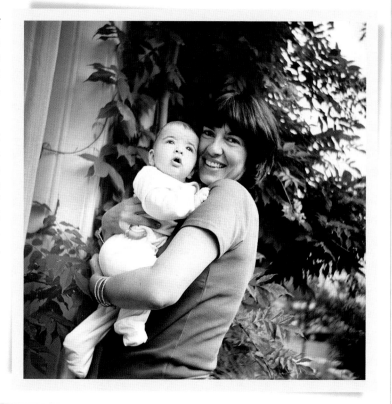

(Right) Christiane and her son, Darius, in July 2000, when he was 3 months old. *(Below)* Christiane and Jamie Rubin at their wedding in Bracciano, Italy, August 1998.

OPRAH: *True. What reporting have you done that makes you proudest?*

CHRISTIANE: Bosnia. That's my most significant, extended body of work. Just by doing my duty as a reporter—along with my colleagues—I believe we made a difference. My proudest lifetime achievement is my son and my family.

OPRAH: *Did the way you told the stories of children change after you had your son?*

CHRISTIANE: It did. In Bosnia, seeing children victims of this genocide was more than I could tolerate. It was really painful to see children who'd deliberately been scoped through a sniper's sights and killed. It's a kind of horror that you don't believe is possible. I'm always moved by the plight of children because they're so defenseless. When I became a mother, it was a thousand times more emotional for me. I cry when I go into hospitals and see children.

OPRAH: *When you became pregnant, did you think twice about whether you'd continue as a war correspondent?*

CHRISTIANE: I was very cavalier when I was pregnant. I was conscious of

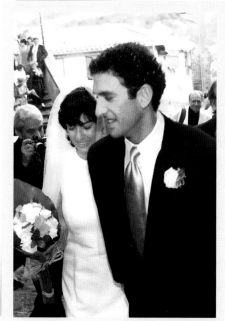

> "I was very cavalier when I was pregnant. I was conscious of being a woman and not letting them say, 'Now you're a mother and you can't do this anymore.'"

being a woman and not letting them say, "Now you're a mother and you can't do this anymore. Let the guys do it." I was a little over-the-top. I was like, "Nothing will change. I'll take my child with me. All I need is some bulletproof diapers." The minute my child was born, everything changed. There's a love inside you that you never knew existed. There's a protectiveness you never knew you were capable of. And there's no way in hell I would take my child to the places I go. That would be completely irresponsible. I'm also much more concerned about my own safety, about surviving.

OPRAH: *You weren't before?*

CHRISTIANE: Not as much. I had a feeling of invulnerability.

OPRAH: *Not everybody has that.*

CHRISTIANE: I couldn't have done the work I did if I'd been married or had a kid. All my energy, my emotion, my intellect went into my work. During the nineties, people would ask me, "When are you going to settle down?" and I'd say, "I don't think I'll ever have a child." But there came a moment where I flipped the switch and said, *Okay, self. You can be proud of the work you've done. You wanted to be a foreign correspondent, you're a foreign correspondent. Maybe now it's time to look for some personal happiness and fulfillment.* It took me a couple of years, but I consciously changed myself.

273

OPRAH: *And then you met Jamie?*

CHRISTIANE: Yes, about six months after that turning point.

OPRAH: *Before that you were fulfilled in giving all your energy to your work. I completely understand that. Now you still seem to be everywhere.*

CHRISTIANE: I'm actually not. I still go to all of these places and try to shine the light on corners that need illuminating. But I can't spend months and months away from my child.

OPRAH: *What's the longest time you've been away?*

CHRISTIANE: I try not to stay away longer than two weeks at a time. For me, 9/11 was a big challenge because I was away for three months. I did come home from Pakistan for a couple of long weekends. My child was just 18 months old. I have been so fortunate. Jamie is a true hero. He was in the Clinton administration, and when that ended in 2000, my husband, a Democrat, didn't have an administration to work for. So he, my son, Darius, and I benefited from the fact that Jamie didn't have to travel much. He moved to London with me and went into private work. That's rare. Jamie is the poster child for good husbands.

OPRAH: *Was moving a hard decision for him?*

CHRISTIANE: Jamie worked for Senator Kerry during this last election. Had Kerry won, we would have moved back to the States. And if Jamie and I were both on the road, I couldn't have traveled as much. I would have had to give up my job. I couldn't have left my child.

OPRAH: *I read that he just gave up everything for you and put on an apron.*

CHRISTIANE: He's not a househusband— that's a myth. He worked for a private company and wrote speeches. Post 9/11, he became Jamie Rubin, the voice of Americans overseas.

OPRAH: *Do you want more children?*

CHRISTIANE: It would be nice. But I'm 47 and a half years old. I think I've come to the end of my natural...

OPRAH: *There's a woman who just had a baby at 66.*

CHRISTIANE: You can believe that was with plenty of aid.

OPRAH: *What makes you happy?*

CHRISTIANE: A lot of things. I love my child. I love my husband. I love my life. I love going out to good dinners and seeing great plays. I love going to hear Eric Clapton, as I just did in the Albert Hall. We saw Cream—they reunited the band. Tell me this isn't amazing: Eric Clapton, Ginger Baker, and Jack Bruce, all over 60.

OPRAH: *Eric Clapton looks good.*

CHRISTIANE: How can you tell them they're old when they're still pulling the young ones into the tent? It's about talent and passion. It's about people believing that you're the real deal. And they are.

OPRAH: *Just like you. You're the real deal, girl.*

CHRISTIANE: Oh, you're sweet.

> "In conventional warfare, I believe America will always win the war. The real challenge is for the United States to win the peace."

OPRAH: *I can tell you still have the fire for your work.*

CHRISTIANE: I do. That makes me a bit of an endangered species. I think we need to stop undermining ourselves and realize that journalism is an incredibly noble profession. Look at Woodward and Bernstein. What heroes! Their Watergate investigation inspired a whole generation of journalists. They've never lost their integrity. One thing that pains me is that public trust of journalists is diminishing. There have been stupid mistakes. But we [journalists] really do have transparent investigations of them. We bring outsiders in and investigate from top to bottom.

OPRAH: *That's at your level. But the truth is that in this country, the lines are so blurred between tabloid journalism and mainstream press.*

CHRISTIANE: Right.

OPRAH: *As you travel, what do you hear about how the world feels about America?*

CHRISTIANE: It's still very tense, though not quite as tense as it was at the height of anti-Americanism post 9/11. A couple of issues remain unresolved. The Iraq war is not going as well as had been expected or hoped. The constant bloodletting there is a source of great fear around the world. Many are saying, "If that's change, are we ready to pay the price in our blood?" In one month, around 700 Iraqis were killed—a huge number for such a short time. There's a lot of work to be done.

OPRAH: *I've noticed that when I'm abroad, I get more international news. Earlier this year when I was in the Oslo airport, I heard the total number of Iraqi deaths. That's not discussed in the United States.*

CHRISTIANE: Iraq is not a foreign news story. It's an American story. Though it's difficult to report from Iraq because it's so dangerous, everything's at stake in this war. The success of the democracy experiment is going to live and die in Iraq; the success of combating terrorism will be proved or disproved in Iraq. For that reason alone, I believe the war should be on the front page of every newspaper every day and at the top of every newscast.

OPRAH: *When you're in Iraq, do you feel fear?*

CHRISTIANE: Oh, yes. It's the scariest place I've ever been. You know that you're personally targeted. You also know you could get caught up in some suicide bomb that was meant for somebody else.

OPRAH: *At any time.*

CHRISTIANE: Yes. I'm one of those people who believe that the Iraq war could have already been won. I was there when Baghdad was liberated. There was a real moment of opportunity when the people were thankful to the United States and so glad to see the back of Saddam Hussein. Because there weren't enough troops and allies onboard to pacify the situation immediately, there was a loss of authority. Then came an incredible orgy of looting and a basic breakdown of law and order. That sowed seeds of possibility among those who would do harm and cause mayhem. They saw that although the superpower was there...

OPRAH: *But there weren't enough troops.*

CHRISTIANE: Which is why they took their chances. Now the reconstruction effort is hobbled by the insecurity. The people still don't have a properly functioning sewage system, they still don't have electricity 24 hours a day, and the medical situation is terrible. Doctors are fleeing because of the violence. It's all very sad.

OPRAH: *How do you see it ending?*

CHRISTIANE: I honestly don't know. I hope for the best. I'm an Iranian. Saddam Hussein invaded my country. My family fought against the Iraqi forces during the Iran-Iraq War. My cousins fought on the front line.

OPRAH: *And your family eventually fled, right?*

CHRISTIANE: We left partly because of that war. So I have no love for Saddam Hussein and his regime, as a human being and as an Iranian. Everybody in their right mind is glad to see the back of that man. We just wish the postwar had been better planned, that there had been more allies onboard and a way to win the peace. In conventional warfare, I believe America will always win the war. It's a superpower that no one can challenge. The real challenge is for the Unites States to win the peace. And it must win, because otherwise we're all at risk.

OPRAH: *How do you define risk?*

CHRISTIANE: Several ways. There's the obvious: physical risk of your life. Every time I go into a scary situation, I weigh its worth—should I or shouldn't I? Then there's what I call intellectual risk. Do you tell the truth? Do you speak out? Do you push the limit with your bosses, colleagues, friends, and family? Do you stand up for what you believe is right? And are you prepared to live with the risks of doing that?

OPRAH: *You are one gusty, ballsy sister. Did you always know you wanted to be a foreign correspondent?*

CHRISTIANE: Oh, yes. I knew when I went to college. I was old enough to understand the revolution in Iran and to know that I wanted to be part of that kind of earth-shattering world event.

OPRAH: *Were you brave as a child?*

CHRISTIANE: I remember being very shy. I was also very curious—some people would say nosy. I always wanted to be around the grown-ups and listen to what they were saying. I rode horses from the age of 5. If I'm asked to trace my...

OPRAH: *Chutzpah.*

CHRISTIANE: I'd have to say it has something to do with falling off a very, very fast horse a lot. I was literally picked up and put back on the horse by the scruff of my neck. My riding teacher gave me no choice.

OPRAH: *Where were your parents?*

CHRISTIANE: They were the kind who sat there and watched, and obviously, they wouldn't let their child be abused. But I was taught courage and sticking power. Then when you lose your country, when you lose everything important to you, when members of your family and friends are executed, when you go

through a revolution, you survive with a certain fortitude.

OPRAH: *How old were you during Iran's revolution?*

CHRISTIANE: That was in 1978, so I was 20 when it all started rumbling.

OPRAH: *How do you relax, for goodness sake?*

CHRISTIANE: Very easily. I have a great family structure and great friends. I've still got friends from childhood. I'm really proactive in the way I keep them around me. When I come back from the road, it's as if I've never gone. We go out to dinners, to movies. I have family lunches every week in London. I order out Persian food, and all ten of us gather.

OPRAH: *Wow. I would think that when you come home from such intensity, you'd need alone time to breathe.*

CHRISTIANE: There's not much alone time when you have a kid. I put a lot of energy into being a good mother and wife. Life is fun, things are good, and I'm really lucky.

OPRAH: *Now that you have a child, do you take fewer physical risks?*

CHRISTIANE: I'm more careful about wearing the bulletproof vest and availing myself of whatever security is available.

OPRAH: *When was the last time you were in Iraq?*

CHRISTIANE: In January [2005] for the elections. I spent nearly three weeks there, which is a long time for me now.

OPRAH: *Even with the level of anxiety there, you still go?*

CHRISTIANE: Yes. When I'm there, I turn off the fear switch. So I'm actually relaxed. Know what I mean?

OPRAH: *No, I don't know what you mean!*

CHRISTIANE: When I board a plane to fly to Baghdad, I do get fearful. I don't know whether I'll get shot out of the sky. Then I don't know whether I'll make it from the airport to the base. I think, *What am I doing here? It's a war zone.* But I always end up going back.

OPRAH: *Good God. All I can say is that the horse worked for you! Do you think you're brave?*

CHRISTIANE: I don't think about it.

OPRAH: *Just like I don't think of myself as being famous, because fame is something that happens outside of yourself. You don't wake up and think,* Gee, what a brave woman I am. *But let me tell you, you're a brave widdle wabbit!*

CHRISTIANE: I wake up thinking about what a scaredy-cat I am these days. After I make it into Baghdad, I high-five my colleagues.

OPRAH: *Five years from now, do you see yourself going around the world wherever there's a need?*

CHRISTIANE: I don't rule anything in or out. I've still got a lot of energy, passion, and commitment. I really believe in the power of mass media to do good. I believe that we are indispensable forces in proper functioning democracies and proper civil societies. If you look around the emerging democracies in the world—like Iran, for instance—it's often the journalists who are on the cutting edge of reform. We have an enormous role to play. Television brought you the abuses at Abu Ghraib. News like this is vital. If we don't respect our profession and we see it frittering away into the realm of triviality and sensationalism, we'll lose our standing. That won't be good for democracy. A thriving society must have a thriving press. **O**

The Hallelujah Chorus

On paper, these boys from war-ravaged Liberia weren't the world's most adoptable orphans. But if you heard them sing (like angels, everyone said), or knew that their orphanage back home lay in ruins, or felt the mysterious tug that drew each boy to his proper family, you'd know why every last one of them found a home. AIMEE LEE BALL reports.

Upon learning that she'd be meeting a dozen boys from Liberia at her church near Charlotte, North Carolina, Lysa TerKeurst consulted a world map—she vaguely thought that Liberia was in South America. The boys, ages 11 to 16, all had parents who had died or disappeared in the brutal civil war ravaging their country. While living in an orphanage outside the capital city of Monrovia, they were chosen for an a cappella choir that would tour the United States, raising money to send home. But in the summer of 2003, while the boys were visiting the Charlotte area, their orphanage was attacked twice, first by rebel forces and then by militia loyal to the warlord-turned-president Charles Taylor. The property was ransacked, caregivers were severely beaten, and several hundred children fled into the jungle, the teenagers carrying toddlers on their backs. The visas of the choirboys in the States were about to expire, and now they were homeless.

Lysa, a 37-year-old motivational speaker, was going to hear the choir with her then 8-year-old's Brownie troop. She decided to take all three of her daughters, imagining no more than a new cultural experience. "It was an ordinary day," she says. "Nothing led me to believe that life was about to be seriously interrupted." But listening to the honeyed voices of the young travelers, she was overwhelmed with a sudden thought: Two of those boys were meant to be hers. She literally put her fingers in her ears to drown out what she assumed was a divine message she didn't want to hear. At the postconcert reception, two boys named Mark and Jackson separated from the crowd, wrapped their arms around her, and called her mom. Fourteen-year-old Mark had a scar on his cheek from the hot poker of a rebel soldier; 15-year-old Jackson had hepatitis B, probably from contamination of a leg wound. Still not knowing exactly what had hit her, Lysa walked up to the choir director and said, "Not that I'm interested at all, but if someone wanted to adopt, how would she do it?" Back in her car, she called her husband, Art, from her cell phone. "I said something like 'Do we need milk and what would you think of adopting two teenage boys from Liberia?' He said, 'Get home now.'"

The idea of adoption was crazy, she understood—not even in the realm of possibility—but she made him promise to hear the boys sing. And "crazy" became a calling for both of them. If the TerKeursts weren't the sort of people who trusted in the power of friendship, the story would end here. But once they'd determined that they could not let any of these orphans return to the danger and poverty of their homeland, the couple knew they had to get their friends involved. They arranged a cookout in their backyard to introduce the choir.

Sitting on the deck of the TerKeurst home listening to the children sing, Genia Rogers started sobbing uncontrollably. "It was their graciousness and joy," says Genia, a 42-year-old nutritional consultant. "Despite what they'd witnessed, these were not broken boys; they were whole and courageous. Some of my reaction came from my own experience: I'd been fighting a pretty significant illness and had started healing. I'd been thinking about redemption and restoration, and I had 12 examples right in front of me. Something shifted in the world—the word *adventure* kept coming to my mind."

Genia and her husband, Rob, were immediately drawn to a lanky, smiling boy named Robert. After two miscarriages, the Rogers already had what Genia calls "a huge heart for adoption, the process and the opportunity"—their son and daughter had been adopted as newborns. Bringing a teenager into their lives would raise a multitude of issues, not least of which was rearranging the family birth order that psychologists say is so significant to childhood development: Twelve-year-old Robert would displace their 10-year-old son as firstborn. "And he's a kid who doesn't transition well," says Genia. "But when we talked to him, he said, 'There's good change and there's bad change, and this is a good change.' Robert was in our house three weeks later. It was meant to be: His birthday is the same as the due date for one of my lost pregnancies."

Having the Rogers family validate their adoption plan gave the TerKeursts confidence to proceed, especially in light of the apprehension that the rest of their circle seemed to share. "I thought all my friends would go 'hip hip hooray' and start planning my teenage boys' baby shower," says Lysa. "But they were all saying, 'It's not safe.' 'Have you thought about the security of your girls?' I started thinking, *I love these boys, but they could stand over my bed with a hatchet one night.* We decided to invite the boys to sing at our church. It was never on our radar that anybody else would be interested in adopting—we did it so that the congregation would have a vision for welcoming our sons. That night the friends who'd had such huge concerns all signed up to be parents of Liberian boys."

Becky Peed was one of those friends who'd reacted with

LIVING IN THE WORLD

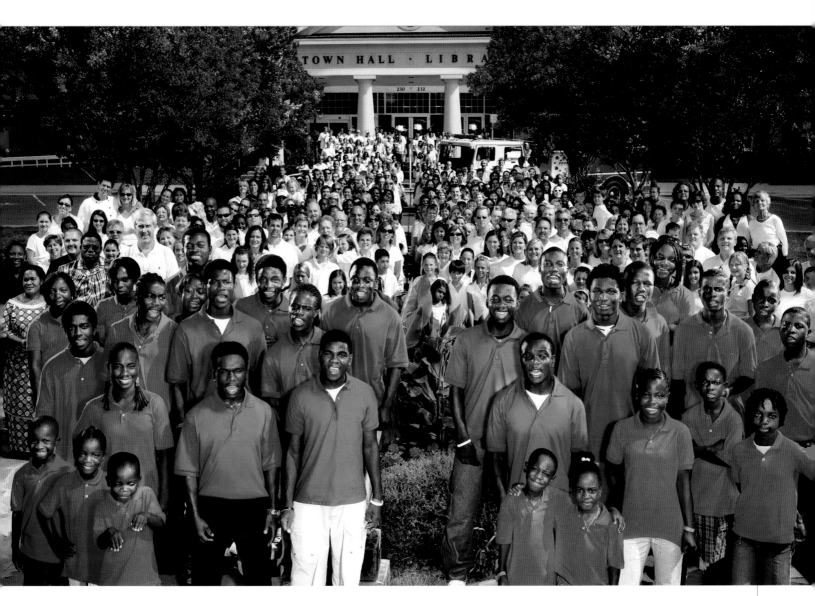

In blue, ten of the 12 original members of the Liberian choir sing alongside their brothers and sisters in red.
First Row: Melvin Covert, Kolu Apodaca, James Gale, Davis Osepchuk, Jada Osepchuk. **Second Row:** Dora Peed, George Brewer, Sam Peed, David Alexander, Patience Apodaca, Justice Haywood, Angel Nemiloy. **Third Row:** Isaiah Haywood, Joe Alexander, Abraham Haywood, Seeboe Alexander, Robert Rogers, Nyan Cianciosa, John Haywood, James Alexander. **Fourth Row:** Teta Alexander, Mala Brewer, Tina Wilkie, Jackson TerKeurst, Mark TerKeurst, Barcon Jackson, Eric Haywood. **Fifth Row:** Roosevelt Haywood, Mercy Alexander, Zinnah Apodaca.

rolling eyes at the idea of adopting teenage war orphans. "I was curious and a little excited about meeting them because of Lysa," says the 41-year-old former flight attendant, "and I went to hear them with an open mind, but I wasn't going to find a son." After the church concert, Becky and her husband, David, had three young children lobbying for an older brother (she reminded them that they weren't talking about a new puppy) but didn't really make a one-on-one connection until a few days later, at a soccer game, when one of the choirboys, a 14-year-old named Sam, sought them out. "He said he felt like he needed to talk," says Becky. "Of course the boys were courting parents—they knew the desperation of their situation. If I were in the same situation, I'd be trying to do that, too. And when we went out to the movies, that's when we saw his sense of humor. He has a contagious laugh and an innocence about him. I knew he was the kind of child who would fit into our home." What she didn't know

until Sam joined their family was that children at the Liberian orphanage were often assigned a "mission brother" or "mission sister" so they would feel less alone. Within months, the Peeds had sent for Sam's 14-year-old mission sister, Dora. "We had room and we had love," says Becky. "How could we say no?"

Debbie Alexander was at church the same night as the Peeds. A 48-year-old empty-nester with two sons in college, she was planning on going back to school herself. But as the music took its hold on her, she felt "like a moth drawn to flame." By the following evening, she knew that she and her husband, David, had to adopt two of the boys, David and Seeboe, both 13, because one might be lonely in a house with no other children. "I'm living my psychology major," says Debbie. The boys did not speak much about the atrocities they'd witnessed, but they did say that they'd come to America without having a chance to say goodbye to brothers and sisters at the orphanage—the choirboys weren't

277

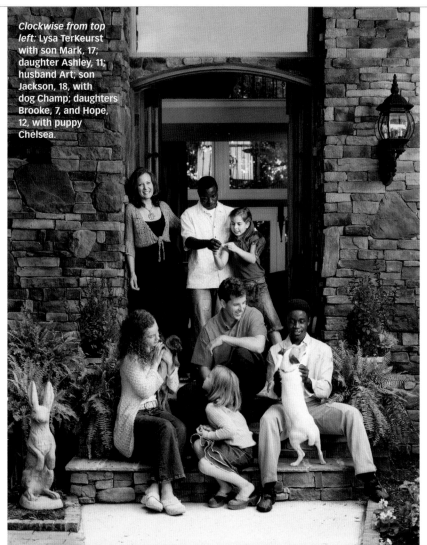

Clockwise from top left: Lysa TerKeurst with son Mark, 17; daughter Ashley, 11; husband Art; son Jackson, 18, with dog Champ; daughters Brooke, 7, and Hope, 12, with puppy Chelsea.

adopting, and once she saw a photo of a toddler named Prince in an ACFI pamphlet, her husband, John, joined a missionary trip to Liberia. He called his wife with good news and a kicker: "You're going to love Prince. And there's a Princess." He left almost everything in his possession at the orphanage, from the money in his wallet to the clothes in his suitcase, and put into place a plan to bring home the 4-year-old twins, renamed Davis and Jada.

By December 2006, there were 15 families with 35 Liberian children in the Charlotte area, and their friendships have sustained them. There have been shared financial issues: In order for the adoptions to go through, the families banded together to hire a lawyer and acquire the heartbreaking death certificates of the children's biological parents. (There was little variety—the words *gunshot wound, beating,* and *drowning* were most common.) There have been shared emotional issues, including the subtle or not-so-subtle racism of extended family members. (One grandmother, presented with the idea of a black teenage grandson, declared, "I don't know how I'll begin to tell people about this.") And there have been shared practical matters, like caring for black skin and hair unfamiliar to these white mothers. Donna Osepchuk was quite proud of the braids she made for Jada until she happened to meet an African-American teacher in the hall of the little girl's school, and the woman offered, "You know, I could help you with her hair."

English is spoken in Liberia, which was founded by freed American slaves in the early 19th century, but the dialect can be difficult to understand—the adopted children have been learning to speak "American," and some have been home-schooled to facilitate their assimilation. One night at dinner, Jada stopped eating because her teeth hurt, and her parents realized that she'd been trying to gnaw on the chicken bones. (Often there was just one meal a day at the orphanage: rice with chicken cooked so long that the bones were soft enough to eat.) And since chores and behavior in Liberia were quite different for girls than boys, says Donna Osepchuk, "Jada didn't know how to hold a pen, but she could fold laundry like nobody's business."

Much of Liberia was without electricity or running water, and the new Americans had to learn how things like elevators, washing machines, and refrigerators worked—they'd help unload groceries from the car without realizing which items were to be kept cold. Many of the children arrived with only the clothes on their back; their parents were

even told where they were going when they were driven to the Monrovia airport, to protect them from anyone who might try to take their place on the plane. The Alexanders kept thinking about those siblings left behind. And about a year after David and Seeboe arrived, four more children joined the Alexander family: Seeboe's 14-year-old mission brother, Joe, and David's three biological siblings: 8-year-old James, 12-year-old Teta, and 15-year-old Mercy.

Every one of the original 12 choirboys found homes. The adopting families say, with a consistent and almost mystical refrain, that it just sort of became clear who belonged where. And their presence in the community drew so much attention to the plight of Liberian children that the African Christians Fellowship International (ACFI), the ministry running the rebuilt orphanage, received inquiries about more adoptions. Donna Osepchuk, a 46-year-old former special education teacher, had four children of her own, but she'd always thought of

"I called my husband and said, 'Do we need milk and what would you think of adopting two teenage boys from Liberia?' He said, 'Get home now.'"

surprised that they didn't always show gratitude for the new possessions that came with life in America. "They imagined we had money trees in our backyards," says Genia Rogers. "Robert literally thought it didn't rain here and was shocked that there are poor people." The parents were counseled that they might sometimes see a "war face" on their child. "It's hard for them to express feelings; for so long there was no one to tell," explains Debbie Alexander. "Talking about feelings was a luxury that couldn't be indulged, so the children would withdraw. The big adjustment has been a matter of trust and learning how to live with structure."

Some cultural differences are more amusing than worrisome. Donna Osepchuk weathered stares in the supermarket when her kids chanted the songs of civil war from their homeland. The TerKeursts' two new sons were horrified at the idea of a pet dog or cat—all four-legged creatures were considered livestock, certainly

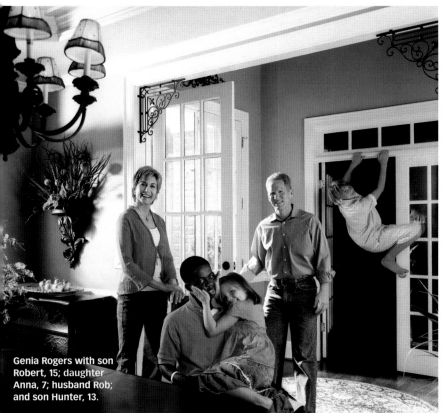

Genia Rogers with son Robert, 15; daughter Anna, 7; husband Rob; and son Hunter, 13.

not deserving of a name, let alone a place in the home. Thirteen-year-old George, who became the son of Judy and Keith Brewer, had the notion that real men are not supposed to smile. And his 12-year-old sister Mala resisted affectionate gestures, informing her new parents, "Hugs and kisses aren't used to me." Mala believes that math is evil and learning is for boys. "These children have to be taught just to ask, 'How was your day?' " says Judy. But when a child has had to walk over dead bodies, as Mala did leaving Monrovia, a longer learning curve is understandable.

The lives of the adopting parents have changed in both prosaic and profound ways. "We pulled all our children out of private school, knowing that it would be a challenge to pay three tuitions

and that it might be an intimidating place for Robert to start his formal education," says Genia Rogers. "We moved to the country, where I never would have ventured in my former life, so that we could be in a lower property tax zone, near the children's new charter school and also closer to the other families that adopted the boys. Our friend base changed considerably. And I went back to work, knowing that we had a tighter time frame to prepare financially for college."

For Debbie Alexander, the logistics of a large family are dramatically different. "We live by schedules and car pools," she says. "We have a schedule for laundry, kitchen cleaning, a sheet that's signed by the children and myself when allowances are given. I am not an overly organized person, but I've had to become one just to survive." Debbie has a new and deeply felt appreciation for what she previously took for granted. "Our children came never knowing what it was like to feel full or be able to sleep in a bed without pulling the covers over your head to keep the rats from biting. The word *struggle* has taken on a very different meaning."

"It's been a stretching experience," Lysa TerKeurst confirms. "And it's not like I sat around before and thought, *I have a lot of white space in my life.* My schedule is fuller, and our budget is tighter." But the more powerful outcome of the adoptions is what she calls a new sweetness for her family. "It's one thing to tell my kids we should have a heart to help the poor, but it's completely different to see it lived out in our home every single day. We recognize that our little peace, our comfortable home, our beautiful car is not what the world is like. In one sense, it breaks my heart because I know the people behind those random faces now. My boys could be in that world news report—my boys that I tuck into bed every night could be in those statistics. It gives me joy to know that I didn't walk away, that I am living my life well and making a difference and doing my part."

Genia Rogers often reminds herself that the experience was a near miss. "This is a story of courageous friendship," she says, "of people saying, 'It doesn't make sense on paper, but we should do it.' All the blessings of my life have come from stepping over a precipice when I could have what-if'd myself out of a decision."

The Liberian boys are now so fully assimilated into their American lives that it seems as if family photos from the time before they arrived are missing something. In fact, the assimilation is so complete that these families have come close to achieving something fairly uncommon in our culture: color blindness. The children themselves often forget that they aren't related by birth. Recently, Seeboe Alexander was describing his urgent desire to grow taller. "Kids generally are tall if their parents are tall," explained his mother, to which Seeboe replied, "But Dad is tall...." ▣

For more information about the ACFI and how you can help, go to acfinet.org.

A Phenomenal Woman

She was just 26, and blind, when she rode into Tibet (on horseback, no less!) to found a school where blind children could learn to read Braille, speak three languages, take care of themselves, teach each other, and put a joyous new spin on the idea of the blind leading the blind. ROSEMARY MAHONEY listens and learns from—and tries to keep pace with—the spectacular Sabriye Tenberken.

Sabriye Tenberken has, among many other things, notably long legs. She walks fast and with authority. Accustomed to walking arm-in-arm with companions, she's hooked her elbow in mine. Linked in this way, I find that for every step she takes through the streets of Lhasa, I'm forced to take a step and a half. I have been in Lhasa less than 24 hours, and its unaccustomed high altitude (at nearly 12,000 feet above sea level, Lhasa is the second-highest capital city in the world) and consequent lack of oxygen have rendered me breathless, lightheaded, and physically clumsy. Not 40 seconds into our walk, I stumble over a pile of granite stones that have been dumped in the middle of the street. Tenberken, who is saying, "People always ask me when did I go blind…" interrupts herself to steady me, then gently guides me to the edge of Chingdol Dong Lu, where heavy Chinese traffic, with an illogic all its own, careers by in both directions. Tenberken lifts her chin a fraction, cocks her head in concentration, waits for a break in the lanes of eastward-rushing traffic, then leads me swiftly to the center of the avenue, where, to my dismay, we pause atop the yellow dividing line. Large vehicles are roaring by so close to us that the wind they whip up tosses Tenberken's long blonde hair across her mouth as she talks. "But I can never say when exactly I went blind," she says, white cane held lightly in her fingers, voice rising to compete with the noise. "It was gradual. I began to realize that a color I thought was green was really blue. I couldn't see words I was writing. I thought I could see, but I couldn't."

A small break appears in the two lanes of traffic rushing west, and at just the right moment Tenberken applies a light pressure to my arm and we plunge forward and cross safely to the far side of the street. There, without breaking her stride, she hops nimbly over a shin-high length of chain that delineates the bicycle lane from the rest of the traffic. She turns left at the next corner, where a woman selling dumplings from a bamboo pot stares at her in wide-eyed astonishment. I can hardly blame the woman, for I'm staring too, mystified as to how Tenberken manages to navigate the city this way. She hurries across an empty lot, turns

> "People tried to put limits on me, but limits always show opportunities. I persisted because I believed it was possible."

slightly left again, straight for a minute, veers around a pile of rubble, expertly dodges the scores of bicycles blowing past us in the narrow alleys, turns left again, then right. I have to maintain a hectic little skipping trot to keep up with her. As we stride up yet another narrow street, a little girl sitting on a stoop spots Tenberken through the crowd, springs to her feet, and crows at the top of her lungs, *"Xia ze lai le!"* A simple Chinese sentence, it means, *Gangway! Here comes an idiot!*

Tenberken laughs, softly repeats the words, and carries on. In the years she's spent living in Tibet—and indeed in the 27 in her native Germany before that—she's been the object of this phrase, and worse, countless times. Sabriye Tenberken (pronounced Sah-bree-yah Ten-BURR-ken) single-handed has brought literacy to the blind people of Tibet. In founding the Lhasa-based Braille Without Borders (BWB) in 1998, the region's first rehabilitation and training center for the blind, she has inspired nothing short of a revolution in their status, their thinking, their future. She and her partner in life, Paul Kronenberg, who handles much of the practical work of the school, have been knighted by the Dutch queen. She has also won numerous honors and awards for her work. She is hardly an idiot. "You cannot insult me with blindness," she says, "because I'm proud to be blind." These days epithets leave her unfazed; they didn't always.

Born with a degenerative retinal disease, Tenberken was blind by 12. In her early years, she was able to make out faces, colors, landscapes, but her vision was highly impaired, and as a result her schoolteachers approached her with what she felt was a patronizing deference that set her apart. Her classmates spurned and taunted her, gave her false directions in order to watch her tumble down a flight of stairs. They told her she was ugly; unable to see her own face, she believed the lie. Determined to fit in, Tenberken denied her blindness to herself and worked overtime to hide it. At a bus stop, she would ask a bystander to read the schedule for her with the excuse that she had something stuck in her eye. Or she simply got on the wrong bus, too proud to ask where the bus was going.

Sabriye Tenberken, at 34, at the school's training farm, 2004. She rode from village to village persuading Tibetans that their blind children could learn.

Sitting in the bright offices of Braille Without Borders, Tenberken leans forward and says, "Not accepting that I was blind was miserable." As she speaks, the delighted shrieks of 20 blind children at recess drift in from the sun-blanched school courtyard beyond the window. "I was constantly compensating and pretending." She pauses to think and with visible emotion adds, "Not until I accepted my blindness did I begin to live."

Tenberken enrolled at a boarding school for the blind, where among academic subjects the students were taught horseback riding, swimming, white-water rafting, Braille, and, above all, self-reliance. "Suddenly, I was one among many," she tells me. "I had friends. I was equal and happy. We had Braille. For the first time in my life, I actually read an entire book. I read *Dr. Faustus* and Shakespeare. I thought, *Okay. I may be ugly and blind, but I have a brain. I can do things.*"

For the record, Tenberken's long, oval face is quite the opposite of ugly—she has a Roman sort of beauty. But perhaps her most appealing feature is her manner. She is genial, direct, deeply focused, and speaks with a great deal of visual description. She will tell you that a person blushed, a landscape was beautiful, a film she "saw" was frightening. There's a refreshing lack of performance in her persona, no overweening eagerness to please, no

calculation, false intimacy, or guile. She looks directly at you and listens with an air of such intelligence and alert expectation that you find yourself regretting you're not a more articulate, more interesting person. Though Tenberken is blessed with a wry sense of humor and a big, appreciative laugh, her natural mien is one of seriousness and quiet conviction. She and Kronenberg are devoted to their cause.

Tenberken majored in central Asian studies at the University of Bonn, the only blind student out of 30,000. There, several professors tried to dissuade her from studying the difficult Tibetan language. There were no Tibetan texts available in Braille. How would she read? How would she keep up? Tenberken ignored their discouragements and immersed herself in her courses. Using the system of rhythmic spelling Tibetans employ to memorize their complex language, Tenberken created her own method of translating the Tibetan language into Braille. With a specially adapted Braille writing machine she found she was able to take notes far faster than her classmates. She compiled a Tibetan-German/German-Tibetan dictionary, and when sighted students began asking for help, she was vindicated and delighted. Eventually, Tenberken helped to devise a software system that enabled her to transpose entire Tibetan texts into formally printed Braille, a feat no one before had ever accomplished.

"I developed this system for my own use," she says, "but when I realized that blind people in Tibet could also benefit from it, I got the idea to bring it here and start a school." In a pattern of skepticism that even now Tenberken faces daily, almost all her professors told her that her idea was absurd—it would be impossible for a blind woman to do. "*Stay on the ground!* is what people always say," she says, smiling ironically. "*Don't give false hope to the blind!*" Rejected by several development organizations, who saw her blindness as too great a liability, Tenberken resolved to make the project happen on her own. In 1997, at the age of 26, much to the dismay of everyone but her immediate family, she traveled alone to China, took an intensive course in Chinese, then proceeded to Tibet, where she learned that more than 30,000 of Tibet's 2.6 million people are blind—about twice the global rate. While poor diet and unhygienic conditions are factors, Tibet's main cause of blindness is its high elevation; at this altitude the intensity of the sun's ultraviolet rays causes damage to the unprotected eye.

Tenberken also discovered a deep prejudice against the blind in Tibet, where blindness is considered punishment for misdeeds perpetrated in a past life. Many Tibetans believe the blind are cursed or possessed by demons; in parts of Tibet it's thought that merely touching a blind person can render one impure. For centuries Tibet's blind have been shunned, vilified, and generally treated as subhuman. When Tenberken first arrived, she found not a single institution or organization geared to provide assistance for the region's blind—clearly a result of this deep-seated fear and opprobrium.

Tenberken decided to travel through remote areas of the countryside, visiting rural villages, spreading the word about her Braille system, assessing the situation of blind children there. When she concluded that the best way to do this was on

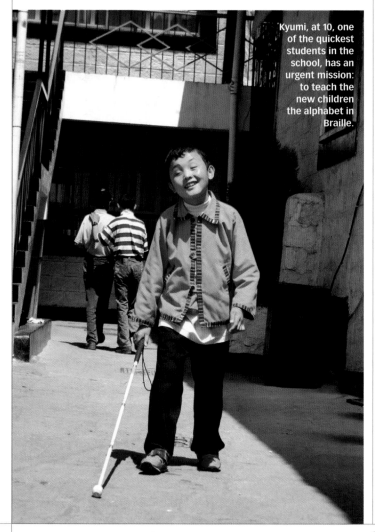

Kyumi, at 10, one of the quickest students in the school, has an urgent mission: to teach the new children the alphabet in Braille.

horseback, there were more howls of protest from the skeptics. Nevertheless she set off with three supportive companions, two of whom were Tibetan, riding from village to village, across high mountain passes, through flooded rivers. What she found appalled her: a small child who, because of her blindness, was tethered to a bed all day, her tiny body withered with misuse; others, barred from the local schools, who regularly had stones thrown at them, who were taunted and jeered at and locked in dark rooms for years. Isolated, disrespected, sometimes beaten, abandoned, or turned out in the streets to beg, almost all were illiterate and uneducated. When villagers saw Tenberken walking, riding a horse, they refused at first to believe she was blind. Tenberken persuaded them that though blind, their children, too, could ride horses, read, and write. One astounded father told her, "The prospect of your school is like a dream for us."

A group of blind children and I are sitting in the dining room at Braille Without Borders, waiting for a beginner's Braille class to start. I'm already acquainted with two, having sat in a car with them on the long ride to Lhasa from Shigatse, where Tenberken and Kronenberg have established a farm to train blind adults in agriculture and farm management. Arriving at the farm, we'd found these two boys sitting alone in the kitchen—hearing about the project, their families had dropped them here a few days earlier. Panden Tsering was 6, Kileh was 14, too young to stay at the farm. Tenberken invited them to attend her school in Lhasa, and without hesitation both boys said yes. We were three unfamiliar foreign adults, yet when it came time to leave Shigatse, they climbed eagerly, smilingly into the car with us. They carried nothing. No luggage, no diverting toys or gadgets, no toothbrush, nothing but the clothes on their backs. Though they knew Lhasa was far and they wouldn't see their families again for months, they made no protest during the arduous ten-hour ride over rutted dirt roads. I marveled at their level of trust and realized I did not know a single American child who would willingly do what they were doing. I asked Panden Tsering if he was happy; the face he made in response said, *Are you nuts! I'm thrilled!* I asked Tenberken why they joined us so trustingly. She said, "They have nothing. No friends, no future. Perhaps they're so low they feel they have nothing to lose."

Now the boys and I are sitting together in Lhasa, waiting to learn the Tibetan alphabet. One tiny boy has his pants on backward. Another is wearing his sneakers on the wrong feet. Some have damaged eyes. One seems to have no eyes at all. Some sit with their eyes closed. Those who can see traces of light with one or both eyes tend to squint a lot and screw up their faces. They tilt their heads at sounds and run their hands over everything within reach, seeing the world in an alternative way. On a shelf near my head, I can see a book: *The Little Mermaid* in Braille, edited by Sabriye Tenberken and printed by Braille Without Borders.

> One astounded father told Tenberken, "The prospect of your school is like a dream to us."

Presently, the door bangs open and Kyumi, the teacher, comes importantly into the room. "Now," he announces, "we learn Tibetan alphabet!" Kyumi is 10, but like many of the children here, he looks four years younger than his age. His pants are three sizes too big for him. He is blind. He has been a student at BWB for the past four years. Kyumi has a large head and big ears that stick out like two handles on a coffee mug. His wide, rosy-cheeked face is roughly the shape of a pie plate. His one open eye is an unnatural glacial blue. At times he shakes his hands in the air in a trembling way, as if they're on fire, a trait known as blindism.

Kyumi moves with great purpose. He has no time to lose in small talk. He crosses the room, puts his hand on the shoulder of a new boy, runs his hand down the boy's arm until he finds the fingers, then plants the tip of the boy's index finger firmly on a Braille text on the table in front of him. *"Ka!"* he cries, the first letter of the Tibetan alphabet. The new boy bends over the table, his nose touching the page, and minutely examining the tiny bumps of Braille he says, *"Ka!"* Kyumi feels his way to the next boy and repeats the process. Eventually, all heads are bent low in concentration. Kyumi's teaching style is both lordly and intimate. Like all the veteran students here, he can operate a Braille typewriter and a computer, can dress and wash himself, is learning to cook, can speak English and Chinese as well as his native Tibetan—in short, Kyumi can do more than most sighted Tibetan children his age. Though his voice is high and piping, his English has a British diplomat's precision and flourish. He speaks in a kind of shriek, wraps his arm around students' shoulders, presses his forehead against theirs, and entreats them as if it's a matter of national importance to repeat after him. He moves from student to student, tsking and sighing as if overburdened with responsibility, yet it's clear he relishes his status as one of the quickest students in the school.

The new children are getting the hang of the alphabet, sounding out the letters and smiling at their own fingers sliding over the pocked papers before them. I ask Kyumi a question unrelated to the class, and he lifts his head at me abruptly, as if he's forgotten I'm there. "Rose?" he says, stepping toward me. His big eyes are slightly crossed. He reaches for my arm, puts his face close to mine, and answers my question. I thank him. He tells me it is his pleasure to help me, then pauses to rest a sympathetic hand on my shoulder. "Rose?" he pipes.

"Yes, Kyumi?"

"Can you listen now and learn while I teach these men and women?" I apologize for the interruption, promise not to do it again. He wags his head and says with a kind of noblesse oblige, "No problem, Rose. But...," and raising a correcting finger at me, he says with undisguised concern about my intellectual abilities, "please, *try* to listen and learn."

Minutes pass. We listen and learn. The door swings open again, and Migmar, a tiny, mischievous girl of 12, flies into the room chewing gum with the insouciant flair of a swindler. From a nearby classroom the sound of communal singing follows her in.

Oprah Talks to
A Phenomenal Man: Archbishop Desmond Tutu

He's a man with an exuberant laugh and a generous heart to match—my friend Archbishop Desmond Tutu. In his seventies, he can tell you about the rise of apartheid, the marches and rebellions in Soweto that led to its collapse, and the AIDS pandemic now ravaging Africa. Just when you think the conversation has turned particularly dismal, he throws back his head and breaks out in laughter.

How does a man who grew up with the indignities of government-sanctioned segregation survive to become a Nobel laureate, the first black Anglican archbishop of Cape Town, and someone who can still laugh and love? Born in Klerksdorp, South Africa, in 1931, Tutu dreamed of becoming a physician, but because his parents didn't have the money to send him to medical school, he became a teacher, like his father. After three years, he resigned in protest of the Bantu Education Act, which mandated that black children be taught only enough to prepare them for menial labor. Tutu decided to study theology; he was ordained by the Anglican Church in 1960. His pacifist crusade for the end of apartheid earned him a place in history—and, on October 16, 1984, the Nobel Peace Prize. Tutu has been married to his wife, Leah, for over 50 years, and together they have four children.

OPRAH: *Your latest book is called* God Has a Dream. *What is God's dream?*

ARCHBISHOP TUTU: God's dream is that we could know that we are members of one family. There are no outsiders—black, white, rich, poor, male, female, gay, lesbian, and so-called straight. Bin Laden. Bush. Sharon. They all belong.

OPRAH: *Can peace between countries exist in our lifetime? Isn't that idealistic?*

ARCHBISHOP TUTU: God is an idealist. Look at South Africa before 1994. Who could have imagined that we would have a country where black and white, the formerly oppressed and their oppressors, would live [peacefully] in one country? I knew it was possible because it is God's will. None of us seems to accept that we are incredibly precious—that when I dehumanize you, I am dehumanized. We saw that in South Africa with those who carried out the awful policies of apartheid. In the end, they actually needed the [forgiveness of the] victims to help them recover their humanity.

OPRAH: *Isn't South Africa still a country of white prosperity and black poverty?*

ARCHBISHOP TUTU: Absolutely. If we do not quickly and dramatically narrow the gap between rich and poor, we can kiss reconciliation goodbye. Aside from poverty, the other issue is AIDS. But when you look at countries like Uganda, where there has been a massive campaign, you see that it's possible to turn the situation around.

OPRAH: *One thing that fascinates me about you and Nelson Mandela is that you could endure the horrors of apartheid and still have a loving spirit. How can you not be bitter?*

ARCHBISHOP TUTU: Human beings are fantastic. During the Truth and Reconciliation Commission hearings [in which apartheid's victims testified along with perpetrators asking for clemency], I was devastated at the revelations of our capacity for evil. But that's not the end of the story, nor is it the most important part. The exhilaration was in discovering our capacity for good. We listened to a woman say, "They undressed me, opened a drawer, shoved my breast into the drawer, and slammed the drawer several times on my nipple." I'd say, "God, how could we possibly have sunk to such levels?" And then I'd hear a victim of such an atrocity say, "I am ready to forgive." South Africa has become a testament to the fact that people are fundamentally good. Yes, there is evil. But it's not the norm. The norm is good. That's why our hearts are uplifted when we meet a Mother Teresa, a Dalai Lama, a Nelson Mandela...

OPRAH: *A Bishop Tutu.*

ARCHBISHOP TUTU: Thank you.

OPRAH: *What were the worst stories you heard during the three years you led the hearings?*

ARCHBISHOP TUTU: "I shot him in the head, and then we burned his body." It takes seven or eight hours for a human body to burn. While the body was burning, they'd drink beer.

OPRAH: *And this person was asking for forgiveness?*

ARCHBISHOP TUTU: Yes. The commission said that if you wanted to be exonerated, you had to accuse yourself.

OPRAH: *How can you hear such stories and then go home and eat dinner with your family?*

ARCHBISHOP TUTU: We were told not to be like vacuum cleaners—taking in dirt and keeping it in a bag—but like dishwashers, taking in dirt, then passing it out. Otherwise, we would have been traumatized. Even so, one goes away from that process amazed at the magnanimity and nobility of humans. The commission gave some victims the opportunity to realize that their heroism had contributed.

> "Our world is going to be okay."

OPRAH: *How we can help to stop suffering throughout the world?*

ARCHBISHOP TUTU: Western governments supported apartheid. I went to the White House in 1984 to say, "Please, can you impose sanctions?" No. Then the so-called ordinary people said, "We're not going to tolerate this." People were prepared to be arrested on our behalf. We shouldn't think of ourselves as impotent. We can change things.

OPRAH: *What can we do now to help in South Africa?*

ARCHBISHOP TUTU: Continue to care. And have your caring translate into putting a hand in your pocket. We shouldn't feel uneasy about mentioning money.

OPRAH: *I met your wonderful wife. I think it would have been difficult to be married to someone whose life is occupied with this struggle. Has it been?*

ARCHBISHOP TUTU: My wife, Leah, is quite fantastic. I remember one of the apartheid ministers saying, "Bishop Tutu talks too much." So I asked Leah, "Would you like me to keep quiet?" I'll never forget her answer. She said, "I'd much rather you were happy on Robben Island in prison than unhappy quiet." I wouldn't be where I am without her. She's a great deal more politically radical than I am. She's a fire-eater. I realized in the Truth and Reconciliation Commission that we would not have gotten freedom without the women.

OPRAH: *In order for there to be real peace in the world...*

ARCHBISHOP TUTU: I want to suggest that women start a revolution.

OPRAH: *Okay! I'm all for that. Tell me: What do you know for sure?*

ARCHBISHOP TUTU: That God loves us—and we're lovable because he loves us. Each of us is of infinite worth.

OPRAH: *And you're hopeful for the planet?*

ARCHBISHOP TUTU: Oh, absolutely. Our world is a work in progress. It's going to be okay. **O**

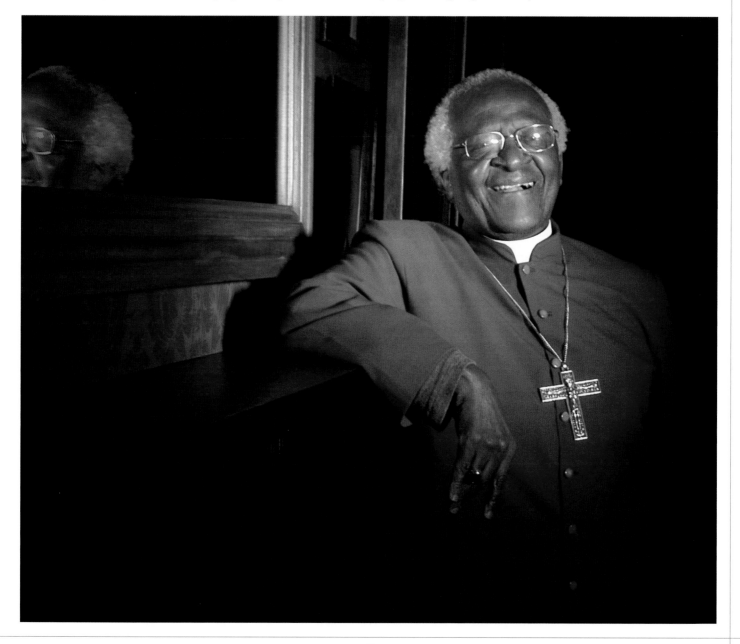

287

A Law Unto Herself

In 2003, in a case that made headlines around the world, Hauwa Ibrahim saved a young woman accused of adultery from death by stoning. In the process, Ibrahim became the first woman ever to stand up, defy tradition, and address a Nigerian Islamic court directly. Since then she's managed to keep scores of women from being stoned and small-time thieves from losing their hands. DINA TEMPLE-RASTON reports on the lawyer reforming justice in Nigeria one defendant at a time.

I n March of 2002, as much of the world still reeled from the image of two planes slamming into the Twin Towers, another chilling vision took hold: A young Nigerian woman, Amina Lawal, was sentenced to be buried in the ground up to her shoulders and, in front of anyone who cared to watch, stoned until she died.

Lawal's crime was having sex while unmarried; the little girl, born more than ten months after she left her husband, the evidence. And in northern Nigeria, where one of the largest concentrations of Muslims on the African continent live, that made her an adulterer—an offense punishable by death. The judges gave her two years to breastfeed her daughter before the execution.

"When I met Amina, she was ready to die," Hauwa Ibrahim, Lawal's defense attorney, tells me on a rainy afternoon in New Haven, where she is a fellow at Yale University until June 2006. "I think she had given up, had lost her faith in life. She is like many victims of Sharia law." Drawn from the Koran, teachings of the Prophet Mohammed, and interpretations by Muslim scholars, *Sharia* literally means "the path to the watering hole" and offers Muslims rules to live by—dictating everything from modest dress to the number of times a day they must pray to how unmarried lovers should be penalized. "The victims of Sharia are very poor," says Ibrahim. "They have no voice; they are powerless."

Head swathed in a flowing scarf, Ibrahim glides into a conversation like the tide—graceful, unstoppable—no hint of sharpness or aggression, yet with the kind of force that won't be denied.

"I understand what it means to have no voice," she says with a smile, and in an instant it's evident how this charismatic 38-year-old just might be the woman to upend hundreds of years of hardened tradition.

Fifty percent of Nigeria's population are Muslim, and though Sharia operated on a local level when the country was a colony, the British did not permit the enforcement of amputations or executions. Even after Nigeria's independence in 1960, its new leaders, fearing Sharia's harsh discipline would inflame tensions between Muslims in the north and Christians in the south, continued to rely on secular courts based on British common law. That all changed in 1999, however, when the first of 12 states in the north adopted Sharia as the formal law of the land for its Muslim residents.

Ibrahim was one of the few women lawyers working in northern Nigeria when a local non-governmental organization (NGO) asked if she would put together a defense team for a pregnant 13-year-old girl who'd been sentenced under Sharia. The girl, a hunchback, said she was raped after men from the village slipped something into her Coke. A judge sentenced her to 100 whips with a leather strap. But when the three alleged rapists claimed she was lying, he added 80 more whippings. "That's when I came in," says Ibrahim.

But she wasn't able to help. Although the state forgave the extra 80 flogs, the teenager still had to face 100. "That was one of my worst cases," says Ibrahim, even now shaken by the verdict, "because the state wouldn't let us appeal."

Ninety cases later, Ibrahim has become the go-to lawyer for Sharia legal matters. More than half of them have involved boys and men charged with stealing, sentenced to have a hand or foot or both amputated. Ten to 15 percent have been adultery cases, mostly women, facing death by stoning.

"These are cases of deep injustice," says Ibrahim, who works pro bono. "People say I am anti-Sharia. I am not. But there is something in me that hates injustice," she tells me, sitting up straight to emphasize her point. "I fight it naturally. And that is what I am trying to do now."

Ibrahim's unique strategy is arguing Sharia with Sharia—because despite its barbaric reputation, she says the Islamic law does contain intricate checks and balances that, when used and recognized in court, can protect the innocent from terrible punishments.

H auwa Ibrahim started life in much the same way Amina Lawal did. She grew up as part of a traditional Muslim family in Hinnah, a small village in the northern Nigerian state of Gombe. Her father had three wives and kept his household under strict rule. As a low-level general officer in the Nigerian customs office, his salary was paltry and the family lived in a hut without water or electricity. Ibrahim's mother collected firewood and sold it in the village market to feed her five children.

Amid such poverty, it was considered an auspicious day when about 50 pounds of salt arrived from a friend of Ibrahim's father. Ibrahim was only 13 when she saw the burlap sack and found out it was payment for her hand in marriage. The man was older than her father. In the family, she explains, her mother didn't have much say. "So I went to my father's favorite wife, who liked me, and I asked her to help me. I said to her, 'I don't think this marriage is a good idea; I want to go to school.' "

How a young girl from rural Gombe came to believe so strongly in education that she was willing to defy family and tradition is hard for even Ibrahim herself to pinpoint. There was the photograph of a woman in a newspaper, though—a graduate of some sort, complete with mortarboard and gown. When Ibrahim saw it, she was entranced. "I wanted to have the confidence the woman in the picture had," she says. "I wanted to have a voice and walk with my shoulders straight. My mother had told me that if I was a little educated, I wouldn't have to sell vegetables in the market. All I knew was that I didn't want to be like my mother."

When Ibrahim refused to marry, her father threw her out of the house. Forced to go live with an uncle, she managed to attend elementary school and then a teachers college, the lowest rung of Nigeria's high school system, earning money while not in class by picking tomatoes and collecting wood. After graduating, however, she was shipped off to live with her older sister and help with housekeeping, as was customary.

Though the move seemed defeating, it delivered her to a town that had electricity—and a house with a television. Watching it one evening, Ibrahim happened to see a woman who said she wanted to help girls in Nigeria go to school. As soon as she could, Ibrahim set off to find her.

When she arrived at the woman's office, however, a security guard held her off. "I didn't look important, so I wasn't allowed to see her," says Ibrahim. But she persisted. "I must have visited that office more than 30 times over two months. And finally the guard said to me, 'Young girl, I am tired of seeing you. Just go up and see her.' "

Ibrahim found herself walking into the office of the state's information commissioner. "I saw you on TV," she said, "and I need your help to get into school." She explained her situation, told the commissioner about her father's opposition to her continued education, and then presented her school transcript. "I want to go to university," she said.

The commissioner looked at her wide-eyed. "You've got guts," she declared in English, a language that Ibrahim—who grew up speaking the native Hausa—understood poorly at the time. She quickly wrote down the word *guts* to look up later in her dictionary.

In fact, her lagging English would plague her. As impressed as the commissioner was by Ibrahim's moxie, she was less supportive when she examined the school records. "Your marks in English aren't good enough," she said to the girl. "You can't go to university."

Ibrahim told the commissioner she'd heard of a remedial university program that allowed students to repeat a year to correct

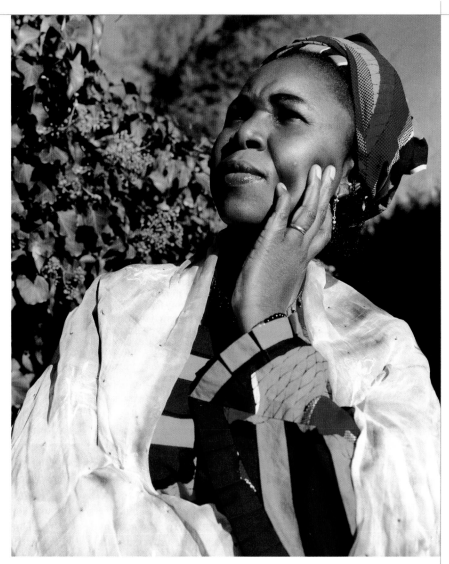

Instead of marrying at 13, Hauwa Ibrahim left home and fought for an education. Sweet, stubborn, like a tree that will not be moved, she's taking to task the harshest Islamic courts and making them rule more justly.

any deficiencies in their studies—perhaps she could take it. Also, she added, she had already signed up for an extra English course.

"Even if you go to the remedial program, I don't think you can make it through the university," the woman said. "I'm sorry I can't—"

"Just try me," Ibrahim said finally.

The woman looked at her a long moment. She took out one of her business cards and wrote something on the back. There were no guarantees, she stressed, handing it to Ibrahim. "It was the first time I had ever seen a business card," she remembers. "And the commissioner put it into a green envelope with a shiny gold crest, which showed how important it was. She told me to go to her friend who was a registrar in the university, give him her card, and make my case to him."

The registrar was at the University of Jos, a two-hour bus ride away. Ibrahim's face fell. She couldn't afford the trip. The commissioner appeared to read her mind. From her wallet she pulled five 20 naira notes, the equivalent of about $60. It was enough to get Ibrahim to the university and back. "The bills were so crisp,"

"You fight for what you've got, even if it's only worth a dime"

The women of West Virginia coal country are taking on a giant industry they say is killing their husbands, sickening their children, ravaging the Appalachian countryside, poisoning the air, and intensifying global warming. With pathetically small resources and dangerously angry forces arrayed against them, the question isn't, *Why are they doing this?* It's, *Where do they find the courage?* JEFF GOODELL reports.

On a cold rainy evening in January 2006, Delorice Bragg left her home in Accoville, West Virginia, and began the half-hour drive to Logan Regional Medical Center, where she had worked as a nurse for the past 15 years. As she drove along the winding blacktop that led out of her hollow and onto the main highway, she passed through a landscape of industrial mayhem—blasted mountains, towering mine silos, sooty black coal trucks careening on the narrow roads. But Bragg, 35, accepted this as the price of progress. Coal, she believed, had been good to her: Both her husband, Don "Rizzle" Bragg, and her 19-year-old son, Billy, worked in coal mines. Bragg and her husband drove new 4 x 4s; they went out to dinner once in a while in Charleston; she could afford to buy him a big new toolbox for his 33rd birthday. They were even getting ready to build a new house. *America needs coal,* Bragg found herself thinking—*thank God West Virginia has it.*

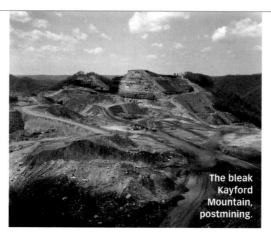

The bleak Kayford Mountain, postmining.

Once, Maria Gunnoe discovered her brake lines had been tampered with. Another day her family's dog was found dead near her kids' bus stop.

mine. He never said a word to her, never stopped to offer her reassurance or even the small kindness of a glass of water.

On Saturday afternoon, the news finally came. She saw it first on the faces of the exhausted rescue workers and mine officials, in the wet eyes of the men in hard hats. Rizzle's body had been found in the mine, as had the body of another miner, Ellery "Elvis" Hatfield.

Bragg now wears Rizzle's wedding ring on a gold chain around her neck. Sitting in a diner in downtown Logan on a rainy spring morning, she says she still doesn't know exactly what happened to her husband—why other miners escaped and he didn't. She acknowledges she may never know the entire story. But she knows that the mine had more than 90 safety violations in 2005, and she believes that the guiding ethos in the operation of the mine was productivity, not safety.

"It wasn't a mine fire that killed my husband," she says, her eyes hardening. "It was greed."

There's a war going on in Appalachia, and it's not just another feud between the Hatfields and McCoys. It's about America's last big reserve of fossil fuel: coal. Most people think coal went out with top hats and corsets, but in fact more than half the electricity in America today comes from black rocks—we burn more than a billion tons of them a year. On one side of the war are the coal industry and its allies, who argue that with gas prices sky-high and soldiers dying in the Middle East, America needs to develop domestic energy sources, especially reliable, plentiful fuels like coal. On the other side are coal miners' widows, wives, and daughters, who believe that the only

She arrived at the hospital at about 6:30 P.M. and was going over her charts when she was called to the phone. It was Rizzle's mom: "Have you heard anything about a fire in Rizzle's mine?"

Delorice remembers the next two days as if they were a hallucination: the ride to the small white Baptist church near the mine; the flashing lights of police cars; the hours sitting on a hard metal chair; the familiar crucifix on the altar; the smell of doughnuts and pizza and coffee; her 11-year-old son Ricky's urgent hugs; the dark, distant look on the face of Don Blankenship, the CEO of Massey Energy, the coal company that owned the

LIVING IN THE WORLD

thing that a renewed push for coal will lead to is more dead miners, destroyed mountains, and economic decline.

As an energy source, coal has always been a devil's bargain: The price per ton may be low, but the hidden cost is high. According to the American Lung Association, air pollution from coal-fired power plants causes 24,000 premature deaths each year; toxic mercury released from power plants—which people are most often exposed to by eating mercury-laden fish—damages the brains of developing fetuses. Most significantly, our addiction to coal is helping to destabilize the planet's climate. Nearly 40 percent of the U.S. emissions of carbon dioxide, the main greenhouse gas responsible for global warming, comes from burning coal.

Nowhere is this devil's bargain more apparent than in Appalachia. In the 20th century, nearly 100,000 workers died in Appalachian coal mines. And despite the coal industry's promise that coal mining creates jobs and economic prosperity, after more than 150 years of mining, the region remains one of the poorest and most troubled in the nation. Mountaintop removal mining— a destructive method of extraction in which instead of removing the coal from the mountains, the mountains are removed from the coal—has devastated large parts of West Virginia and Kentucky. More than 700 miles of streams have been destroyed and 400,000 acres of hardwood forest transformed into barren wasteland. Underground drinking water reservoirs have been poisoned. Air pollution in the region is among the worst in the nation.

Not all the soldiers in the war against coal are women, but a surprising number are. In part this is because

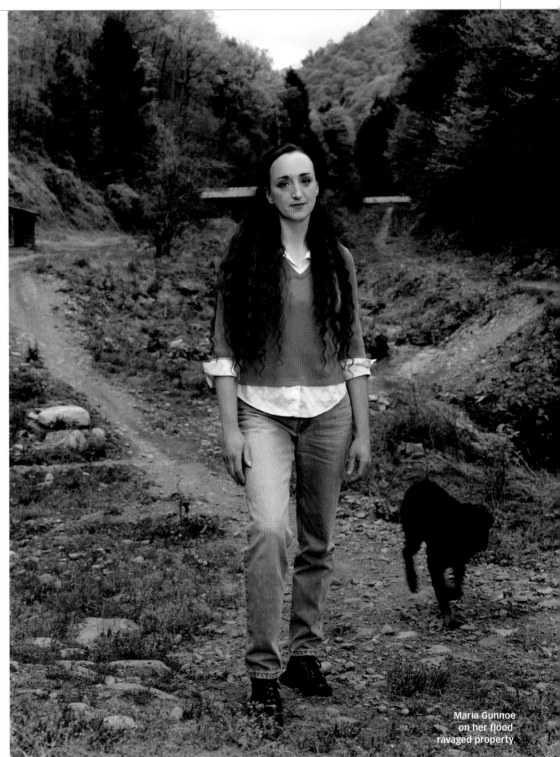

Maria Gunnoe on her flood-ravaged property.

men in Appalachia are silenced by the fact that they work for the coal industry, and these days, with the unions battered and broken, anyone who speaks out against the industry quickly finds himself stocking yo-yos at the mall. Teri Blanton, a longtime Kentucky activist, believes the disparity also reflects different priorities of men and women in Appalachia: "Women traditionally focus on their children's welfare and their long-term future, while men are more concerned with putting bread on the table. They work too hard to think about the big picture." Some

women, like Bragg, are battling for tougher mine safety laws; others are most disturbed by air pollution, toxic mercury poisoning, global warming, or mountaintop removal mining. These women are bound together not by religion or ideology but by a feeling that the people and place they love are being destroyed in the name of cheap energy.

One of the most passionate foot soldiers in this war is Maria Gunnoe. Her grandfather, father, and brothers were (or are) coal miners—and like Bragg, Gunnoe always took it on faith that the

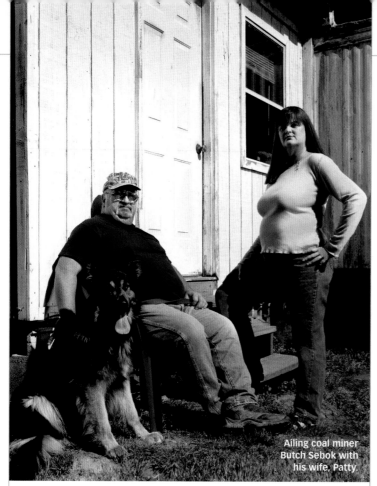
Ailing coal miner Butch Sebok with his wife, Patty.

coal industry was good for the state. Then, during a torrential rainstorm, a 20-foot-high wall of water came rushing down from a mountaintop removal mine located in the hollow above her, nearly washing her and her family away. Flooding is common around big mines after the mountains are stripped of trees, but Gunnoe believes the wall of water came over the dam at a large impoundment pond (coal companies often build reservoirs, usually held back by earthen dams, to store wastewater). The flood galvanized Gunnoe. She gave up her waitress job and is now one of West Virginia's most outspoken activists, tirelessly campaigning on university campuses and addressing political groups about the dangers of unrestrained coal mining in Appalachia.

When I tried to visit Gunnoe, she insisted on meeting me in Madison, the nearest good-size town, "because my place is buried so far up in the hollows, you'll never find it on your own." Gunnoe is 36, thin and muscular, with long, wavy black hair and a habit of speaking her mind. Driving with Gunnoe, I discover, is a good way to see the everyday courage it takes to speak out against coal in a place like southern West Virginia. More than once, she yanks the wheel to evade a loaded coal truck that swerves suspiciously close to the yellow center line. "They all know my truck," she explains coolly. "Ever since I started talking in public about what the coal companies are doing, I've noticed that I'm not real popular with some folks around here." Once, she discovered her brake lines had been tampered with. Another day her family's dog was found dead near her kids' bus stop.

We turn onto a smaller road, approaching the Pond Fork River, then stop at a washed-out bridge. Gunnoe points to a small blue and white house about 500 yards away on the other side of

the river. "That's my place up there," she says proudly. "I used to call it my little piece of heaven."

There is not much heavenly about it anymore. To get there, you have to walk on narrow planks over the washed-out bridge. Besides wrecking the bridge, the flood cut a mean, nasty gash about 20 feet deep and 70 feet wide in Gunnoe's front yard. As we walk toward her house, Gunnoe explains that her paternal grandfather, Martin Luther Gunnoe, a full-blooded Cherokee, built the place himself. He had labored underground in nearby coal mines for 32 years. He earned $18 a week, and after years of struggle, he was able to save enough to buy these 40 acres. "I carried lumber, fetched the nails," Gunnoe recalls. "We were proud of it. It was always real peaceful here." Before we start up the mountain, we stop inside to change into our hiking boots. The house is small, neatly kept, with a collection of knives—pocketknives, hunting knives, military bayonets—framed above the couch. Gunnoe disappears into another room and returns carrying a silver 32-caliber Colt pistol. "It was my grandfather's," she explains. "In case we run into bears." Or angry coal miners? "Unlikely," Gunnoe says matter-of-factly. "But you can't be too careful."

She tucks the pistol in her belt and we head up the hollow, following the steep cut of Big Branch Creek. You can see where the flooding has overturned trees and unearthed boulders. As we hike, I ask her the obvious question: Instead of staying put and fighting against the industry, as well as risking the lives of her children by continuing to live below the mine, why not just move out?

"If I leave, where am I going to go? This is my place; it is who I am. My memories are here, my life is here," she says. "I love this place. Who am I if I give all this up? My feeling is, you fight for what you've got, even if it's only worth a dime." It wasn't just the blasting of the mountains and the floods that woke her up to the dangers of rampant coal mining, Gunnoe says. It was the dead fish in the streams and the startling number of people she knew who had been diagnosed with cancer and the kids with asthma. And most of all, it was the hopelessness and fear she saw all around her. Whenever she pulled up at a gas station and saw a man with a particular look of sadness and desperation in his eyes, she wondered which coal company he worked for, and if more than 100 years of taking orders from mine superintendents and coal barons had crushed something essential in West Virginia's soul.

A half hour or so later, the hollow broadens. We pass several NO TRESPASSING signs that mark the mine border. To Gunnoe, these signs mean less than nothing. On one occasion she heard that a group of miners, apparently unhappy about her frequent treks up the mountain, had spread the word about how dangerous it is for a woman to be walking alone in the woods. If the remarks were supposed to scare her, they backfired: "The next day, I hiked up here with my shotgun and said, 'Who's first?' They left me alone after that."

We walk through a stand of pine and poplar and then abruptly confront a wall of rock maybe 500 feet high, barren of trees but with thin patches of grass growing here and there. We have arrived at the edge of the mine.

"Ain't it pretty?" Gunnoe says wickedly.

I had seen many of these rock fills before—they're known in coal country as valley fills—but never quite from this angle. It was, quite literally, the top of a nearby mountain that had been cut off and dumped in this narrow valley that had once been the headwaters of the Big Branch. In the distance, we could hear the grind and roar of heavy machinery digging out coal.

"They can bury me in these hills," Gunnoe says, facing the wall of rock above us, "but I ain't leavin'."

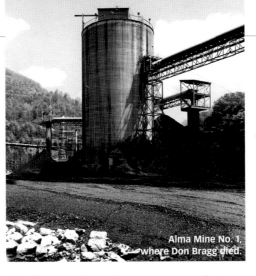

Alma Mine No. 1, where Don Bragg died.

W hitesville, West Virginia, a once-prosperous coal town, is broken and nearly abandoned. The main street is mostly boarded up. The movie theater is closed. The roof on the old high school is burned out. The old union hall is covered with graffiti. The only flash of life is at the edge of town, where a colorful mountain mural is painted on the wall of the old post office. Inside is the office of Coal River Mountain Watch, an organization founded

"They do the same thing to these miners that they do to the mountains and the planet," says Patty Sebok. "Use them up and then throw them away."

in 1998 to fight against outlaw coal operators in the region. The group's outreach coordinator is a former Pizza Hut waitress and coal miner's wife named Judy Bonds. When I visit, Bonds is sitting at a long Formica table, going over the schedule for an upcoming road trip to Ohio. If anyone in West Virginia has been able to channel the spirit of turn-of-the-century labor activist Mother Jones, it's Bonds. She's 53 years old, a fast-talking and fiery coalfield Baptist, with short gray hair, a gray sweatshirt, jeans, and hiking boots. Five minutes after I arrive, she has already launched into a critique of President Bush's energy policy, mourned the death of Don Bragg and the 13 other coal miners who died in West Virginia that January, and compared the state's relationship with the coal industry to battered wife syndrome: "We know they're going to beat us to death and leave us, but still we can't muster up the courage to change our ways." It's blunt talk like this that won Bonds the prestigious Goldman Prize in 2003, the environmental equivalent of a Pulitzer.

Bonds sees herself as a commander in an increasingly complex and deadly war. "I think we're going back to the 1920s," she says. "We're in a struggle here for basic human rights. It's us against the industrial machine." The offices of Coal River Mountain Watch even look like a war room: There are topographic maps all over the walls, pictures of explosives detonating on mine sites, even a black-and-white image of Mother Jones taped to the refrigerator.

After a quick lunch of sloppy joes and Cokes at a nearby drugstore—where Bonds engages the ladies in the lunchroom in a spirited debate over how many cemeteries the coal companies have secretly plowed through—she and I jump into her Toyota Camry and drive out to Marfolk Hollow, where her family lived for generations. Along the way, we pass more broken glass and boarded-up buildings. "The coal industry likes to talk about all the jobs and prosperity they are responsible for—well, where is the prosperity?" Bonds asks, waving her hands as she drives. "Where are the jobs? Do you see jobs and prosperity around here?"

We turn up a dirt road and immediately are confronted with signs warning us that this is private property—we are entering a mining site. A railroad cuts through the hill beside us, and mining trucks blow dust at us as they grind by on the narrow road. Bonds idles up beside a neglected patch of dirt. "This used to be the ball field," she says; a little farther up, we come to a concrete walk that leads nowhere, "and this is where our house used to be," and then a little farther up, a small house that is now turned into a mining office, "and this is where my grandparents lived"; and finally we get to a chain-link fence across the road: "and I was born right up there," she says, pointing to what is now a forbidden zone.

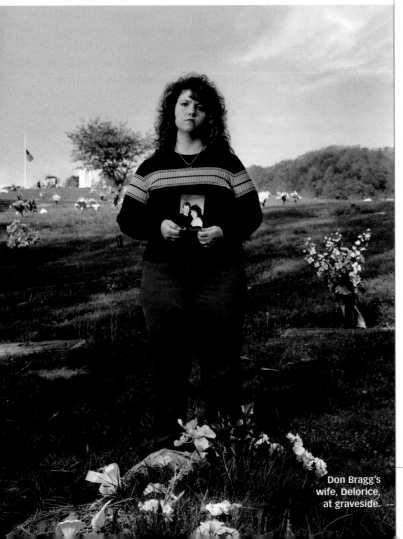

Don Bragg's wife, Delorice, at graveside.

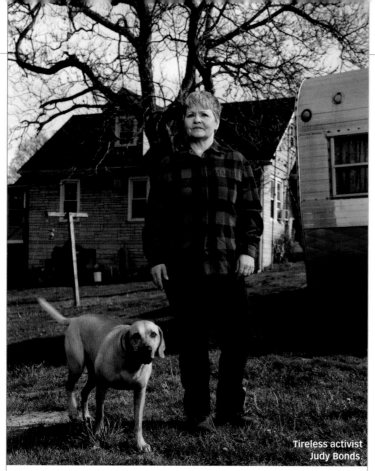

Tireless activist
Judy Bonds.

Before they started coal mining up this hollow, it was a peaceful place. Bonds's memories are of gardens, clear-running streams, and blossoming fruit trees. After high school, she married and settled into her own house in the hollow. When that relationship fell apart, she and her young daughter moved back in with her parents. A few years later, she married a coal miner.

Like everybody else, I was happy for the paycheck and didn't bother much with what was going on around me," she says. But eventually that marriage also went bad, and Bonds found herself (along with her daughter and grandson) living in a trailer on her parents' property. Soon after, A.T. Massey Coal (now Massey Energy) moved in. "That's when the creek started running black and the air was full of dust and the blasting started in the hills. They were blowing my homeplace apart." Bonds eventually sold out to Massey, found a job at Pizza Hut, and brooded about what the coal industry was doing to the mountains and people she loved. In 1999 she attended a reenactment of the historic 1921 labor battle on Blair Mountain. To her shock, a group of coal industry supporters, angry that anyone would be celebrating the rights of miners, began shoving around an 84-year-old West Virginia politician who was in the march. Bonds joined Coal River Mountain Watch, she says, "because I couldn't just stand by and watch the coal industry take over. I couldn't give up everything I love without a fight." Today the group has more than 1,000 members and is the nexus of a growing pan-Appalachian movement to speak out against the crimes of big coal.

We drive out of the hollow and continue down the highway along the Coal River. She points out her favorite swimming hole, an old abandoned playground where she used to take her kids, the burned-out high school. Across the road, you can see the top of a huge mountaintop removal mine, a lunar landscape of gravel and rock. After a few miles, we come to what, for Bonds, is the front line in her battle against the coal industry: Marsh Fork Elementary School.

Bonds parks her Camry and we step out. The school sits close to the road, on the banks of the Coal River. Across the river, several hundred feet away, is another big Massey mine, and less than a quarter mile from the school is a 385-foot-high earthen dam holding back at least two billion gallons of black water and sludge. If this dam were ever to give way, the more than 200 children in this school wouldn't have a chance. And flooding isn't the only danger the children face: Coal dust often drifts over the school; water behind the school turns black. Students are frequently ill with asthma, bronchitis, and other respiratory problems. A group of concerned residents told Governor Joe Manchin recently that three teachers and one 17-year-old former student had died of cancer. Adding to the politically charged debate is the recent revelation that one of the silos may be illegally sited beyond the mine permit boundary.

In Bonds's view, the Marsh Fork school has become a flash point because it symbolizes what's at stake here: commerce over public safety, the protection of a rich, old industry over the health and welfare of hundreds of children. "I mean, can you imagine this kind of thing going on anywhere else? If this school isn't a symbol of political corruption and the failure of democracy, I don't know what is. We like to pretend we live in a modern world, but the truth is, West Virginia is just as much a coal colony today as it was a hundred years ago. The Bible tells us we will be held accountable for what we are doing to these mountains and the people who live here, and I believe we will. I believe we will have a lot to answer for."

As we talk, a man in a white pickup drives by and, recognizing Bonds, guns his engine.

She turns and gives him a hard stare as he drives off.

"You gotta look 'em in the eye," she says. "If you show them any fear, they'll crush you."

In the late afternoon, I follow Patty Sebok, who works with Bonds at Coal River Mountain Watch, to her homeplace in Prenter Hollow, about 20 miles outside of Whitesville. She lives in a 30-year-old mobile home on a flat patch of ground beside a creek. There is a chain-link fence in the front; their German shepherd has run bare a path within it. Old tires, newspapers, and tools litter the yard. Sebok steps out of her beat-up Ford Bronco—the bumper sticker says REAL COAL MINERS DO IT DEEP IN THE DARK—and I follow her into the house, where her husband, Butch, sits on the couch, an ice pack against his back, a pair of rifles on the wall above him, and pain in his eyes.

Sebok, 50, does not look very tough, with her pageboy bangs, dainty nose, and schoolteacher smile. But she has been fighting the coal industry as long as anybody in West Virginia. Starting in 1989, she led a long, difficult, and emotional battle against overweight coal trucks that regularly terrorize the backroads of Appalachia. She lobbied in Charleston, led protests against mountaintop removal mining, and petitioned the federal government to enforce the Clean Water Act in West Virginia. Over the years, her views about what is going on in Appalachia have steadily broadened. She talks now at town meetings and colleges around the country about the big picture—how America's voracious demand for energy is linked not just to the destruction of the mountains around them but also to the destabilization of the earth's climate from global warming. In response, Sebok has been run off the road by coal trucks, videotaped by strangers, and publicly heckled more times than she can remember. (In her vehicle, she carries a big stick; in her bag, pepper spray.) And if it were up to her, she would spend all her time working to raise awareness of what's at stake in America's sudden lust for coal. She would help Bonds organize rallies in Appalachia, work with the United Mine Workers of America to demand a higher ethical standard for the coal industry, and maybe even travel to New York City with Gunnoe and other activists who will be testifying before the United Nations Commission on Sustainable Development.* Unfortunately, Sebok has a more urgent task at hand: trying to keep her family fed and Butch from becoming a cripple.

For nearly 27 years, Butch toiled in an underground mine. He was lucky: It was a union mine, so his pay was better than most. The years of labor took their toll: bruised ribs, worn-out knees, back pain, morning cough (a harbinger of black lung). But Butch, a 240-pound former U.S. marine, could handle all that. Then in October 2004, he picked up a heavy timber and pain shot down his arm and into his hand. He thought it was a minor injury. He reported the injury to his supervisor, then went to the doctor, who sent him for an MRI scan. For about a month, he received workers' compensation. Then he got the results of the MRI—he had a herniated disk in his neck. His doctor told him that if he went back to work, one fall or hard knock could further injure his neck and lead to permanent paralysis. The company sent him to see another doctor, who concluded that Butch had "attained maximum medical improvement," and his workers' comp was cut off. Because they had no savings to fall back on, Butch wanted to return to work, but Sebok insisted that he stay home and fight for workers' compensation.

A year and a half later, Butch has still not received another dime. "The company is fighting us every step of the way," says Sebok, holding up a thick plastic binder full of paperwork. "They claim that because he didn't initially tell them it was a neck injury—how was he supposed to know?—they are not responsible. I spend four or five hours a day on this, writing letters to lawyers, to the coal company, to doctors. I've tried to call the governor. It's impossible to get anyone to listen. He's just an old coal miner. Who cares?" In response, Pine Ridge Coal argues that Butch is seeking "additional compensation for a preexisting condition unrelated to the original claim."

Sebok, who has stood in the middle of the road and blocked 100,000-pound coal trucks with her body, suddenly gets wet-eyed.

"They're trying to starve us out," Butch says.

"They want him to go back to work so they don't have to pay," Sebok explains. "And because he's dared to question them, they'll put him on the worst job. They don't care if he ends up paralyzed." Earlier, Sebok had told me that the family had survived the winter on food stamps and donations from friends.

"In the beginning," she says, "it seemed like a good job. But then—"

"It was a good job," Butch interrupts. "I liked the work. I liked my friends. Coal miners are good people."

"But look what it's done to you," Sebok says.

Butch rearranges the ice pack on his back and glances over at the TV that is playing silently in the corner of the room. "At some point, I may have to go back to work," he says. "Just take the risk. We have to live somehow."

"You will not!" Sebok interjects, sitting bolt upright. "You're not going back. We're going to fight this thing to the end."

On CNN, images flash by of New Orleans residents who are still recovering from Katrina—a hurricane whose intensity, many climatologists argue, was increased by rising sea temperatures related to global warming.

"They do the same thing to these miners that they do to the mountains and the planet," Sebok says, getting up from the couch to play with her dog. "Use it up and then throw it away. It's all disposable." She tosses a ball. "But I got my claws into them, and I'm going to make them pay."

Later, when I leave Sebok's home and drive down the hollow, I think about what she and the other women I'd spoken to are up against. What they are fighting, after all, are not just rich, powerful coal companies well armed with lawyers but a nation of consumers who remain willfully ignorant of where their energy comes from and what it really costs to produce it. Sure, these women have had their successes: Thanks to the lobbying of widows like Bragg, West Virginia has passed tougher mine safety regulations; Sebok and Bonds are largely responsible for new laws cracking down on overweight coal trucks; Gunnoe—who once drove 11 hours in her truck from West Virginia to Connecticut to speak to students at Yale University—is one of many women (in Ohio, Kentucky, and Tennessee as well) who are helping to ensure that the coal industry's rape and pillage of Appalachia is no longer America's dirty little secret. Still, they are just a ragtag bunch of women, deeply rooted in a land they love, and determined to protect the welfare of their families and communities against an all-devouring industrial machine. And like other famously overmatched American rebels—the New England patriots of the 1770s or the Freedom Riders of the 1960s—they are armed with little more than their courage, their passion, and a great moral clarity.

"The battle," Bonds assured me earlier that day in her office in Whitesville, "has only just begun." **◘**

> "You gotta look 'em in the eye," says Judy Bonds. "If you show them any fear, they'll crush you."

Gunnoe and nine other activists testified before the United Nations in May 2006.

Oprah Talks to
Paul Rusesabagina

His country had gone totally, blood-in-the-streets mad. Neighbors attacking each other with machetes. A million slaughtered. So how did this soft-spoken, unarmed man manage to rescue so many of his countrymen from a rageful death? Now, years later, the real-life hero of *Hotel Rwanda* tells Oprah about the art of talking yourself (and 1,268 others) out of danger (a bottle of wine helps), why the world turned away, and what it's like to start all over again in exile. Oprah can't get over his spirit....

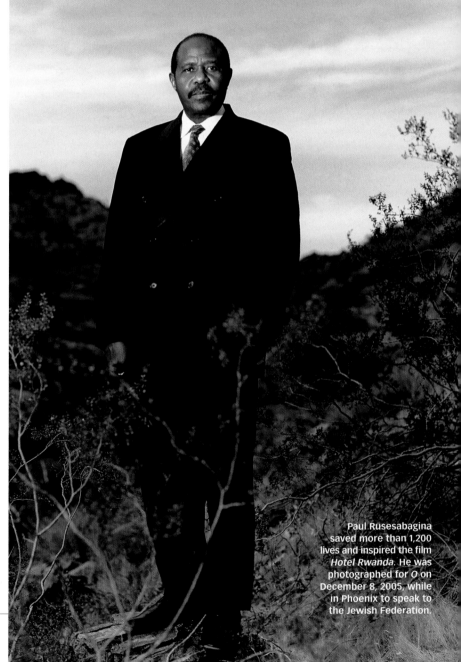

Paul Rusesabagina saved more than 1,200 lives and inspired the film *Hotel Rwanda*. He was photographed for *O* on December 8, 2005, while in Phoenix to speak to the Jewish Federation.

I n 1994 in the African country of Rwanda, nearly one million people were slaughtered in exactly 100 days. Our world—with its 24-hour news stations—chose to turn its head. This is the story of one man who couldn't.

Paul Rusesabagina, whose courage inspired the 2004 film *Hotel Rwanda*, grew up with the tensions that exploded in 1994, but the hatred had been simmering for nearly a century. In 1916 Belgian colonists deemed the Tutsi ethnic group superior to the Hutus, giving them better education and jobs while the Hutus were relegated to dirty work. But when Rwanda became independent in 1962, the Hutus took power, and that, in turn, led to a Tutsi rebel movement. On April 6, 1994, a plane carrying Hutu president Juvénal Habyarimana was shot down, killing him along with the president of neighboring Burundi. Although no one could prove who ordered the attack, retaliation was immediate: Opposition leaders were murdered, and suddenly civilians were slaughtering every Tutsi and moderate Hutu they could find.

Paul, who is of both Hutu and Tutsi descent, and his wife, Tatiana, a Tutsi, fled with their four children to the Hotel Mille Collines, where he had once been the manager. There, with no water or electricity and despite constant threats on his life, he sheltered 1,268 people, saving them from the massacre.

Paul's memoir, *An Ordinary Man*, hit bookstores in April 2006. Just before Christmas 2005, he and I talked about what it feels like to watch your neighbors turn into killers and to survive a horror that I pray our world will never forget.

OPRAH: *In your book, you write that you walked out of your house the first morning of the killings and saw your neighbors armed with machetes.*

PAUL: That was a terrible day. Men I'd known for years

were carrying machetes, grenades, guns, spears—any weapon you can think of. Neighbors I'd seen as gentlemen had suddenly become killers in military uniforms.

OPRAH: *How do the people you've shared barbecues with become the personification of evil?*

PAUL: I've never understood. Some of our neighbors were murdered that morning. My son found a mother, her six daughters, and her son slaughtered. Some of them weren't completely dead yet. They were still moving slightly. After my son came running home, he didn't talk for four days. We couldn't understand how our country could just go mad.

OPRAH: *Would the violence have erupted if that plane hadn't been shot down?*

PAUL: That added oil to a burning fire. Since the sixties, Hutus and Tutsis have been in heavy tension.

OPRAH: *Here's why I found your book so fascinating: It shows what role radio played in inciting the masses.*

PAUL: In 1993 a station called the "radio-television of the thousands of hills" was started. It was funded by Rwanda's then president, Habyarimana, and his *akazu*—his closest friends, including leaders and businessmen. When the president was threatened by armed rebels, he decided to fight and keep power by all means.

OPRAH: *So media was his tool.*

PAUL: To do evil.

OPRAH: *It's interesting how quickly propaganda can change the commonsense thinking of everyday people.*

PAUL: In Rwanda people don't buy newspapers or magazines. They prefer radio. Every peasant on the plantation, everyone on buses, in cars, listens. It was a planned strategic manipulation to use radio for evil. [Once the violence started] people were hiding in the bushes. On the radio, leaders encouraged people to clear the bushes and kill their neighbors.

OPRAH: *I marvel that you remained so resilient in the face of such terror.*

PAUL: You would have been strong enough to do the same thing.

OPRAH: *Weren't you afraid for your life, or were you secure because you're mostly Hutu?*

PAUL: Here's what we have to make clear: The million people who were killed included both Hutus and Tutsis. Because the president was a Hutu from the north, all Hutus elsewhere in the country were considered opposition.

OPRAH: *After you looked out to see your neighbors' machetes dripping with blood, you decided to hide people.*

PAUL: That was on April 7, 1994. By the end of the day, I had 26 people in my house.

OPRAH: *Why did they come to you?*

PAUL: I have always wondered—and I have never found an answer. Maybe they trusted me. When I got a chance to evacuate, I took them with me as my own family.

OPRAH: *The day you took everyone to the Hotel Mille Collines, where you'd once been the manager, someone put a gun to your face....*

PAUL: He was a Tutsi army captain sent by the new government

that was put up on April 9. They decided to take over the hotel. The manager who'd been working there had already fled.

OPRAH: *Why did the army captain come after you?*

PAUL: Because I'd gotten hold of the keys to the hotel cellar and all the unoccupied rooms. The government wanted those rooms and supplies.

OPRAH: *But the captain also ordered you to shoot your family!*

PAUL: Yes. And this guy wasn't joking. All along the road there were dead bodies; some missing their heads, others with their bellies open. I was speechless. He handed me a gun, and I told him I didn't know how to use it.

OPRAH: *I'm surprised he bought that.*

PAUL: He didn't. But I also told him that I understood him. "You're tired," I said. "You're thirsty. You're stressed by the war. I don't blame you for this. But we can find other solutions. Your enemy isn't the old man driving my car or this baby over here."

OPRAH: *But Paul, I'm surprised he'd even listen to you after slaughtering so many!*

PAUL: I've noticed that any person who can open his or her mouth and talk to you can also listen to you. This man did. When I saw that the appeal to morality wasn't working, I offered him cash. Then I told him I needed to go to the hotel safe to get it.

OPRAH: *You kept 1,268 people alive in that hotel.*

PAUL: For 78 days. In a hotel designed to hold 200 people.

OPRAH: *You've said the only thing that saved those people was words—not money, not liquor, not the UN. Just ordinary words directed against the darkness. How did you bargain for those people's lives?*

PAUL: In Rwandan culture, we say that two men can never sit down and deal without a drink. So I'd always bring a drink to sit and talk. And certainly, any person who came to talk with me arrived at a positive conclusion.

"If we want to change things in the world, we must first change ourselves."

OPRAH: *How did you survive those days when killers were coming to the hotel?*

PAUL: It was complicated. If you want to control someone, you've got to keep him close, talk to him. That's what I did [with the armed men constantly threatening to take over the hotel]. The people inside were frightened. There was no water, no electricity, and we were cooking any corn and dried beans we could find with firewood. But it's surprising how quickly people adapt to a situation, however dangerous. Women were giving birth, young couples were getting married by a bishop from St. Michel Cathedral next door.

OPRAH: *In the middle of a genocide?*

PAUL: Yes. The hotel became a home, a lifestyle. People got used to sleeping in conference rooms and corridors.

OPRAH: *Was there fighting?*

PAUL: No. Everyone was so respectful.

OPRAH: *Were they aware of the slaughtering?*

PAUL: Oh, yes—but they weren't always aware of the assaults on our hotel. I didn't make them aware. But on April 23, when I awakened to find soldiers with guns at my head, everyone was informed. Three days later, I got a call saying that we were going to be attacked again. That's when Thomas Kamilindi, a Rwandan journalist staying there, managed to ring Radio France International. He described how the rebels were advancing and asked for help. I saw a colonel come up to the hotel just as the journalist ended his plea. From the main entrance, the colonel shouted that he'd come to pick up that "dog"—meaning Thomas. I took the colonel to my office, offered him a drink, and convinced him that it wasn't the job of a colonel to run after a dog. "Small boys are supposed to run after dogs," I said, appealing to his ego. "Leave that dirty dog to others." I talked with him for hours. He finally left without the journalist—but he promised that others would return to kill the man. Thankfully, that never happened. Thomas is now at the University of Michigan.

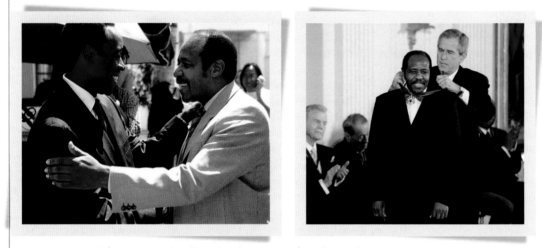

(*Above, left*) Actor Don Cheadle and Paul on the set of *Hotel Rwanda*, 2004. (*Above, right*) Receiving the Presidential Medal of Freedom, November 9, 2005.

OPRAH: *He owes his life to you, as do 1,267 other people.*

PAUL: They owe their lives to their God.

OPRAH: *Where was God in all of this?*

PAUL: That's a big question mark for Rwandans. In our tradition, we say that God wanders around the world before returning to sleep in Rwanda in the evenings.

OPRAH: *Because the sunsets are so beautiful?*

PAUL: Everything was so beautiful. But since 1994, we ask ourselves, "Where is God?"

OPRAH: *God was in all the so-called serendipitous occurrences. I don't believe in happenstance. In your story, I feel the power of something bigger than you or me.*

PAUL: That's how I see it. But after Rwandans watched a million of their people killed in 100 days, they asked, "Did God do that—or did people? And why us? Are we the most criminal in this world? Why did God let people suffer this way?"

OPRAH: *I understand the questions, and there are others: Like where was the rest of the world?*

PAUL: The world simply decided to close its ears and eyes, stand back, run away. Maybe the world didn't think Rwanda was worth an intervention. Maybe that's because Africa is far away from America and Europe. Perhaps it happened because Rwanda did not have oil. Or maybe it's because people were focused on South Africa. [*At the time, Nelson Mandela was being elected president in South Africa's first democratic elections.*]

OPRAH: *You were once given a chance to leave the hotel on a UN truck for a safer location, but you sent your family without you.*

PAUL: The day before, some of my people had come to me and said, "Listen, Paul, we've heard you're leaving us. If it's true, tell us so we can go to the roof and jump. We don't want to be killed with machetes." Later that day, I made a decision. I had to tell my wife and children that I would send them to a safe place—but without me.

OPRAH: *In the movie, you didn't tell them. So it happened differently in real life?*

PAUL: That's right. Tatiana and the children were angry that I wasn't going with them. I told them I was the only person who could negotiate for the people in the hotel. If I left, they would be killed, and I would never be a free man. I'd be a prisoner of myself, never able to eat and feel satisfied or go to bed and rest. I'd be a traitor. But imagine me escorting my wife and children to the evacuation trucks! There's real footage of that—we found it while we were filming *Hotel Rwanda*. It was heartbreaking. I wasn't sure I'd ever see my family again.

OPRAH: *Then their truck was intercepted.*

PAUL: They were ambushed and beaten. When Tatiana came back to me, she was lying in blood in the back of the truck. My son was beaten by his former classmate, a young boy who screamed, "You cockroach! Remove your shoes and give them to me."

OPRAH: *After you finally escaped from the hotel and were taken to the Tutsi rebel camp, was life ever normal again?*

PAUL: Life wasn't normal until September 1996, when I sought asylum in Belgium. I narrowly escaped with my life. I fled my own country as a refugee.

OPRAH: *Yet you saved 1,268 people—which you say in your book was the number being killed every three hours.*

PAUL: So small a number to save!

OPRAH: *It really wasn't, Paul.*

PAUL: To me, it was.

OPRAH: *What happened to those people?*

PAUL: They're living all around the world—in America, Europe, Rwanda. Some became prominent leaders in our country.

OPRAH: *You must get lots of Christmas cards.*

PAUL: [*Laughs.*] You can't imagine how many thousands of e-mails I get every day.

OPRAH: *Your book is called* An Ordinary Man, *yet you took on an extraordinary feat with courage, determination, and diplomacy. You talked your butt off, Paul!*

PAUL: An ordinary man is one who does his job. That's what I did.

As a hotel manager, I simply catered to a different clientele.

OPRAH: *How did you rebuild your life after escaping?*

PAUL: That's difficult to do after you've been terrorized. In Rwanda we were like a bird's nest near a passageway. Each time someone passed the nest, we wondered whether we'd survive. Every moment was a threat.

When I arrived in Belgium, my friends at Sabena Hotels offered me a job, but not as a general manager. They offered me a lesser job. I've never liked to beg. So I instead chose to raise enough money to buy a taxicab in Brussels. A year later, I bought a second car. Three years after that, I opened a trucking company, which is based in Zambia. I love it. And since 1999, I've had a Belgian passport.

OPRAH: *Do you miss Rwanda?*

PAUL: Every day.

OPRAH: *Will you ever be able to go back?*

PAUL: I believe.

OPRAH: *Couldn't you go back with protection?*

PAUL: With some GI's around me! [*Laughs.*]

OPRAH: *How is your life now?*

PAUL: It's completely different from what it once was. Now I deliver speeches all over the world. In Boston I've started a foundation to care for orphans of the genocide, as well as AIDS orphans. Did you know that the genocide and its aftermath left Rwanda with half a million orphans? AIDS added to that figure. All these people need medical care, psychological follow-up, tuition for the kids.

OPRAH: *In the movie, you reunited with your orphaned nieces in a refugee camp.*

PAUL: Right—and my wife and I waited until they were 7 and 8 to tell them that their parents had been murdered. They didn't believe it. They'd been only 2 years old and 9 months old when they lost their mother and father. We told them before the movie came out. They cried and said, "No, no, no. We do not have any other parents." The first time my wife saw the movie, she couldn't finish it—nor could she finish it the second or third time. Always in tears. She finally finished it the fourth time.

OPRAH: *How did you react the first time you saw it?*

PAUL: I was able to finish it because I'd been involved in the filming in Johannesburg. I met the actor who played my role.

OPRAH: *Don Cheadle.*

PAUL: He didn't really understand me until we met, sat down, shared wine, and spent almost a week together. He'd expected me to be a shell-shocked man who hid in alcohol after all I went through. But when he met me, a real person, he noticed that I was different from his preconception.

OPRAH: *After the horrors you've witnessed, how can you and your family carry on with life?*

PAUL: Our days are so few, our existences so complicated. As long as we're breathing, we shouldn't further complicate our lives. If we want to change things, we must first change ourselves. If we want to play—if we want to change the world—we must first show up on the field to score.

OPRAH: *Have your children recovered from the trauma?*

PAUL: At one point, I noticed that my children were becoming aggressive. Our solution was to get them talking around a table. The best therapy is talking.

OPRAH: *Was it difficult at first for them to speak about it?*

PAUL: Yes. The children said, "You love your country, but we don't need it." Until I convinced them to talk about Rwanda, they were hardly even willing to mention it. We'll never forget what we went through—the torture, the frustration. But we're recovering well. It's much better now than it was in 1995, 1996.

OPRAH: *Have your children gone to college?*

PAUL: Yes. My eldest daughter is an accountant and married with two daughters. My eldest son studied management and is now looking toward a master's. My second daughter is married and working on a BS in accounting. My younger son is in boarding school near Boston. My two nieces are attending primary and secondary school.

OPRAH: *After living through such a horror, does it take a lot to upset you?*

PAUL: Yes. Whatever I see in life, I take it to be so small and simple compared with what I've witnessed.

OPRAH: *What was the worst thing you saw?*

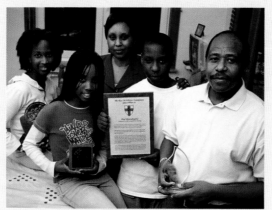

At home with *(from left)* nieces Anaise and Carine Kahimba, wife Tatiana, and son Tresor.

PAUL: Many days I went to the roof of the hotel and saw people being killed in the streets. The killers would pile up their bodies to form roadblocks. They'd then sit on the bodies as they drank beers.

OPRAH: *That's what happened during the Holocaust. In the concentration camps, Jewish bodies were thrown into a hole as the guards sat nearby, smoking cigarettes. Did you have nightmares?*

PAUL: I did, and so did my children. But since I started speaking about the genocide almost every day and since I began calling my children around the table to talk, our healing has come through our sharing.

OPRAH: *During your three months in that hotel, did you wake up every morning thinking you would die?*

PAUL: I was sure I'd be killed. I just didn't know how, when, or by whom. For years after the genocide, I was still afraid I'd be found and murdered. That was almost the case in September 1996, when I finally escaped from Rwanda. Since that day, I've referred to every hour of my life as a bonus.

OPRAH: *Why do you think you survived?*

PAUL: My day, my hour, my minute had not yet come. I believe I lived so that I could tell the world this story. That is my mission. **O**

Giving Back

"What have you done today to make you feel proud?"

Getting three new pups at the same time wasn't the smartest decision I ever made. I acted on impulse, charmed by their cute little faces, intoxicated by that sweet puppy breath and the underbite on Puppy Number Three (Layla). Then I spent weeks getting up at all hours of the night with them. I picked up pounds of poop and am still in the throes of puppy training so they can have good manners. It's a lot of work. A month in, I had to hire some help because I was so sleep deprived—and trying to keep three at a time from destroying my worldly goods was making me constantly frazzled. Whoa, did I gain *big* new respect for mothers of real babies! I see now how the day can get away from you, with no time to shower because you're off and running from the first cry.

All this puppy love was starting to get on my nerves, so I had to make a paradigm shift. One day while walking them through the woods, I stood and watched them frolic—and I do mean frolic: rolling, tumbling, chasing, laughing (yes, dogs laugh), and leaping like bunnies. They were having so much fun, and seeing them that way made my whole body sigh, relax, and smile. New life discovering a field of grass for the first time: What a wonder! We all get the opportunity to feel wonder every day, but we've been lulled into numbness. Have you ever driven home from work, opened your front door, and asked yourself how you got there?

I know for sure that I don't want to live a shut-down life—desensitized to feeling, seeing, and the possibility of experiencing joy on every level. I want every day to be a fresh start on expanding what is possible. And I also know that one person can make a huge difference. One of our themes on the show for the 2006 season was "What have you done today to make you feel proud?"

The surest way to bring goodness to yourself is to make it your intention to do good for somebody else. Years ago I started a gratitude journal. In 2006, I started keeping a "proud" journal. Every day I make a conscious effort to extend kindness, grace, comfort, and peace. It doesn't take a lot to have an impact on someone's life.

I've often told the story of Tish Hooker, a pretty woman who visited my church while she was campaigning for her husband, who was running for governor. I was 8. She stopped me and told me I was pretty as a speckled pup. I never forgot it, and I make it a point to tell every

other little girl I see who may not know her own beauty the same thing.

I know for sure that when you shift your paradigm to what you can do for others, you begin to accelerate your own evolution and trigger a bounty of blessings. What have you done *today?* O

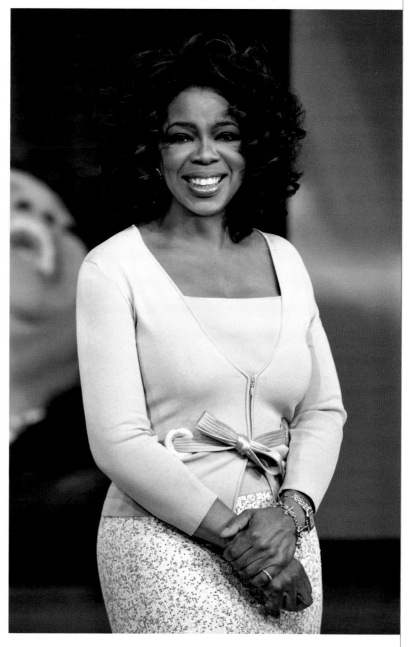

How to Stop Being Overwhelmed by the World's Troubles

Five experts tell you how to make a difference—one small good deed at a time.

HELENE GAYLE, MD, *president and CEO of CARE, working to fight global poverty*

There are a lot of ways to make a difference—contact a congressman, get involved with a charitable organization, even write a check. It's a matter of looking at your talents and asking what you have to give. My overarching goal was to find practical ways to create change, so I went into medicine and public health, and developed concrete tools to address social inequities and injustice. Now I look for specific, short-term objectives and just chip away.

ERVIN STAUB, PhD, *cofounder of the Advancing Healing and Reconciliation Project, focusing on the 1994 genocide in Rwanda*

As a boy, I survived the Holocaust in Hungary. My family suffered tremendously, but we lived because other people helped us. So my work is clearly influenced by my past. I tell people to choose a personal cause and make one ongoing commitment to help. There was a period when I went through a crisis because I'd been working so long and the world was still full of violence. But I realized that engagement is a matter of principle. Even if the effects are not always evident, it's very worthwhile in the long run.

AL GORE, *environmental activist, author of* An Inconvenient Truth, *and former vice president*

I've always been concerned with the environment, but it wasn't until my wife and I almost lost our son in a very serious car accident (he recovered completely) that global warming became my focus. Suddenly, I understood that just as we'd almost lost our precious child, our civilization was in danger of losing what was most precious to it. But we have a chance to change the course. What keeps me going is my optimism that once people really become aware of what's needed, we will all get busy. I've seen this before— like during the civil rights movement, when awareness of a wrong reached a level that caused the majority to rise up and make big changes. I'm convinced that's going to happen with global warming.

GEOFFREY CANADA, *president and CEO of Harlem Children's Zone, helping children and families in New York's inner city*

When I was growing up in the South Bronx, my mother and I took some friends who had never been outside our neighborhood to the zoo. Witnessing their joy that day was more exciting for me than seeing the animals. Since then I've loved improving children's lives. Feeling that kind of passion is the first clear indicator of how you can change the world. And searching for your cause should be like shopping for groceries: You won't necessarily like everything you see, but it doesn't mean there's nothing in the supermarket you'll enjoy. Most people just give up before they've gone down enough aisles.

SALLY FISHER, *president of Intersect Worldwide, combating HIV and violence against women and girls*

Every time a new problem arises, my first reaction is: "I can't change this." And then I realize I'm feeling overwhelmed because I haven't chosen a course of action. Once I've made a decision, I find that there is always time to help. I pick causes that I care about, and I know I never have to go it alone. I can't stop AIDS or end violence against women on my own. It was such a relief when I realized that. You have to remind yourself: You can do only what you can do. **O**

LIVING IN THE WORLD

"If you empower women, you can change the world"

Can the women of richer nations unite with the women of third world nations?
Meg Ryan thinks so—and during a recent journey through an impoverished region of
northern India, she was delighted, moved, awed, and heartened by a cadre
of young women eager to educate their peers about sex, HIV, contraception, and
substance abuse. As ROSEMARY MAHONEY found out, female voices carry.

Sitting in a car caught in tangled traffic on the outskirts of Agra, India, Meg Ryan is speaking about the dismal status of the world's women. Beyond her delicate profile, beyond the window of our SUV, a tiny bare-foot girl not more than 3 years old, with long, matted hair, flies in her eyes, and a tattered red rag for a dress, sifts through a fuming pile of garbage at the side of the road. Now and then the girl plucks a dusty, rotting object from the trash, puts it in her mouth. Her sole companions are two soot-streaked piglets who, like her, are rummaging through the garbage for any-thing remotely edible. Women in flip-flops and brightly col-ored saris and veils cross the highway carrying big tin buck-ets of water on their heads, hauling them home to their houses at the edge of the highway—flimsy huts constructed of sticks and string and black plastic sheeting. The Agra air is dense with the noxious smoke of factories, brick kilns, and burning rubble. Our car is air-conditioned, yet all day I've found myself faintly short of breath. With her camera in her lap, Ryan looks silently out the window, then turns and says quietly, "If you empower women, you can change the world. And I think it's important for the women of the first world to hold hands with the women of the third."

This Hollywood icon, the star of *When Harry Met Sally...* and *Sleepless in Seattle,* is making a four-day trip across northern India with representatives from the international aid organization CARE. In notably casual attire—baggy green army pants, worn clogs, a brown pullover, no makeup, no fussy hairdo—Ryan has been humble, observant, polite, and reserved. She has brought no

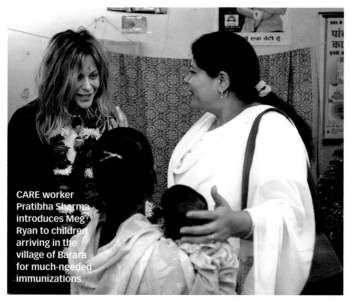

CARE worker Pratibha Sharma introduces Meg Ryan to children arriving in the village of Barara for much-needed immunizations.

fanfare, no glitter, no Hollywood ego or trumpery. In the hope of calling to the world's attention their stories and their needs, she's spent four days literally and figuratively holding hands with some of the world's most disadvantaged women.

In Jehangirpuri, north of New Delhi, a vast slum of rickety brick buildings and makeshift shanties, where raw sewage runs in the gutters and half-naked children play in muddy dirt lanes, Ryan was welcomed on the first day of her trip by a group of Indian women engaged in CARE's HIV prevention pro-gram, which focuses on young women ages 15 to 24. That sex is a forbidden topic here has proved one of the biggest hur-dles in preventing the spread of AIDS. With more than five mil-lion HIV-positive citizens, about 40 percent of whom are women, India has more HIV infections than any other country but South Africa. CARE staff are working to prevent new infections by training teenage girls to talk with each other about issues of sex and sexually transmitted diseases.

Six women welcome Ryan, Anne Goddard (CARE's chief of staff), and me into a small room with garlands of flowers, rose petals, dots of red grease paint applied to our fore-heads. The small room in a cement building is home to a family of four, lit only by a candle at the center of a low table. "We never have electricity for a full 24 hours!" one woman apologetically tells our interpreter, CARE's Sunita Prasad. We huddle around the table and meet 18-year-old Rani, 16-year-old Ruby, and their mothers, Manorama and Savitri. Other women with multiple gold bangles on their forearms stand in the doorway in orange and red saris and shawls. Their long black hair, pulled into buns or ponytails, is so glossy, it looks, in the candlelight, positively lacquered. At the table, the women's dark eyes glitter with excitement and pride. Ruby and Rani are two of some 80 girls who have volunteered to spread information about HIV/AIDS to their friends in the neighborhood. Mature and self-possessed, decorative studs in their nostrils, they are not shy about discussing sex, substance abuse, and contraception.

Ryan leans forward to get a better look at dark-eyed Rani and asks, "What's the most common question your friends ask?"

"Well!" Rani says eagerly, "Girls ask mostly about menstrual cycle and hygiene. When we answer, sometimes they are offended. But! We don't let them off the hook! We pester them until they understand the problems of poor hygiene and sexually transmitted disease."

Visibly charmed, Ryan smiles and asks the girls how the work makes them feel. Rani says, "I'm very happy. It gives us a chance to go out of our houses and empower other girls. I don't like always sitting within the same four walls." Rani is engaged to be married to a boy her parents have chosen—she's seen only his photograph. Asked if the boy is handsome, Rani suddenly goes shy. She wags her head and giggles: "Yes. I like him!" What if her husband wants her to stop the work she's doing? Rani straightens up. "I will use my persuasion and my love! I will inform him of the good work I am doing, and he will understand." Rani would like to have two children, one boy, one girl. But what if she ends up with two girls?

Rani's mother, Manorama, peers at her. "Rani," she says, "daughters are much better than sons! Two girls is good!" Delighted by the mother's boldness, Ryan laughs and claps her hands, and suddenly the lights flicker on and the starkness of the

> "Women are socialized to be docile. I call it 'shrink to fit,'" says Meg Ryan.

room is fully revealed. On a cracked lettuce green wall hangs a clouded mirror, two photos of elderly ancestors, and a cheap electric clock. The blankets on the neatly made beds are threadbare. There's a small refrigerator in a corner and a battered TV and a vase of plastic roses on a dresser. The room is spare but spotless.

We walk down the alley to the community youth center, one of the few places in Jehangirpuri that girls may visit without a chaperone. Here we meet a group of barefoot teenage girls. Among them is Lakshmi, a fiery, high-voiced 18-year-old in a jean jacket. A born performer with dancing hands, Lakshmi shows us her book recording the reactions of the girls and boys she has spoken to about sex and disease. Before this program, she tells us, girls were easily influenced by pressure from boys. "But now they learn to say no, to trust themselves and make their own decisions." Lakshmi says conversing with boys is easier than she thought it would be, "but when we mention abstinence, they become wary. They say, 'Don't teach our girlfriends that!'"

Lakshmi attests to a great change in her own life since she began her awareness work. In the past, she rarely left her house except to go to school. "Before, my mother would object when I talked to boys. But now she trusts me to go out in the world." Boys, too, once skeptical, have begun visiting the youth center and encouraging their parents to let their sisters come. "There's more openness between mothers and daughters," Lakshmi says, "more camaraderie between girls and boys."

Ryan asks Lakshmi what she hopes for her future. Lakshmi cracks her knuckles, then slowly waves her palms at us, as if wiping mist from a windowpane. "I want to be completely free," she pipes. "Freedom is a big responsibility, but I want it. I don't want even my husband to stop me later in life. I want to use my skills to make a career."

Later, as we're leaving the community center, Ryan snaps a few photographs of the girls and says, "Oh, what that little girl who wants total freedom can do!"

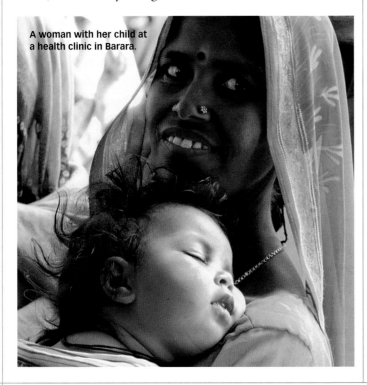

A woman with her child at a health clinic in Barara.

Consider these facts: One out of every six people in the world lives on less than a dollar a day. Seventy-five percent of those people are women. Women produce 50 percent of the world's food, yet own only 1 percent of its land. Of the 876 million illiterate adults in the developing world, two-thirds are women. Every year more than half a million women die from pregnancy-related causes. CARE aims to empower the disenfranchised, particularly women and girls. Anne Goddard tells me that women have proved to be a more efficient avenue than men for effecting change. "Microfinance programs used to focus a lot on men, but we've found that men use what they earn from these small loans to benefit themselves—buying cigarettes, for instance—while women use it to benefit their families. In the end, if you invest in women, you benefit the whole family." Women are a better financial risk as well: "We have 99 percent repayment rates with women." Education, too, has proved more effective in the long term when directed at women. "Educate a

306

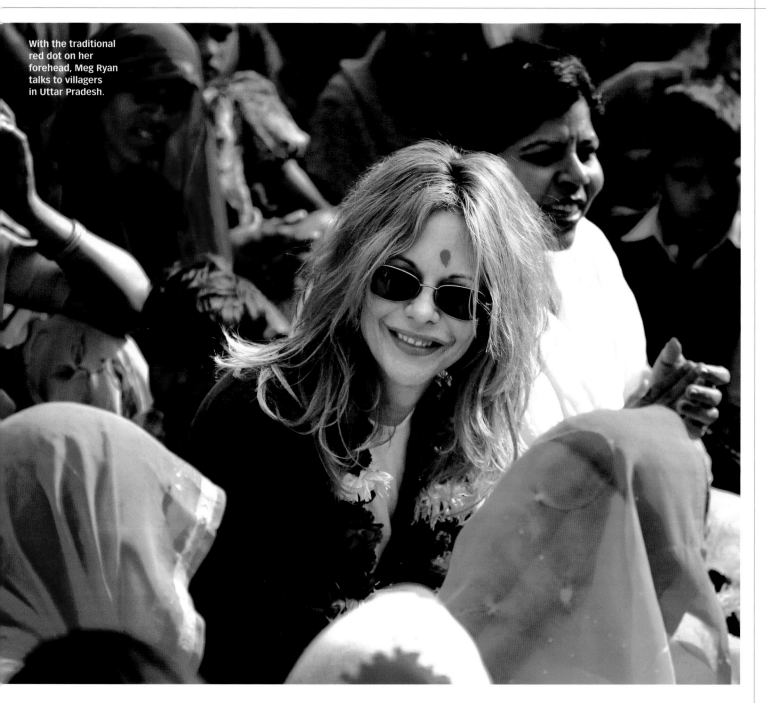

man and you educate an individual," says Goddard, "but educate a woman and you educate a nation." Why? Because women raise the children. "And research shows that the longer a girl stays in school, the fewer children she will have, the healthier those children will be, and the higher her family income. First we need to help women feel powerful, then we need to get them to organize, to use their voices."

At the entrance to a straw-roofed hut in the village of Barara in Uttar Pradesh, a young mother takes Meg Ryan's hand and invites her to step inside. In the dimness of the one-room hut, the woman is radiant in her red sari. Her husband's smile is expectant and generous. He earns 25 rupees,

approximately 50 cents, a day at his job in Agra. In the shadows, the children hide, shyly staring. There is no electricity here and no running water. The woman asks if we're hungry, proffers a jar of spicy pickles and a tin of chapatis. On our way out of the hut, our interpreter points to a clay cylinder the size of a paint can in the dirt by the front door: "This is her stove, her kitchen."

Poverty in Uttar Pradesh is dire. More than half the women here are illiterate, 70 percent don't regularly visit health clinics or hospitals, and 40 percent of the children are not immunized. CARE worker Pratibha Sharma says, "The greatest number of children who die in this country die on their very first day of life. After that they die in the first month, the first year." The most common causes are diarrhea, malnutrition, and pneumonia—

easily treatable, easily preventable ailments. Perhaps the most startling statistic in the Agra area is the ratio between the sexes—a dismal 852 women per 1,000 men. Where are northern India's missing girls and women? Poor nutrition and healthcare, selective abortion of female fetuses, and female infanticide are all too common here. "Baby girls," Sharma says, "have a very deprived childhood."

As we cross the village square, Ryan, who has a loose, ambling way of walking, raises her long-lensed camera to her face and snaps a series of photos. I ask whether she does a lot of photography. She answers modestly, "Well, I do, but I'm bad at it! Out of 60 pictures I might get only *four* that are any good." She laughs, and the laugh is clear as a carillon. Distinct notes trip from her throat in a descending melody, like a lark fluttering out of the sky.

At the clinic, infant immunizations are under way. A rainbow of brilliant saris twists toward the door; a long line of young

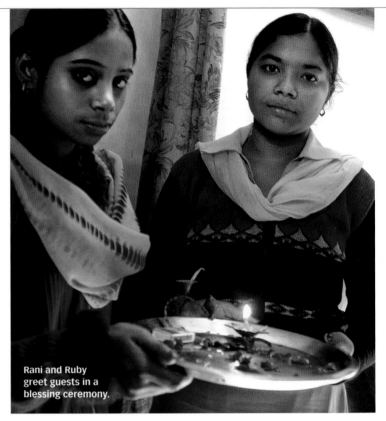

Rani and Ruby greet guests in a blessing ceremony.

"Daughters are much better than sons!" says Rani's mother.

mothers, most with veils drawn across their faces, await their turn with the visiting healthcare worker overseen by CARE. Their infants, bundles of cloth held lightly in the crook of the arm, are tiny, heads wobbling on tender necks, huge brown eyes staring vacantly, fine black hair damp with sweat. At a desk in front of the clinic, two poker-faced men distribute free sanitary pads and condoms. Inside—one room lit by a single window—a nurse weighs an infant on a meat scale sus-

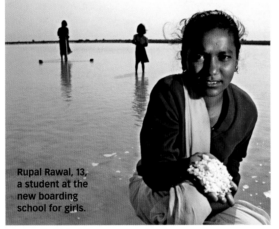

Rupal Rawal, 13, a student at the new boarding school for girls.

pended from the ceiling; another pricks a baby in the arm with a hypodermic needle. The infant lies wide-eyed and silent as the needle pierces his skin; there's a three-second delay before he lets out a howl of pain and outrage. Ryan bends to coo at him. "Oh, you are so *cute*," she murmurs. With genuine relief in her voice, Sharma says, "More and more village women are bringing their children for immunizations." On the clinic wall is a picture of 19-year-old Sania Mirza, India's top-ranked female tennis player. Below her image are the words "Save the girl child."

Leaving Barara, Ryan absently twists a lock of her shaggy blonde hair around a finger and ponders the status of women. "Women are socialized to be nice, to be docile," she says. "I call it 'shrink to fit': Shrink yourself to fit what others expect of you." Sharma says, "Yes. Here they often tell young women, 'Don't take a promotion at your work; it will be harder for you to find a boy.'"

"But the moment you hide your light," says Ryan, "you're throwing a burqa over your head. You have to give *yourself* power and confidence." When I ask Ryan what moved her to make this trip with CARE, she says, "I came here because I wanted to help make a change. Celebrity is such a random assignment that you might as well do something useful with it. Whatever light shines on me, I want to share it, to stand next to something that really matters. Giving internationally to a group like CARE is a way for Americans to build up goodwill in the world." Paraphrasing *New York Times* columnist Nicholas Kristof, Ryan adds, "The 19th century was about the eradication of slavery, the 20th century was about the eradication of totalitarianism, and the 21st century is about finding equality for women." She falls silent for a moment, then says, "I was apprehensive about going into all these poor people's houses. But the moment you go in, you realize there's God in everyone's eyes. Mother Teresa said there is wealth in poverty and poverty in wealth. When you look through the doors of these mud-brick huts, you don't see squalor; you see beauty. That woman who offered us pickles and chapatis in her hut! Did you smell the pickles? Beautiful!"

On our last day, driving across the mud desert outside Surendranagar in western Gujarat, we see no houses, no trees, no vegetation whatever, no clouds or birds, cars or people. In the course of half an hour there is only a milky blue sky and a terrifyingly huge expanse of cracked beige earth that stretches to the horizon and seemingly beyond. This desert is flat as a griddle and nearly as hot. From time to time, Ryan and the other passengers in the car lift magazines and pamphlets to the sides of their faces, shading themselves from the menacing sun. We're on our way to visit the migratory salt-pan workers, among the poorest and most socially stigmatized castes in all of India. I cannot imagine anyone living and working in this hellish place, let alone for eight months at a time. Another quarter of an hour passes and suddenly Ryan says, "What are those little red flags I'm seeing way over there?" Our guide, CARE's Veena Padia, replies in her calm, stately way, "The flags are indicators of the human beings' existence." Soon a dark speck appears in the distance and slowly grows—a man riding toward us on a bicycle hauling an impossibly huge bundle of sticks and twigs on his back. Padia points to a white van far in the distance. "That is the visiting doctor. CARE arranged for him to come here once a week."

We learn from Padia that salt workers put in ten- to 12-hour days; families of seven subsist on a dollar and a half a day. Conditions are harsh—there is blindness due to the sun and salt, skin disease, a high rate of tuberculosis and alcoholism.

We pull up to a make-shift school—the workers built it themselves by digging a ten-by-ten-foot pit, with walls of bamboo and a ceiling of burlap. Inside, children are sitting cross-legged on the floor on burlap bags—25 boys but only seven girls. Many walk an hour to get here in the morning; all bathe only once every 15 days, when water is trucked in. Their sunburned cheeks are dry and flecked with a faint, mottled tracing that echoes the pattern of cracks in the earth beneath their feet.

Next door is a family of seven in a handmade hut with a dirt floor and beds made of rope and sticks. Labhubhai, the head of the household, is wearing a rag wrapped around

his head, trousers mended in seven different places, and salt-encrusted rubber boots on his feet. "The boots," Padia explains, "are a new feature in his life. Before, everyone in the salt pans worked barefoot. The government first agreed to provide boots for the men, then we pressed them to provide boots for the women as well." His wife, Leelaben, and the other women are saving their money so that together they can buy new machinery for more efficient salt collecting. "I save 30 cents per month," she says proudly.

Our last stop is the experimental Ganatar school, which was begun with support from CARE to encourage the daughters of salt-pan workers to seek a life beyond the oppressive salt pans. In contrast to the hideous mud desert, the campus of this small residential school is graced with trees, grass, and a flower garden. Padia tells us that in the past, the salt workers didn't want to send girls to a boarding school such as this. "They would only send the boys. They could not see the point of spending money on their girls." When we meet with the 25 girls enrolled at the school, Ryan asks them what they like about their new school. A beautiful, short-haired little girl in a pretty purple sari stands up and says, "Before we came here, we were never brushing our teeth or cutting our nails. We were not bathing or cleaning our clothes or even wearing them properly. Now we do. Before, we didn't know even A, B, C, and we could not speak Hindi. Now we have learned and we are able to read."

When Ryan tells them they should all be very proud, the girls burst into spontaneous applause. Clearly moved, Ryan claps with them. She asks them what they'd like to do with their future. Some want to become beauticians, some want to go to design school, others are interested in studying tailoring and embroidering. Curious, they ask Ryan what she does for work. She tells them, "I work in Hollywood." They look puzzled, and one asks, "Hollywood? Is that like Bollywood?" Ryan laughs. "Yes, but it's much smaller than Bollywood." The girls want to know what movies Ryan has starred in. Diffidently, she says, "Oh, I don't think you'd know my movies." Another girl asks, "Why are there so many people accompanying you today?" Ryan laughs and points to the CARE workers in the room and to the cameraman who's been recording her trip. Shyly she says, "They're not accompanying me; I'm accompanying them."

Ryan asks the girls if there's anything they'd like to ask us, anything they'd like to tell us. The short-haired girl stands up again and says intently, "I would like to give this message to other children: They should study hard and become something in their life, just as we have studied and tried to come forward in our life. May all girls do the same. Come forward." ◉

"Educate a woman and you educate a nation," says CARE's Anne Goddard.

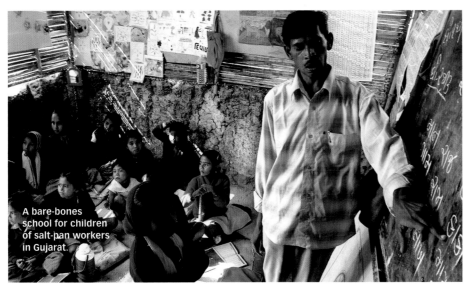

A bare-bones school for children of salt-pan workers in Gujarat.

Julia Louis-Dreyfus's Aha! Moment

Dirty air. Grubby water. Just sit back and take it?
Nuh-uh. The actress goes from green living to red-hot action.

About 13 years ago, my first son and I began to take walks along the beaches in Los Angeles, and some days he couldn't swim because the water was too polluted. By the time my second son was born, I'd joined the California environmental organizations Heal the Bay and Heal the Ocean.

Several years later, some "green" friends invited me, my husband, and a few other people to dinner at their house. The activist Bobby Kennedy Jr., another friend of theirs, would be joining us.

On the way to dinner, I nearly turned around and went home. I mean, wasn't I already a big-time enviro-activist? Was it really worth it to leave the kids on a school night? Hadn't I already sacrificed enough? My husband and I had been to many a rubber chicken evening of do-gooders and dull-ass conversation. And *The Sopranos* was on! But we had committed, so there we were, smug in our eco-superiority.

After we'd mingled for a while, we settled in the living room to listen as Bobby spoke—for an hour, in beautiful, precise sentences, without pause, without notes. He was revelatory, funny, spiritual, profound. He connected all the causes I've most cared about since I was a child: poverty, civil rights, racism, education, and conservation. "The greatest assets the average American has, regardless of her race or class, are clean air and clean water and safe food and enriching places to bring her children," he said. "If we want to give our children the same opportunities for dignity and enrichment that

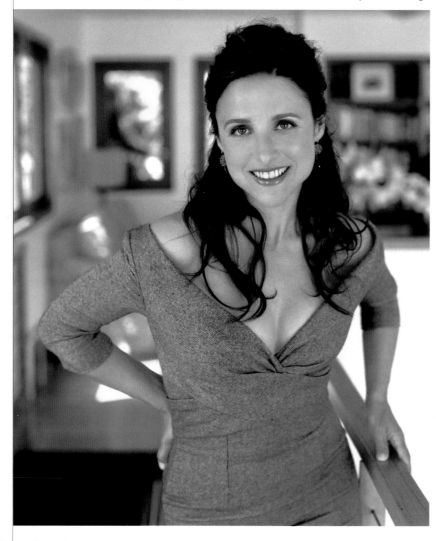

"I realized an essential irony: Fighting for the planet is fighting for the little guy."

our parents gave us, we have to start protecting the public lands, the wildlife, the water." Listening to Bobby made me see an essential irony: Fighting for the planet is fighting for the little guy.

When he stopped talking, I lifted my jaw from the floor. All my holier-than-thou eco-green feelings were replaced with the realization that I had done nothing. I knew that I had to do so much more. We *all* do.

Since that night, I've redoubled my efforts. I've tried to spread the message that we all must get involved with spectacular organizations like the Natural Resources Defense Council, the Waterkeeper Alliance, and the countless local organizations whose brilliant, underpaid, overworked, wildly dedicated staffs work day in and day out to save our planet from ourselves. Working with these people is a great privilege and it keeps you very, very humble, believe me. And while I know I don't do nearly enough, I sure am glad that I didn't turn around and go home the night I met Bobby Kennedy, because now at least I know where to start. 🇴

Elizabeth Perkins's Aha! Moment

One girl had all the opportunity in the world.
The other didn't. For the actress, it was a call to freedom—and fairness for all.

I was helping my friend plant herbs in her backyard garden one perfect, smog-free Los Angeles Wednesday, and I had just patted down the soil around a bunch of basil when I heard the sound of a lawn mower. At the far end of the property, I saw a very small person pushing a very large machine.

I said to my friend, "Is that a child?"

Whoever it was continued to mow the lawn, moving closer to us, and we confirmed that it was indeed a young girl. Clear, open face, deep-set eyes, long chestnut hair in two neat braids. My friend's new gardener told us the girl was his 14-year-old daughter, Alicia. She was born in Mexico and spoke little English.

"Why isn't she in school?" we asked.

"She has to work," he said. "To support the family." Then he patiently explained his predicament: Of course he would love for Alicia to spend her days in school, but money was scarce and sometimes everyone had to work so that they could all survive.

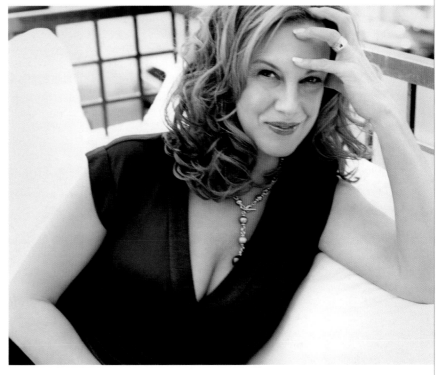

For a while, I stood on the lawn, watching Alicia. She was carrying bags of mulch and digging holes with heavy shovels. Eventually, she took a break and sat on the grass to eat a sandwich she'd brought. I thought of my daughter, the same age, dressed in her brand-name jeans, leaving science class, laughing with her friends. Although this wasn't news—that there are children in this country who cannot get the education that is their only hope of improving their state, while others have every advantage imaginable—the stark contrast, the terrific unfairness of it, took my breath away.

When my daughter got back from school, she started to complain about her homework.

"Come with me," I said, and we went down the street to meet Alicia. I told my daughter that Alicia had been working in the garden with her father most of the day.

"Why aren't you in school?" my daughter asked her.

"Because this is what I do," Alicia said. My daughter nodded slowly.

As I went inside to say hello to my friend, I noticed my daughter follow Alicia to the front of the house. And then they began to move plants together. I couldn't hear their voices, but I could see them talking as they worked, fumbling for words and giggling. For a second, through that window, they looked like a couple of best friends doing chores outside, having fun on a lovely California afternoon—not strangers from vastly different backgrounds trying to comprehend each other's situation. It was an ordinary scene, but I wondered why it was only a "scene." Why couldn't it simply be ordinary? Why should two 14-year-old girls have such disparate hopes for a future?

I realized that afternoon that while it's important to be thankful for how fortunate I've been, it's even more pressing that I take things in with a broader perspective. As a person, as a citizen, it's my duty to ensure that Alicia enjoy the same rights as my daughter; she mustn't be denied the chance to pursue her dreams. It falls to me as the granddaughter of Greek immigrants to call my political representatives, to rally in support of immigrants' rights when I can. It's my responsibility to extend the wealth of opportunity I've been given by this country to those just beginning their fight here.

Right now America is grappling with its "immigrant problem." I struggled with it, too. But I know where I stand. This country's history is bound up with migrants and refugees who fought through prejudice and carved out their version of the American dream. Now is no different. And where better to learn that lesson than in my own backyard? ◑

The Legends Who Lunch:
A Weekend of Glory
at Promised Land

The setting: Oprah's place in California. **The honored guests:** Cicely Tyson, Maya Angelou, Diahann Carroll, Coretta Scott King, Leontyne Price, Diana Ross, Tina Turner, and the other breakthrough women Oprah wanted to thank for building a "Bridge to Now"— women without whom her life and work wouldn't have been possible. **The celebration:** A luncheon, a white-tie ball, and a rousing, heart-bursting gospel brunch. The food, the love—the outfits!—and just plain joy in the air…don't get us started. LAURIE WINER has the details. But first a word from OPRAH…

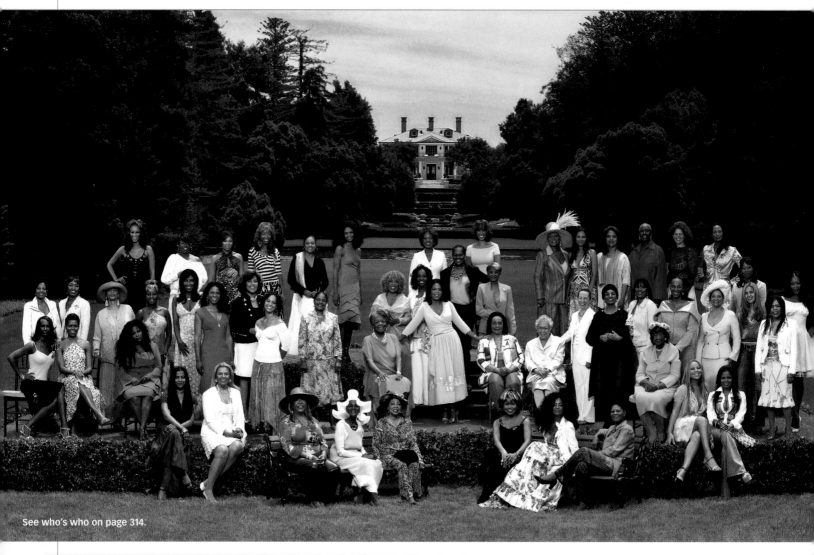

See who's who on page 314.

OPRAH: "HEAVEN IN MY LIVING ROOM"

I forgot to invite Cicely Tyson to my 50th birthday party. I have always admired her, though I didn't know her well. When I turned 50, she sent me a lovely gift she had knit herself. I was so touched by her thoughtfulness that I chided myself for not including her among the 50 women around my birthday luncheon table.

I decided to make up for it by inviting her to lunch alone, and then thought, Wouldn't it be even more special if Ruby Dee could come?

And thus began the idea of Legends. I started thinking about all the women who'd come before me, many of whom have now passed on—women whose steps created a journey of no boundaries for my generation. I wanted to thank them, celebrate them, and rejoice in their spirit.

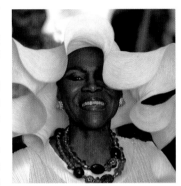

I wanted the best for this occasion, so I called in Colin Cowie, the most creative entertaining expert I know. We planned for a year: I delighted in every detail, then handed it over to God and let it become what it was meant to be—one of the greatest experiences of my life.

I sent out 25 invitations to women who had been a "Bridge to Now" for me. Eighteen were able to attend. I sent a separate invitation to 45 "young'uns," women like myself who'd benefited from crossing that bridge. Most of them said, "Yes, I'll be there." They rearranged tours, changed plans, and traveled from Los Angeles, the East Coast, and even Europe, not knowing who else was invited. It was a hallelujah moment when all of us came together for the first time.

Alicia Keys said, "It was like going to heaven and seeing everybody you've always wanted to meet."

Heaven in my living room! Such squealing and laughing I've never heard from grown women. We were giddy. So much energy, talent, and power in one place. It was electrifying, and every one of us felt the current. The joy, pride, and deep appreciation we held for one another was overwhelming and humbling.

I've always had fierce respect and reverence for those whose names made history and for the millions whose names did not. People who were so resourceful, resilient, and remarkable in their will to keep moving forward. These are the roots from which I've grown. This weekend was the fulfillment of a dream for me: To honor where I've come from, to celebrate how I got here, and to claim where I'm going.

THE LEGENDS CELEBRATION

BY LAURIE WINER

Pam Grier was the first to arrive. "I'm from Colorado," she said by way of explanation. "We're always on time."

She was wearing a lime green pantsuit. Oprah greeted her in a sea green, tea-length dress, cinched at the waist. Soon Maya Angelou appeared in an apple green gown, loose and flowing. For a moment, green seemed to be the color of the day.

Before long, Oprah's large front room was alive with dozens of fabulous outfits in every shade of the rainbow as guests poured

(Left) Cicely Tyson, the inspiration for the party, arrives wearing beads Oprah left each Legend in her hotel room. *(Above)* Alfre Woodard looks on as Oprah embraces Judith Jamison.

Dr. Maya Angelou and Oprah relish the moment in front of Oprah's favorite painting, *To the Highest Bidder,* by Harry Roseland. "Isn't it ironic," Oprah said, "that all of these free women are celebrating our lives under the gaze of a woman who is about to be sold into slavery and separated from her young daughter."

Who's Who at the Party

(Legends in red, young'uns in purple)

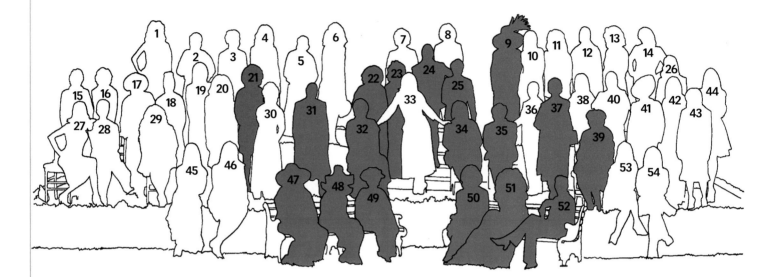

1. Tyra Banks
MODEL

2. Missy Elliot
RAP ARTIST

3. Ashanti
SINGER

4. Brandy Norwood
ACTRESS-SINGER

5. Kathleen Battle
OPERA SINGER

6. Kimberly Elise
ACTRESS

7. Alfre Woodard
ACTRESS

8. Gayle King
**EDITOR AT LARGE,
O, THE OPRAH MAGAZINE**

9. Patti LaBelle
SINGER

10. Halle Berry
ACTRESS

11. Phylicia Rashad
ACTRESS

12. Judith Jamison
DANCER-CHOREOGRAPHER

13. Anna Deavere Smith
ACTRESS-PLAYWRIGHT

14. Beverly Johnson
MODEL

15. Melba Moore
ACTRESS-SINGER

16. Angela Bassett
ACTRESS

17. Terry McMillan
AUTHOR

18. Mary J. Blige
SINGER

19. Natalie Cole
SINGER

20. Audra McDonald
ACTRESS-SINGER

21. Diahann Carroll
ACTRESS-SINGER

22. Roberta Flack
SINGER

23. Gladys Knight
SINGER

24. Naomi Sims
MODEL

25. Nancy Wilson
SINGER

26. Yolanda Adams
SINGER

27. Iman
MODEL

28. Michelle Obama
COMMUNITY AFFAIRS EXECUTIVE

29. Chaka Khan
SINGER

30. Alicia Keys
SINGER

31. Shirley Caesar
SINGER

32. Dr. Maya Angelou
AUTHOR

33. Oprah Winfrey

34. Coretta Scott King
CIVIL RIGHTS ACTIVIST

35. Elizabeth Catlett
ARTIST

36. Pearl Cleage
POET-PLAYWRIGHT

37. Leontyne Price
OPERA SINGER

38. Pam Grier
ACTRESS

39. Dr. Dorothy Height
CIVIL RIGHTS ACTIVIST

40. Susan L. Taylor
**EDITORIAL DIRECTOR,
ESSENCE MAGAZINE**

41. Debbie Allen
ACTRESS-DANCER

42. Darnell Martin
DIRECTOR-SCREENWRITER

43. Valerie Simpson
**SINGER-
COMPOSER**

44. Naomi Campbell
MODEL

45. Suzan-Lori Parks
PLAYWRIGHT

46. Suzanne de Passe
PRODUCER-WRITER

47. Della Reese
ACTRESS-SINGER

48. Cicely Tyson
ACTRESS

49. Ruby Dee
ACTRESS

50. Tina Turner
SINGER

51. Diana Ross
SINGER

52. Dionne Warwick
SINGER

53. Mariah Carey
SINGER

54. Janet Jackson
SINGER

---

*The Legends Unable
to Attend*

Katherine Dunham
**CHOREOGRAPHER-
DANCER**

Aretha Franklin
SINGER

Nikki Giovanni
POET

Lena Horne
ACTRESS-SINGER

Toni Morrison
AUTHOR

Rosa Parks
CIVIL RIGHTS ACTIVIST

Alice Walker
AUTHOR

The Legends Lunch

into her California home, Promised Land. There were fantastic hats: Leontyne Price wore a black-and-red-patterned turban, Patti LaBelle sported a tall straw number with feathers the color of cornhusk, and Cicely Tyson's face could just be seen under a floating white cloud of cotton. Dr. Dorothy Height wore a crownless hat (no hat hair!). Hatless were Diana Ross, Tina Turner, Dionne Warwick, Nancy Wilson, and many others.

It was a Friday and one of those temperate, untroubled, clear days that are so unfairly plentiful here, setting off Promised Land's 42 acres to dazzling advantage. "I live between the mountains and the sea," Oprah told a guest, using what seemed to be a metaphor for something mysterious and wonderful. Today was a long-awaited day: the beginning of a weekend of festivities honoring the African-American women Oprah calls Legends.

A couple of months earlier, Oprah took a break from planning this party to explain the inspiration for it. "I wanted to honor the women who have been a bridge to my life, to this moment, to now. This is such a great moment for African-American women. But we're so interested in progress and moving forward that we've lost the remembering. So I made a list of women who broke through barriers, women I wanted to thank and honor."

I n preparation for the three-day feast of gratitude, Oprah and her best friend, Gayle King, spent hours refining every last detail—examining every napkin and plate (the soup bowl—"too deep"), tasting every course. Along with feast-planner Colin Cowie, they sampled ten different desserts for the ball to be held on Saturday night, and when they couldn't decide which was more delicious, they threw up their hands and chose to serve ten. They considered the manner in which the fresh gardenia blooms

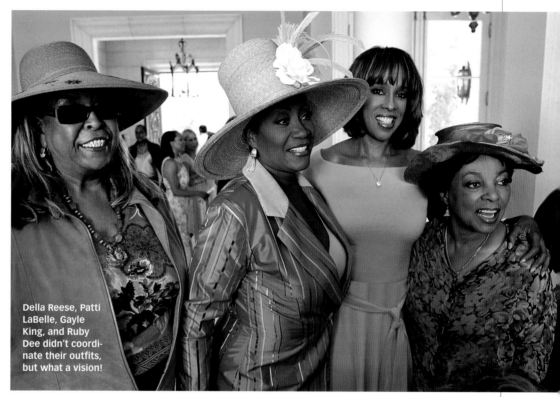

Oprah welcomes Halle Berry and Tina Turner to her home for preluncheon cocktails.

Della Reese, Patti LaBelle, Gayle King, and Ruby Dee didn't coordinate their outfits, but what a vision!

"So much energy, talent, and power in one place. It was electrifying, and every one of us felt the current."
—*Oprah*

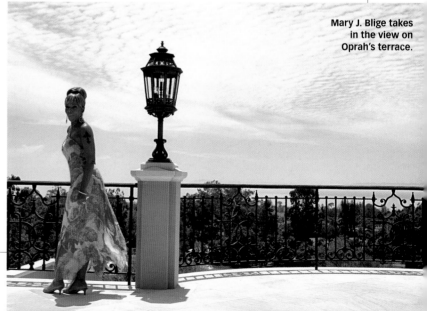

Mary J. Blige takes in the view on Oprah's terrace.

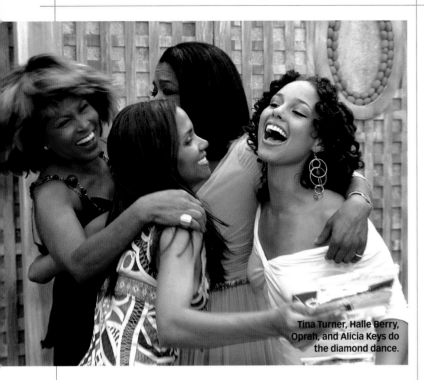

Tina Turner, Halle Berry, Oprah, and Alicia Keys do the diamond dance.

And now the long-planned-for weekend had started. Many of the women had never met and were nervous and excited. Halle Berry, looking about 16 in a simple flowered dress with her hair long and straight, approached Leontyne Price with great shyness. Both women seemed touched that the other recognized her and knew about her work. Singer Brandy Norwood sat chatting literally at the feet of Coretta Scott King. When she got up, all she could say was, "I'm just overwhelmed." For Della Reese, who had performed in the past with Nancy Wilson and Dionne Warwick, and who'd been moved to tears when she'd gone to hear Leontyne Price sing opera, the day was unforgettable. She stood off by herself, just taking it all in. "There are a lot of people here who pulled themselves up from the bottom," she said. "This is a magnificent thing, to bring these particular people together. This is love."

A green trolley was waiting to take everybody to the garden. "Oh, of course there would be a trolley!" said four-time Tony winner Audra McDonald. "Everyone should have a trolley!" Down the rolling hills of Promised Land, they crossed the bridge that had just been completed the day before ("We had, like, 127 people here finishing it," Oprah said) and came to an arbor flooded with roses. When they were seated, an army of waitstaff emerged single file—white shirts, green ties, khaki pants—one for each guest. After the minted pea soup, the pistachio-covered chicken paillard, and the chocolate cake with truffle cream designed to look exactly like little flowers in a terracotta pot, complete with chocolate soil, Pearl Cleage stood to present the poem Oprah had commissioned for the occasion. Helping Cleage were young'uns Angela Bassett, Alfre Woodard, Phylicia Rashad, and Halle Berry, who recited the tribute directly to those being honored.

"We celebrate your courage," Halle Berry read. "We celebrate your spirit. / We celebrate your genius.... / We thank you for the dues you've paid, / and the prayers you've prayed. / We thank you for showing us how to fly *by flying.*"

would be tied to each of the "tribute books" for the guests, as well as the tabletop arrangements. "Every flower on every table is an expression of my love for these women," Oprah said.

Each of the women she was honoring meant something very specific to Oprah, most of them since childhood. "Diahann Carroll—I remember the first time I saw her TV show *Julia.* It was so exciting. I thought, *She's not on welfare! She's not a maid!* Then I saw Diana Ross on Ed Sullivan, and I thought, *Whatever this is, I want to be some of that!*

"Leontyne Price comes from Mississippi, as I do," she said. "She sang in the major opera houses and concert halls around the world, and opened doors to those who came behind her. The artist Elizabeth Catlett—I was attracted to her sculptures before I could ever afford them. I've chosen remarkable women who have been remarkable to me."

Oprah decided to make a bridge not only from her past to the present but from the present to the future, inviting a group of brilliant "young'uns"—women like Valerie Simpson, Debbie Allen, Kathleen Battle, Alicia Keys, Mary J. Blige, Mariah Carey, Natalie Cole, and Anna Deavere Smith. The idea of a bridge was so crucial that Oprah built a real one for the women to walk across on the way to the Friday luncheon.

> "This is a magnificent thing, to bring these particular people together. This is love."
> *—Della Reese*

Angela Bassett read: "You could not have known that your collective example of the limitless possibilities / that were open to us are what allowed us to look into our mother's eye and say: / '*Mama,* I want to be a singer. / *Mama,* I want to be an actress. / *Mama,* I want to be a dancer, or a sculptor, or a lawyer, or a leader, / or a world changing force for good, loose in the world, *and whirling....*' "

All the younger women joined in the chorus: *"We speak your names. / We speak your names."* As they recited the names of the Legends, sunglasses came off, eyes were dabbed with napkins. Occasionally, a moan or a sob could be heard in the otherwise rapt and quiet crowd. There can't have been many gatherings anywhere in the world where so many famous, gifted, and powerful people have willingly found such a deep and open connection to the pain of the past. But there was something else there, too. This was a meeting of women who felt the full measure of how blessed they are.

"All of us have a debt of respect and responsibility," she said. "I see a lot of young stars who have the benefits of wealth and fame and think very little about everyone who changed the world for them before they were even born. I see them acting as if it were all created for them and by them. It wasn't. It was paid for by generations of people. You cannot move forward unless you acknowledge where you came from."

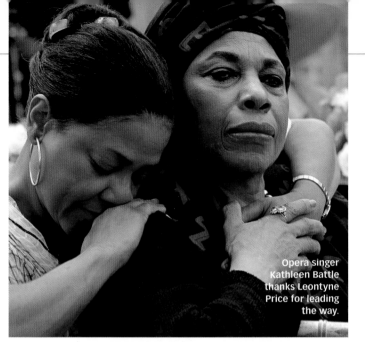

Opera singer Kathleen Battle thanks Leontyne Price for leading the way.

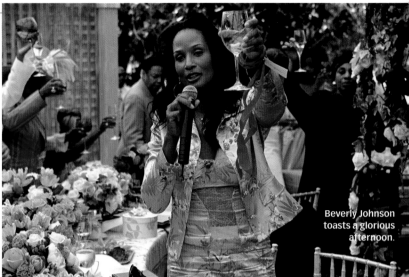

Beverly Johnson toasts a glorious afternoon.

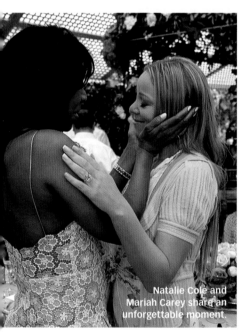

Natalie Cole and Mariah Carey share an unforgettable moment.

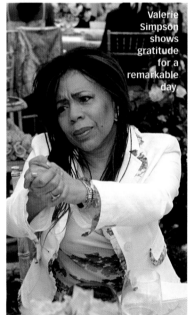

Valerie Simpson shows gratitude for a remarkable day.

We Speak Your Names

Excerpt from the poem by Pearl Cleage

"My sisters we are gathered here to speak your names. We are here because we are your daughters as surely as if you had conceived us, nurtured us, carried us in your wombs and then sent us out into the world to make our mark, and see what we see *and be what we be, but better, truer, deeper* because of the shining example of your own incandescent lives."

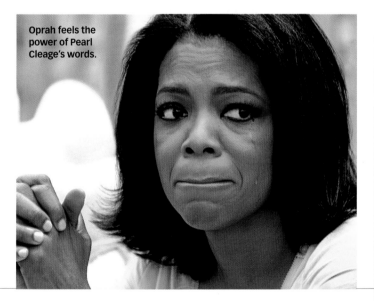

Oprah feels the power of Pearl Cleage's words.

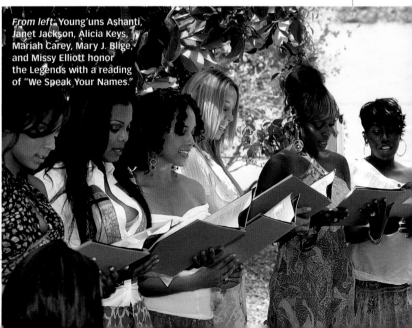

From left: Young'uns Ashanti, Janet Jackson, Alicia Keys, Mariah Carey, Mary J. Blige, and Missy Elliott honor the Legends with a reading of "We Speak Your Names."

The Ball

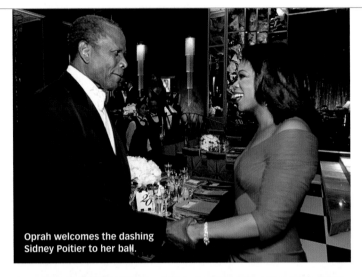

Oprah welcomes the dashing Sidney Poitier to her ball.

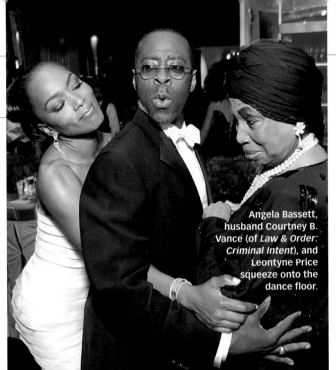

Angela Bassett, husband Courtney B. Vance (of *Law & Order: Criminal Intent*), and Leontyne Price squeeze onto the dance floor.

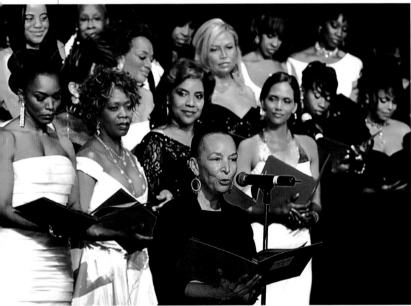

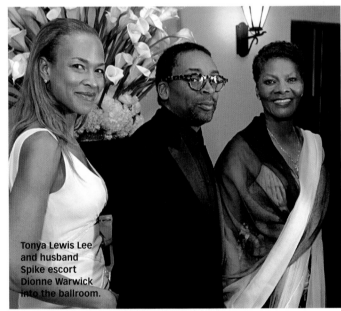

Tonya Lewis Lee and husband Spike escort Dionne Warwick into the ballroom.

(*Above*) At Saturday's ball, Pearl Cleage and the "young'uns" read "We Speak Your Names" (*back, from left:* Suzan-Lori Parks, Judith Jamison, Natalie Cole, Gayle King, Yolanda Adams; *middle:* Melba Moore, Suzanne de Passe, Missy Elliott, Janet Jackson; *front:* Angela Bassett, Alfre Woodard, Phylicia Rashad, Halle Berry).

"Creating the Legends celebration will forever be one of the great highlights of my life."
—*Oprah*

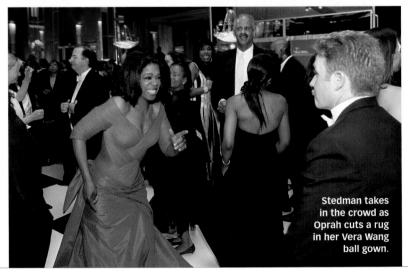

Stedman takes in the crowd as Oprah cuts a rug in her Vera Wang ball gown.

The Gospel Brunch

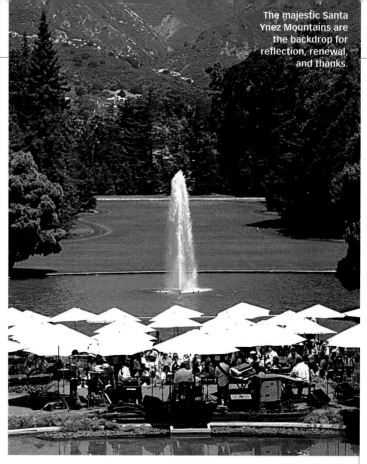

The majestic Santa Ynez Mountains are the backdrop for reflection, renewal, and thanks.

Oprah had one more announcement to make. She brought out Dorrit Moussaieff, the first lady of Iceland, who had helped her design a present for each of her guests.

The army of waitstaff reappeared, this time carrying red alligator boxes. Oprah asked that all her guests open their gifts at once. There was a moment of silence. Then Angela Bassett let out a scream, Debbie Allen a fantastic shriek. Under her cloud-like hat, Cicely Tyson covered her face with her hands. Diahann Carroll stood up and exclaimed, "You have lost your incredible mind!" Inside each box was a pair of diamond earrings: A large hoop dripping with diamonds for the younger women, an elegant double teardrop for the Legends.

Once the excitement subsided a little, Maya Angelou said she would like to speak to the young'uns. Her mellifluous voice filled the air. "In 20 years, there will be young women who will be doing this for you," she told them. "You are all extraordinary. There is nothing greater than 'thank you.' That is what we say to God. In 20 years, someone will be saying it to you."

The rest of the weekend was still to unfurl. There was a magnificent white-tie ball for 362 guests on Saturday night and an invigorating gospel brunch on Sunday. On that final day, guests sipping Bloody Marys and Bellinis walked among the giant redwoods on Oprah's front lawn. The mood now was friendly and elegiac; everyone had shared something extraordinary, and they were sad it was almost over. New and dear old friends chatted, and all were irresistibly drawn to a temporary bandstand when the singing started. BeBe Winans belted "Oh Happy Day" with the Hawkinses—Edwin, Walter, Lynette, and Tramaine. Then a gorgeous testimonial called "Changed" brought Bebe into the audience, looking for a few golden throats to join in. Dionne Warwick took the mic, as did Chaka Khan, Patti LaBelle, Valerie Simpson, Gladys Knight, and Yolanda Adams; they brought down the house.

Jesse Jackson roamed through the crowd, while Spike and Tonya Lewis Lee and Barack and Michelle Obama sat and listened. John Travolta, Barbra Streisand, and James Brolin moved into the shade of some nearby trees, as did Diane Sawyer and Mike Nichols, where they could stand and sway to the astounding voices emanating from the stage and the audience. It was "church," as Oprah said, and it was rousing and beautiful.

Eventually, the guests headed back to earth, and filled their stomachs for the journey home with chilled lobster and stone crabs, fruit, homemade mini-doughnuts, lemon waffles, and Art Smith's perfect fried chicken. It had been a weekend of great food, but everyone knew the real nourishment had come from all that had happened between the meals. O

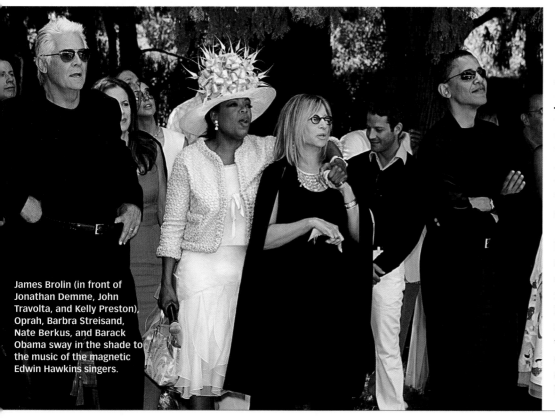

James Brolin (in front of Jonathan Demme, John Travolta, and Kelly Preston), Oprah, Barbra Streisand, Nate Berkus, and Barack Obama sway in the shade to the music of the magnetic Edwin Hawkins singers.

Make a Connection

The End of Hatred

BY SHARON SALZBERG

Recently, traveling by train to New York City, I found myself sitting between a woman having a moderately loud conversation on a cell phone and a man growing increasingly agitated at the volume of her call. As the ride went on, accompanied by the unremitting sound of her voice, he wriggled and sighed, then finally exploded. "You're making too much noise!"

She turned to glare at him over my shoulder, as I hunched further down in my seat. Sandwiched between them, I glanced over at him and reflected, *Well, the same could be said about you, too!*

A saying I once heard came into my mind: "The problems we face cannot be solved by the same level of thinking that created them." It takes strong insight and often a good deal of courage to break away from our habitual ways of looking at things, to be able to respond from a different place. Imagine if we dropped our need to be right, our easy perpetuation of what we're used to, our urge to go along with what others think, and tried to practice what the Buddha taught: "Hatred does not cease by hatred at any time: hatred ceases by love."

Shouting to drown out someone else's noise, returning belligerence for belligerence may be automatic, but it tires us out. Rigidly categorizing people as good or bad or right or wrong helps us feel secure; yet relating in that way doesn't allow us to really connect to anyone, and we actually feel alone.

Risking a new level of seeing enables us to try out new behaviors and find ways to communicate that convey our feelings without damaging ourselves, or those around us.

That would kick off an enormous adventure of consciousness—a readiness to step into new terrain, redefine power, see patience as strength rather than as resignation. Instead of yelling at the woman on the train, the man might have made his request before his anger built to unmanageable proportions and he saw her only as an irritant, not as a person. He might have asked before insisting and spoken before shouting, just as he might like to be spoken to himself.

My seatmates on the train settled down, but we see elements of that ride every day: frustration, carelessness, an effort to be in control, rage, fear—and the chance to be different. Can we see it all and seize the chance to operate from new levels of thinking?

Even in horrible circumstances, we have that opportunity—and the prospect for meaningful change. I saw it after the metro bombing in London in July 2005, when, like most people, my initial response was sorrow for the lives lost and some anxiety about getting on a subway in New York. This was all natural and appropriate, but limited by "us versus them" thinking.

> Imagine if we dropped our need to be right, our urge to go along with what others think.

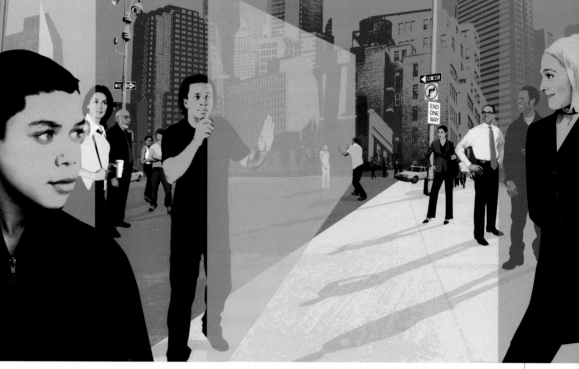

Willa, the 7-year-old daughter of a friend, had another perspective. On being told what had happened, her eyes filled with tears, her mother wrote me, and she said, "Mom, we should say a prayer." As she and her mother held hands, Willa asked to go first. Her mother was stunned to hear Willa begin with, "May the bad guys remember the love in their hearts."

Hearing that, my own heart leaped to another level altogether. ◐

321

The Devils Wear Sneakers

KATHERINE RUSSELL RICH wrote a provocative memoir about surviving cancer in her 30s. Years later, to her amazement, she learned that her book was inspiring an incredible group of people to help breast cancer patients through thick, thin, sickness, and health. Was this the final stage in her own recovery?

This is a story about angels and devils, and a woman who managed to make flowers bloom in the rocky place that lies between them. It's a story that begins with two coincidences, one terrible, the other fortuitous.

The terrible one first. In October 2000, a Baltimore lawyer named Lark Schulze was in the middle of a breast cancer fund-raising walk when she turned to a friend and said, "You know what? I am so lucky. I don't know one person with breast cancer." A month later, those words haunted her. On a climbing trek in Bhutan, she got a frantic message from her husband. Her daughter, Jessica, 30, had just been diagnosed with breast cancer. Lark scrambled to get home. Nineteen months later, Jessica died.

Cut ahead to this year: A friend of mine, driving back from vacation, was derailed by engine trouble outside Baltimore. During the long wait for the garageman, she picked up a newspaper and read about a group raising money for Maryland breast cancer patients. Their idea was to use the money to provide milk-of-human-kindness services: foot the bill for transportation to treatment, housecleaning, and massage; pick up drugs for women sunk by the costs. My friend looked at the group's name: the Red Devils. She blinked. She made a note to call me.

Seven years earlier, I'd published a book called *The Red Devil: To Hell with Cancer—and Back,* an account of how I'd gotten sick at 32 with a form of the disease that was, at the start, relentless. It cracked bones, brought me to the point of death, and then spookily—and wondrously—receded. In low moments, I imagined that if I ever got well, I'd start an organization something like the one my friend was now describing on the phone. But by the time I was in one piece again, I'd beaten a retreat from the world of illness— far as I could go.

I went onto the group's Web site. I caught my breath. There

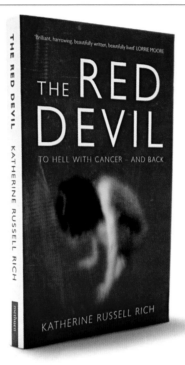

THE RED DEVIL

KATHERINE RUSSELL RICH

'Brilliant, harrowing, beautifully written, beautifully lived' LORRIE MOORE

THE RED DEVIL

TO HELL WITH CANCER – AND BACK

KATHERINE RUSSELL RICH

methuen

Her daughter died at the age I'd been when I got sick. Lark was so glad to know I "made it through."

was my picture. There was a line about my book and how it had inspired their name. "The red devil," the Web site explained, was slang for the most corrosive of the chemotherapy drugs.

I quickly sent an e-mail cheering them on, and just as quickly got one back from one of the founders, Lark Schulze. They'd been trying for four years to track me down, she wrote. Her daughter, Jessica Cowling, had had the same stage-four diagnosis that I had, and she died at nearly the same age I was when I got sick. Lark wrote that she'd been desperate to know what a young woman in that situation would think or feel but hadn't found any other book that might tell her. When I read that, I froze. Old sorrow spiked. There was a practical reason she hadn't found one: In young women, the disease tends to be vicious. Young women who get it often die quickly. They don't have time to leave their voices in print.

She'd been so glad, Lark told me, to come across a magazine story I'd written and to know "you'd made it through." Our e-mail exchanges kept up. I was afraid to be drawn back into that world. But I was suddenly hungry to comprehend the experience from the mother's side—my own mother had been so careful to mask her fear for me—to try to imagine the terrible grief, to understand the grace and drive it would take to transform that experience into healing.

As the e-mails continued, a hard knot I'd carried inside me for years began to soften. Large portions of my book had come from journals kept when I was given a year or two to live and was plunged into a terrifying loneliness. At the time, it seemed impossible that anyone would ever hear me again. Now I found it astonishing that the isolated, scared person I'd been had, in fact, connected with a woman in the fight of her life to save her daughter. That choking loneliness was being retroactively erased.

Such a deep and bizarre connection, I thought, the day Lark and I were to talk on the phone about my coming down for a fund-raising

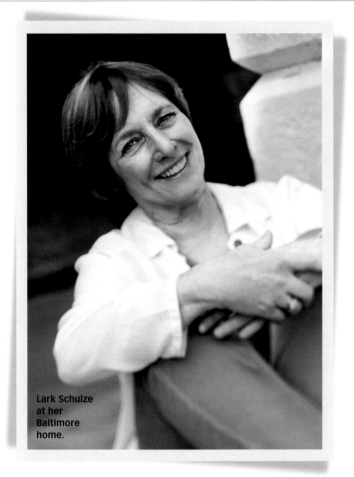

Lark Schulze at her Baltimore home.

"stroll" the Red Devils were doing. She'd helped me, I'd helped her, across a strange disjuncture of years. Yet we'd never met.

I was nervous about calling. Her Southern accent put me at ease. She had a lovely, self-deprecating sense of humor. "I can't lose the 20 pounds, and it's too late for the facelift," she said after mentioning that a photographer was shooting her for a story about the group. "When we started out," she said, "I thought I'd do this for five years and quit. I didn't want my life to be about breast cancer. But the pleasure is in the creation. I could be creating anything: a group to fight hunger in Maryland, say." She told me how, at first, she and a board member had butted heads over a position paper, and how the model they worked out became what she was proudest of. "It wasn't her idea. It wasn't my idea. It was the result of the process. At 63 I've learned to listen."

The board of the Red Devils convened in late 2002, Lark said, three months after Jessica died. Their mandate was to "improve the quality of life for breast cancer patients and their families." Money would be spent on catered meals, grocery deliveries, household help, and transportation to doctors. None of these services would be performed by volunteers; early on, the group decided it made more sense to use professionals, and hospital social workers and nurses could identify people in need. Money would come in from the stroll registration fees and philanthropic donations and grants.

After telling me how excited she was that we'd be meeting soon, Lark said: "But you've already changed my life." She caught

me off-guard—I didn't have time to say what I thought: *The feeling is entirely mutual.*

At the founders' party the night before the stroll, the atmosphere was giddy: kids running, shrieking, in and out the back door; adults, only slightly more subdued, congregating in the kitchen of Lark's brick row house. I'd brought a friend, and as soon as we walked in, we were presented with feathered devil-horn headbands.

We ate buffalo chicken wings and chocolate cake, and people clamored to tell me about Lark and Jessica, and how the group had come into being. "We made it up as we went along," observed Lark, who kept getting drawn in to side discussions. She seemed both wonderfully distractible and laser sharp, with a stealthy beauty that crept up on you. "What do you do at your board meetings?" I asked her when she circled back. "We hug and we eat," she said.

Rebecca Berger, cherub-faced, Jessica's best friend, talked about where the money goes. "Our biggest seller is transportation," she said. "Seventy-five percent of our costs go to that. One nurse said, 'This is truly a lifesaver.' There are people who couldn't have kept up treatment. Think of people nauseous, with radiation burns, having to take three hours of buses."

Later I met one of the women who'd been helped. Marilyn Foster, 40, lives in a two-story house with five of her children and had had such a rough time of it on chemo, she'd lost 30 pounds. "I'd get up as fast as I could to do things, fix the little ones something to eat; then I just wanted to get back in bed," she said. The Red Devils arranged for vans to the hospital, for vouchers from Jamba Juice in the lobby. "Lark steps in like your grandmother

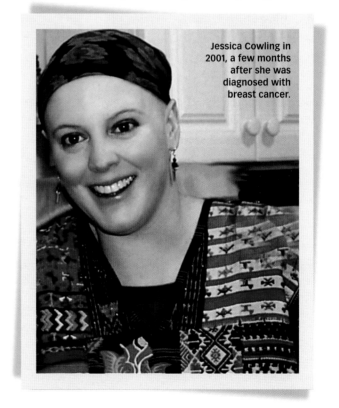

Jessica Cowling in 2001, a few months after she was diagnosed with breast cancer.

would," the nurse who'd put me in touch with Marilyn had said.

In the kitchen, a calico cat curled through our legs. "There were two things we agreed on when we started," Lark remembered. "That it wasn't just going to be about need but also about family. Cancer is a family disease. It affects everyone." Nearly everyone on the board had a family member or close friend with cancer.

Conversation turned to Jessica. After she'd gotten too sick to work, she started a cookie company at home, sold triple ginger, citrus pecan, and chocolate chip macadamia. The adjectives *ebullient* and *sardonic* came up. "We fancied ourselves the Ab Fab girls," Rebecca said. "We joked about motoring in a scarf. It's been pointed out to me that if Jessica could see the Red Devils, she'd be like, 'What the hell are you doing? You have a fanny pack on! Why don't we eat spaghetti and watch TV?'"

A woman wandered over with a plate of party dinner: brownies alongside artichoke dip. "Tell her about the tutus," she said. "Oh right," Lark said, grin crooked. This was on a day when Jessica had gotten one more piece of grim news. They all decided to dress up in costumes and go bowling. "Then we came back and had a party," Lark said. Her voice dropped. "Later a woman said to me, 'How can you throw a bowling party in tutus when your daughter is terminally sick?'"

> "What do you do at meetings?" I asked. "We hug and we eat," Lark said.

the Red Devils went from working with one hospital to 21, from raising $3,000 the first year to nearly $300,000 this year.

"We've been flying by the seat of our pants," a quiet man named Christopher Schardt observed on the subject of their evolution. Christopher had been married to Ginny, who was in a cancer support group with Jessica and died six weeks after her. The two women formed a tight bond and buoyed each other through their illnesses. Now Ginny's family and Jessica's form the nucleus of the Red Devils. "I'm from a large family," Christopher said. "Ginny was, too. In the chemo room, we'd see many women having infusions by themselves, sometimes in tears. We knew one guy, he was the only caregiver for his wife, 24 hours a day. We didn't want people to go through that."

People cleared out. They had to be up early to get to the park. Lark watched them go. She was standing under a small laminated sign that at any other time might have struck me as overly sweet: FRIENDS ARE ANGELS WHO LIFT US WHEN OUR WINGS HAVE TROUBLE REMEMBERING HOW TO FLY.

The next morning, there were signs all up and down the highway, urging be a devil's advocate. Six hundred people turned out for the stroll. The atmosphere was small-town wholesome and fierce: people in red devil horns and tails, in red boas. There was a booth for face paints (most popular motif: red devils), another to get your hair sprayed (red). Red balloons everywhere, Boy Scouts directing traffic in red berets, dogs in red bandannas. I walked around feeling off-kilter and happy and something else diffuse—not quite sharp enough to be pride, more like a hardness dissolving. I alternately considered that you can never know how the seeds you plant will flower and worried I was going to end up bawling

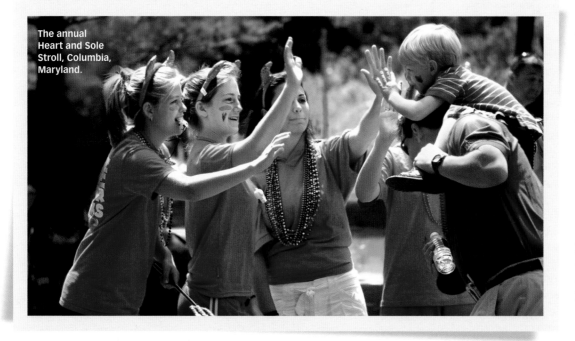

The annual Heart and Sole Stroll, Columbia, Maryland.

It was getting late. The board members and their families were reminiscing about other strolls, about the time a consultant said, "No one's going to come out on a July morning and give you money," and that they'd never raise the hoped-for $50,000. "But there are two times you can," Lark said, eyebrows arching. "If you don't *know* you can't, you can. And if someone *says* you can't, you can do it." That year's tally was more than $50,000. In four years,

in front of a bunch of children with devils on their faces, and how would that look?

A gong sounded. A voice on loudspeaker said, "Okay, strollers, let's stroll." The group took off at a meander, with children racing into adults, mothers scolding them, fathers pulling toddlers in various conveyances—a little like one big family outing if half your relatives up and painted themselves red. ◻

Five Pieces of Unsolicited Advice That Saved My Butt

A few of our favorite writers on the spontaneous, indispensable bits of wisdom that changed their lives.

1 BREAK THE RULES
LILA KEARY

I was raised to believe that the only time to call Daddy at the office was if someone in the house was on fire, and though it was never stated explicitly, you got the definite sense that it'd better be the whole bathrobe and not just the hair going up in flames. Men weren't to be disturbed or questioned: No back talk! Those were the rules and following them served me well, but at 28 I got cancer and the rules no longer applied. "You mustn't ever be afraid to make a scene," Marion said. "The meek shall inherit nothing." She was my fellow patient, my guardian angel, my partner in crime, and she did not suffer arrogance, catatonic indifference, or incompetence gladly. She died 14 years ago this month, but not before teaching me that "trying to find help in a hospital should not be like trying to find a clock in a casino." Hell, the woman actually came out of a coma to tell her doctor he had "the interpersonal skills of a wolverine." I remember her words every time I'm sitting on a steel table in the middle of a heavily trafficked hallway, spilling out of a gown made from a Handi Wipe and an English muffin twist tie, and you'd better believe I make a scene.

2 LIVE LIKE THERE'S NO TOMORROW
DANZY SENNA

That was the year I was dying of a million different diseases. Which was tragic, given that I was 22, just out of college, my whole life ahead of me. I didn't have any evidence, but I could feel it, a mysterious illness growing inside of me. I searched medical books for the correct diagnosis. Lupus. AIDS. Cancer. I didn't know its name, only that it was something serious and deadly.

It wasn't just illness that obsessed me in those days. I lived in a constant state of dread. My fear was like a stray dog, roving the neighborhood of my life, looking for a new source of worry. I secretly wanted to write fiction, but my state of anxiety had led me to take a job that I cared nothing about. It was the kind of job that would look good on my résumé, the kind that, boring as it was in the moment, might come in handy someday.

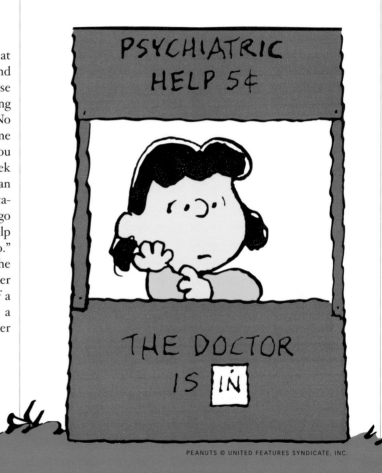

PEANUTS © UNITED FEATURES SYNDICATE, INC.

> My fear was like a stray dog, roving the neighborhood of my life, looking for a new source of worry.

One day my mother, concerned, I guess, by my anxious phone calls, sent me a book in the mail. It was called *The Tibetan Book of Living and Dying,* by Sogyal Rinpoche. I began to read it on that long ride from Brooklyn into Manhattan, crushed between morning commuters.

The book asked me to imagine that I was going to die tomorrow. Not the way I had been imagining but calmly, fearlessly. It asked me: Are you living today in the spirit that you would like to be living on your last day on earth? Instead of fearing death, the book told me to prepare for its inevitable coming. Begin the process of becoming the person you want to be when you die.

When I finished the book, I didn't reach enlightenment. But the book gave me a new, decidedly un-Western way of thinking about life and death and how the two connect. And one thing was for certain: When I imagined dying tomorrow, I didn't want to be working at my job. The résumé wouldn't do me much good after I died. So I quit my job. The next year, I went back to graduate school. I began to write fiction, my secret passion, rather than putting it off for the mythical future. I stopped thinking of my life as an anxious sprint toward some fixed finished line. It wasn't that I knew I was not dying, but rather that I knew, paradoxically, that of course I was dying, as was everyone else on earth, and so I had better learn how to live.

3 NEVER COMPROMISE
AMY BLOOM

If you want advice, ask a smart failure, not a smug success. The best advice I ever got about love was from a man who had been divorced once, after marrying too young, and was long separated from a second wife. He spent the rest of his life unable to file the final divorce papers and unable to make that marriage work. His other romances came and went, after six months or a couple of years, whenever the lady in question wanted a commitment. He was committed to his friends, to me, and to his son, and as far as I could tell, for 30 years, that was it. I went to him for advice when I was 14. My best friend was in love with me, and I loved him so. I loved his sense of humor and his kindness. I loved how smart he was. I loved being with him every day, all the time. I never got tired of him. But. Of course. Not in love. I was trying. We were making out, standing up and lying down.

We were unbuttoning tops and getting sweaty. It wasn't bad is what I told my adviser. "Honey," he said. "It's not going to get better. Love is a dance, and either you are moving to the same music or you're not, either your heart feels what his heart feels or it doesn't. Yours doesn't. Let him go and do it fast. Slower and kinder never feels better."

Right on every count.

Given that my visceral reaction was to lob a large ceramic vase at the side of his head, it was not easy advice to follow.

4 TRUST YOUR GUT REACTIONS
FRANCINE PROSE

There's advice that saves your life at the moment you get it (Don't get in that car with that lunatic! Don't accept that free ticket on the *Titanic!*), and then there's advice that just keeps on saving you. The best advice I ever got, of the latter sort, was given to me more than 30 years ago by a friend, the California filmmaker Freude Bartlett. We were discussing the nature of friendship in general and love in particular, and she said, "If you want to know who your friends really are and whom you should be hanging around with, all you have to do is follow this simple test. Whenever you've just finished spending time with a particular person, ask yourself, *Do I feel better or worse than I did before?* No long explanations, no equivocations. No excuses. Just 'better' or 'worse.' Then tally up the results, and pretty soon everything will begin to seem very clear." Over the years, that advice has given me the courage to stay in relationships and to leave them; it's inspired me to extricate myself from unproductive professional associations, destructive friendships, disastrous love affairs. It's helped me surround myself with friends whom I love, and who love me. For three decades, that simple question—*Do I feel better or worse than I did before I saw this person?*—has saved my butt, and my heart, in more ways than I can possibly begin to count.

5 THINK BEFORE YOU SHRIEK
LISA KOGAN

He loved me. He needed me. He couldn't see a way to make it work. There might've been more—he was not in a position to give me the things I deserved, we lived on two separate continents, etc., etc.—but at a certain point, I became too focused on not throwing up to hear anything else. I was furious and wounded and more than a little bit shrill—a lethal combination if ever there was one. I ranted. I sobbed. I blurted. Finally, I called my oldest friend. "You're going to have to live with whatever you do next for the rest of your life," she said. "How you choose to say what you want to say is crucial, so think very carefully about who you want to be when you look back on this story." Given that my visceral reaction was to lob a large ceramic vase at the side of his head, it was not easy advice to follow. But ever so gingerly, we talked. With great deference, we listened. Slowly, slowly, we got clarity. And then we got better. That was 11 years and one daughter ago.

I don't believe that if a relationship is meant to be, it'll be. I believe that the heart is a fragile little critter and it's alarmingly simple to let love slip away. Had my friend handed me a pint of Ben & Jerry's and the standard men-are-dogs speech, things might've ended not so happily ever after. ◖

"Whenever you've been touched by love, a heart-print lingers"

What I know about love I mostly learned on TV. In 20 years of hosting my show, I've seen what love can do in the most ordinary moments (watching a mother take her child to the first day of school) and the most extraordinary (strangers offering their homes to strangers in the aftermath of Katrina). Whenever you've been touched by love, a heart-print lingers, so that you're always reminded of the feeling of being cared for, knowing that, to someone, you mattered.

I remember leaving the Houston Astrodome early in the morning eight days after Katrina hit. Most people were still sleeping as we finished taping our show. A young father in a clean white T-shirt was carrying his sleeping 6-year-old daughter over his shoulder, and I stopped to ask, "How ya making out, sir?"

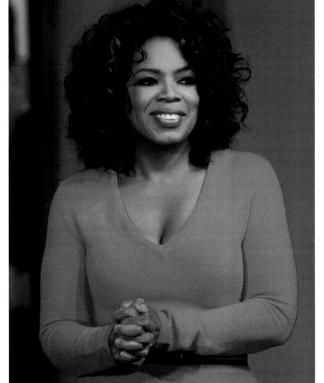

He replied, "I'm gonna make it, 'cause I've already survived Katrina and now I'm just moving on love—and I ain't never felt so much love in my whole life."

"Wow," I said. "You *are* gonna make it."

Lots of guests over the years have left heart-prints on me. Mattie Stepanek, a child poet whose only goal was to spread peace, was one of the wisest people I've ever met. If angels come to earth, he was definitely one of them. He came to remind us of who we are: love incarnate. When he died at age 13, I made a book of all the e-mails we exchanged. He was love to me.

Erin Kramp was an "ordinary" mother. She discovered she had breast cancer, and while she was fighting to live, she prepared her 6-year-old daughter, Peyton, for life the best way she knew how. She started recording tapes, more than 100 total, about everything she could think of to tell her daughter as she grew up, knowing there wouldn't be enough time to say it all: how to put on makeup, get boys to like you, choose friends, and dress well; stories about herself; her favorite songs, foods, and movies. Her most awesome gift, I thought, was this message: "If God decides to take me to heaven, I'm going to be looking for another soul to bring to Daddy. So I want you to know that I would very much bless Daddy remarrying."

Four years later, when Peyton's father wanted to remarry, he went to his daughter first. The 10-year-old said she needed more time to get to know her father's bride to be, so he waited. When Peyton said she was ready, Doug proposed. That same night, Peyton wrote a letter welcoming her new mom. Awesome! The love exchanged among Peyton, Doug, and his new wife, Cheryl, was so authentic it made us all rejoice when we witnessed it on the show.

That's what love does: It fills you up, mends the tattered and broken spaces in your spirit. It makes you feel whole. Not everybody has an Erin Kramp in her life, but love is all around and ever available. I know this for sure.

Sometimes in the thick of life, when my call list is longer than the day and people are lined up waiting for meeting after meeting, I just stop. I still myself. And look at a tree. A flower. The sun's light reflecting off the window. And I remember love is available. I inhale it, exhale, and get back to work.

I recently reread an e-mail from Mattie, dated 11/22/2001. He was 11 at the time. He'd recently seen *The Color Purple* (the movie), and he wrote, "This year my mom and I are both wearing purple for Thanksgiving. I'm thankful for things like safety during terrorism, for food and material things like that, and for the people in the circle of my life, like my mom and Sandy, the Moxes upstairs, and you. For things that God has given us, just because we are loved. Purple. Gentle breezes. Crickets. Shooting stars. Laughter. Feathers. I'm thankful that things *are*, so while we are, we can have gifts every day if we just open our hearts and spirits to them."

Words of wisdom from an 11-year-old.

Look around, feel the love. **O**

About the Contributors

Brent Atkinson, PhD, is a therapist at The Couples Clinic in Geneva, Illinois, and the author of *Emotional Intelligence in Couples Therapy.*

Aimee Lee Ball is the coauthor of four books, including *Changing the Rules* with Muriel Siebert.

Russell Banks is the author of the novels *Affliction* and *The Sweet Hereafter,* among many others. His most recent book is *The Darling.*

Martha Beck writes a monthly column for *O.* She is a life coach and the author of *The Four Day Win, Leaving the Saints,* and other books.

Elizabeth Bern is a contributor to *O.*

Amy Bloom's books include the novels *Away* and *Love Invents Us* and the short story collections *A Blind Man Can See How Much I Love You* and *Come to Me.* She has written for *The New Yorker, The Atlantic Monthly,* and *The New York Times* and is a frequent contributor to *O.*

Ariane de Bonvoisin is the founder and CEO of first30days.com, a Web site that offers advice on navigating the first month of any new enterprise.

Liz Brody is *O*'s health and news director.

Sarah Broom works as a correspondent for Radio Publique Africaine in Bujumbura, Burundi. She is writing a book about New Orleans, her hometown.

Michelle Burford, *O*'s contributing features writer, teaches at the Columbia University Publishing Course. She is a founding member of a multiracial community house in Harlem.

Nina Burleigh is the author of *The Stranger and the Statesman.* She has written for *Time, People, The Washington Post,* and *New York,* among other publications.

W. Bruce Cameron is the author of *How to Remodel a Man* and *8 Simple Rules for Dating My Teenage Daughter,* which became the basis for the ABC sitcom.

Betsy Carter's most recent novel is *Swim to Me.*

James Carville is a Democratic party consultant and CNN contributor.

Madeleine Chestnut is a contributor to *O.*

Tom Chiarella, *Esquire*'s fiction editor and writer at large, teaches creative writing at DePauw University.

Nancy Comiskey teaches journalism at Indiana University.

Madelyn Pugh Davis, one of television's first women writers, worked on *I Love Lucy* throughout the show's six-year run. She is the author of *Laughing with Lucy: My Life with America's Leading Lady of Comedy.*

Trish Deitch is a writer living in Brooklyn.

Lisa Dierbeck, author of *One Pill Makes You Smaller,* is working on a second novel.

Simon Doonan is the creative director of Barneys New York. His memoir, *Nasty: My Family and Other Glorious Varmints,* was published in 2005.

Lesley Dormen is the author of the short story collection *The Best Place to Be* and other books.

Jancee Dunn's memoir, *But Enough About Me,* was published in 2006. She is a contributing editor at *Rolling Stone.*

Tish Durkin has written for *The Atlantic Monthly, Rolling Stone, The New York Times Magazine,* and *The New York Observer.*

Nora Ephron has written fourteen films (including *Bewitched, You've Got Mail,* and *Sleepless in Seattle*), directed six of those, and produced numerous others. She is the author of the novel *Heartburn.*

Joni Evans has written for *The New York Times, The Washington Post, Vanity Fair,* and *New York,* among other publications. She is currently creating a Web site for women over the age of 40.

Anne Fadiman is the Francis Writer in Residence at Yale University. Her most recent book is *At Large and At Small: Familiar Essays.*

Bonnie Friedman is the author of *Writing Past Dark* and *The Thief of Happiness: The Story of an Extraordinary Psychotherapy.*

Lise Funderburg is a journalist and the author of *Black, White, Other: Biracial Americans Talk About Race and Identity.*

Elizabeth Gilbert's most recent books are *Eat, Pray, Love* and *The Last American Man.*

Jeff Goodell, a contributing editor at *Rolling Stone* and a frequent contributor to *The New York Times Magazine,* is the author of *Big Coal: The Dirty Secret Behind America's Energy Future.*

Jan Goodwin writes for *The New York Times Magazine* and *The Nation.* Her most recent book is *Price of Honor: Muslim Women Lift the Veil of Silence on the Islamic World.*

Barbara Graham is the author of *Women Who Run with the Poodles: Myths and Tips for Honoring Your Mood Swings.*

Amy Gross is the editor in chief of *O.*

Mamie Healey is the editorial projects director for *O.*

Roger Housden's most recent books are *Dancing with Joy: 99 Poems* and *How Rembrandt Reveals Your Beautiful, Imperfect Self.*

Margo Jefferson is a Pulitzer Prize–winning cultural critic for *The New York Times* and the author of *On Michael Jackson.* She teaches creative nonfiction at Columbia University.

Robert Karen, PhD, a clinical psychologist in Manhattan, is the author of *The Forgiving Self: The Road from Resentment to Connection.*

David L. Katz, MD, a professor at Yale University School of Medicine and a medical contributor for ABC News, is the author of *The Flavor Point Diet.*

Lila Keary is a contributor to *O*.

Gayle King is the editor at large of *O* and the host of *The Gayle King Show* on XM Satellite Radio.

Walter Kirn has written for *New York, The New York Times Magazine,* and *The New York Review of Books.* He is the author of *Mission to America,* among other books, and the Internet-only novel *The Unbinding,* which appeared in *Slate*.

Lisa Kogan is *O*'s writer at large. Her column appears monthly.

Anne Lamott's newest book is *Grace (Eventually): Thoughts on Faith*.

Jonathan Lethem's books include *Motherless Brooklyn, The Fortress of Solitude,* and *You Don't Love Me Yet*.

William Henry Lewis teaches English at Colgate University. His latest short-story collection is *I Got Somebody in Staunton*.

Mark Leyner has written several novels and short-story collections, and is the coauthor of the health guides *Why Do Men Have Nipples?* and *Why Do Men Fall Asleep After Sex?*

Julia Louis-Dreyfus stars in the CBS sitcom *The New Adventures of Old Christine*.

Rosemary Mahoney is the author of *Down the Nile: Alone in a Fisherman's Skiff* and other books.

Mary Matalin is a Republican party strategist and the editor in chief of the conservative publisher Threshold Editions.

Phillip C. McGraw, PhD, hosts the daily television show *Dr. Phil* and is the author of six books, including *Love Smart: Find the One You Want—Fix the One You Got.* He writes a monthly column for *O*.

Cathleen Medwick is the author of *Teresa of Avila: The Progress of a Soul* and is a regular contributor to *O*.

Carol Mithers is a frequent contributor to the *Los Angeles Times* and the author of *Therapy Gone Mad*.

Valerie Monroe, *O*'s beauty director, is the author of *In the Weather of the Heart,* a memoir.

Julie Morgenstern is an organizing and time management expert. Her latest book is *Never Check E-Mail in the Morning and Other Unexpected Strategies for Making Your Work Life Work*.

Catherine Newman, a columnist for wondertime.com, is the author of the memoir *Waiting for Birdy*.

Suze Orman, host of CNBC's *The Suze Orman Show,* is the author of several books on personal finance, including *Women & Money: Owning the Power to Control Your Destiny.* She writes a monthly column for *O*.

Mehmet Oz, MD, is Vice-Chair and Professor of Surgery at Columbia University, as well as the director of the Cardiovascular Institute and Complementary Medicine Program at New York-Presbyterian Hospital. He is a health correspondent on *The Oprah Winfrey Show* and host of *The Dr. Mehmet Oz Show* on XM Satellite Radio. His most recent book (coauthored with Michael Roizen, MD) is *YOU: On a Diet*.

Elizabeth Perkins is an actress appearing in the Showtime series *Weeds*.

Francine Prose's many books include *Reading Like a Writer, A Changed Man,* and *Caravaggio: Painter of Miracles.* She regularly writes book reviews for *O*.

Dawn Raffel is the editor at large of *More.* Her most recent book is *Carrying the Body*.

Terrence Real, a couples therapist, is the author of *The New Rules of Marriage*.

Katherine Russell Rich is the author of *The Red Devil: To Hell with Cancer—and Back*.

Michael Roizen, MD, is Chair of the Division of Anesthesiology, Critical Care Medicine, and Comprehensive Pain Management at the Cleveland Clinic. He is the cofounder of RealAge, Inc., a consumer-health media company that provides personalized health information. His most recent book (coauthored with Mehmet Oz, MD) is *YOU: On a Diet*.

Jeffrey B. Rubin, PhD, practices psychotherapy in New York City and Bedford Hills, New York. He is the author of *The Good Life*.

Sharon Salzberg has led meditation retreats worldwide since 1974. Her latest book is *The Force of Kindness*.

Danzy Senna is the author of the novels *Symptomatic* and *Caucasia*.

David Servan-Schreiber, MD, is Clinical Professor of Psychiatry at the University of Pittsburgh School of Medicine. He is the author of *The Instinct to Heal*.

Daniel Shapiro, PhD, is a lecturer at Harvard Law School and director of the International Negotiation Initiative. He is the coauthor of *Beyond Reason: Using Emotions as You Negotiate*.

Lynn Sherr is a correspondent for ABC's *20/20* and the author of *Outside the Box,* a memoir.

René Steinke has written two novels: *The Fires* and *Holy Skirts.* She teaches creative writing at Fairleigh Dickinson University.

Elizabeth Strout is the author of the novels *Abide with Me* and *Amy and Isabelle*.

Dina Temple-Raston's latest book is *Not Just Another Buffalo Soldier: America's First Battle Against Homegrown Islamic Terrorism*.

Ellen Tien is a columnist for *The New York Times* Sunday Styles section. She is the coauthor of *Prime Time Style* and *The I Hate My Job Handbook*.

Patricia Volk's books include *To My Dearest Friends* and *Stuffed: Adventures of a Restaurant Family.* She has written for *The New York Times* and *The New York Times Magazine*.

Suzy Welch is the coauthor of *Winning* and a contributing writer at *O*.

Sarah Wildman is a senior correspondent for *The American Prospect.* Her work has appeared in *The Washington Post, The New York Times, Rolling Stone,* and *The Advocate*.

Laurie Winer writes regularly about food for the *Los Angeles Times*.

Lisa Wolfe is a writer living in New York City.

Emily Yoffe is a contributing writer to *Slate.* She is the author of the memoir *What the Dog Did*.

Photography & Art Credits

Cover Matthew Rolston. **Page 2** Matthew Rolston; 4 Carmichael Lynch Thorburn; 6 Cliff Watts; 8 Matthew Rolston; **11 #1, #3 right, #4, #5 left, #6 left,** and **#8** Chris Eckert/Studio D; **11 #2 left** Brian Leatart/FoodPix/JupiterImages; **11 #2 right** and **#9 right** Lew Robertson/FoodPix/JupiterImages; **11 #3 left** Burke/Triolo Productions/FoodPix/JupiterImages; **11 #5 right** Renato Marcialis/Stockfood; **11 #6 right** Rubberball/MedioImages/JupiterImages; **11 #7 left** and **#9 left** Lew Robertson/Stockfood; **11 #7 right** Peter Rees/Stockfood; **11 #10 left** Bumann/Stockfood; **11 #10 right** Renee Comet Photography, Inc./ Stockfood; **12–13** and **15–17** Eric Ogden; 18 and 20 George Burns/Harpo Productions, Inc.; 23 Rob Howard; 26 Ruth Marten; 29 Art Streiber; 33 Patitucci Photo; **35–37** and 39 Nigel Holmes; **40–41** Rubberball/MedioImages/JupiterImages; **43–44** George Lange; 46 Maggie Taylor; **49–52** Elinor Carucci; 55 and 57 Dean Kaufman; **59–62** Alexandra Compain-Tissier; **63 top** Patrick Lichfield/Retna; **63 bottom left** Everett Collection; **63 bottom center** Giovanni Coruzzi/Rue des Archives/The Granger Collection; **63 bottom right** AGIP/Rue des Archives/The Granger Collection; **64 top** Elisabetta Catalano; **64 bottom** and 65 Courtesy of Simon Doonan; 68 and 69 Istvan Banyai; 72 David Lewis Taylor; 73 Michel Arnaud/Lachapelle Representation; 74 David Lewis Taylor; 77 George Burns; 78 Images.com/Corbis; 80 Oksana Badrak; 83 Ellen Goodman; 85 Gary Isaacs/Getty Images; 86 Courtesy of Hilary Offenberg; **87 top** John Coolidge; **87 bottom** and **88–89** Fernando Bengoechea; **90 top left** John Coolidge; **90 top right, bottom left,** and **bottom right** Fernando Bengoechea; 91 Fernando Bengoechea; 93 Philip Gould/Corbis; **94–95** Sarah Broom; **97 top** Oprah Winfrey; **97 bottom** Bob Greene; 101 Alison Gootee; 102 Fredrik Broden; **107–109** Caroline Shepard; 110 Martin Parr/Magnum Photos; 113 Vincient Nichols; 115, 117, and 120 Cig Harvey; 125 George Burns/Harpo Productions, Inc.; 127 C.J. Burton; 128 Courtesy of Raytheon Company; 130 Kam Mak; 133 Ann Cutting; 138 Robert Maxwell; **140–141** Stephen Lewis; 142 Troy Word; **144 top** Courtesy of Sharon Salzberg; **144 second from top** Getty Images; **144 third from top** Courtesy of Rachel Naomi Remen; **144 bottom** Sigrid Estrada; **145 top** Courtesy of Abigail Thomas; **145 second from top** Dion Ogus; **145 third from top** Brad Barket/Getty Images; **145 bottom** Courtesy of Florence Falk; **146 top** Courtesy of Joan Borysenko; **146 middle** Courtesy of Joan Hamburg; **146 bottom** Courtesy of Olga Sliverstein; 149 and 151 Tim O'Brien; 153 Mark Hooper; 157 Mark Hooper/Getty Images;

158 Marc Royce; **160–161** Michel Arnaud; **163–164** Guy Billout; 167 Art Striber; **171–172** Greg Miller; 173 Keith Carter; 174 Turbo/Zefa/Corbis; 175 Everett Collection; 177 Stephanie Violette; 180 Courtesy of Kate Burton; **183–184** King Features Syndicate; 185 Antonio Amaduzzi/Keith de Lellis Gallery, NYC; 189 David Harry Stewart; 195 Cathrine Wessel/Corbis; **198–199** Brett Ryder; 201 Andrea Shaker/Courtesy of Daniel Cooney Fine Art, New York; 202 Chris Buck; 205 Susan King/Veer; 208 David Lewis Taylor; 212 Teun Hocks/Courtesy of Blind Spot Artist Representation, blindspot.com, and PPOW, New York; 214 Kenneth Rittener/Getty Images; 216 Hugh Kretchmer; 219 Davies & Starr/Getty Images; 220 Mark Hooper; 221 Alex Wong/Getty Images; 222 Art Streiber; 225 Courtesy of Elizabeth Gilbert; 226 Paul Davis; 227 Courtesy of Anne Fadiman; 229 Dudley Reed; 231 and 233 Michal Rubin; 235 Lauren Greenfield/VII Photo Agency; 238 Daniel Hennessy; 239 Courtesy of Karyn MacVean; 241 Michael Edwards; **242–243** Courtesy of Barbara Graham; **245 left** Olan Mills/Courtesy of Jackie Lawrence; **245 middle** Courtesy of Vesta Johnson; **245 right** Patricia Ash; **246 left** Courtesy of Elizabeth Ritter; **246 middle** Courtesy of Kathy Atkinson; **246 right** Joy Elizabeth Page; 251 Michel Arnaud; 252 Courtesy of Gayle King; 253 Courtesy of Oprah Winfrey; 254 George Burns; 255 and 257 Courtesy of Gayle King; 259 Bettmann/Corbis; 260 Courtesy of Nancy L. Comiskey; **263–265** Courtesy of Patricia Volk; **266–267** Cliff Watts; 269 Jake Chessum; 270 Alexandra Boulat/VII Photo Agency; **273 top** Leila Amanpour; **273 bottom** Domenico Stinellis/AP Photo; **277–279** Neal Slavin; **281–282** and 285 Paul Kronenberg; 287 Cambridge Jones/Getty Images; **289–291** Susan Meiselas; **292–296** Jeff Riedel; 298 Misha Gravenor; **300 left** Everett Collection; **300 right** Shawn Thew/EPA/SIPA; 301 Yves & Droeshaut/Reporters/Redux; 303 George Burns/Harpo Productions, Inc.; 304 Joe McKendry; 305 Courtesy of Meg Ryan and CARE; 306 Meg Ryan; 307 Josh Estey/CARE; **308 top** Allen Clinton/CARE; **308 bottom** and 309 Josh Estey/CARE; 310 Jim Wright/Icon International; **311–312** Kwaku Alston; **313–318** George Burns and Bob Davis/Harpo Productions, Inc.; **319 top** Garett Holden/Courtesy of Colin Cowie Lifestyle; **319 bottom** George Burns and Bob Davis/Harpo Productions, Inc.; 321 John Ritter; 322 David Turner/Studio D; **323 top** Mark Swisher; **323 bottom** and 324 Courtesy of Lark Schulze; 325 United Feature Syndicate, Inc.; 327 George Burns/Harpo Productions, Inc.

Index

Published by Oxmoor House, Inc.
Book Division of Southern Progress Corporation
P.O. Box 2262, Birmingham, Alabama 35201-2262

ISBN-13: 978-0-8487-3121-2
ISBN-10: 0-8487-3121-2
Library of Congress Control Number: 2007927883

Printed in the United States of America
First printing 2007

To order more books, call 1-800-765-6400.

O, The Oprah Magazine

Founder and Editorial Director: **Oprah Winfrey**
Editor in Chief: **Amy Gross**
Editor at Large: **Gayle King**
Design Director: **Carla Frank**
Executive Editor: **Catherine Kelley**
Associate Editor: **Brooke Kosofsky Glassberg**
Assistant Photo Editor: **Kathy Nguyen**
Production Director: **Kristen Rayner**

HEARST BOOKS

VP, Publisher: **Jacqueline Deval**

OXMOOR HOUSE, INC.

VP, Publisher: **Brian Carnahan**
Editor in Chief: **Nancy Fitzpatrick Wyatt**
Art Director: **Keith McPherson**
Managing Editor: **Allison Long Lowery**

O's Guide to Life

Editor: **Terri Laschober Robertson**
Senior Copy Editor: **L. Amanda Owens**
Editorial Assistant: **Amelia Heying**
Director of Production: **Laura Lockhart**
Senior Production Manager: **Greg A. Amason**
Production Assistant: **Faye Porter Bonner**

CONTRIBUTORS

Designer: **Tanya Ross-Hughes**
Graphic Artist: **Carol Damsky**
Indexer: **Mary Ann Laurens**
Interns: **Tracey Apperson and Amy Edgerton**

"The Anxious Woman's Guide to Financial Serenity": First published in *O, The Oprah Magazine* March 2005 ©2005 by Anne Lamott, permission of The Wylie Agency
"The Best Makeup": First published in *O, The Oprah Magazine* April 2006 ©2006 by Anne Lamott, permission of The Wylie Agency
"The Binge from Hell (and Back)": First published in *O, The Oprah Magazine* July 2006 ©2006 by Anne Lamott, permission of The Wylie Agency
"How to Steal a Show": First published in *O, The Oprah Magazine* May 2006 ©2006 by Elizabeth Gilbert, permission of The Wylie Agency